Organ	Range
SPLEEN	136-149
LIVER	130-157
PANCREAS	146-155
GALL BLADDER	146-151
DUODENUM	144-163
LEFT ADRENAL	144-147
RIGHT ADRENAL	146-147
LEFT KIDNEY	146-167
RIGHT KIDNEY	148-167
AORTIC BIFURCATION	180-181
PROSTATE	214-219
SEMINAL VESICLES	212-213
PENIS	218-229
MALE BLADDER	202-213
FEMALE BLADDER	238-251
OVARIES	236-239
UTERUS	238-247
VAGINA	246-257
HIP JOINT	206-215 244-251

CROSS-SECTIONAL ANATOMY
–an atlas for computerized tomography

prepared with the assistance of

FAUSTINO R. SUAREZ, M.D.
Assistant Professor, Department of Anatomy
Georgetown University Schools of Medicine and Dentistry
Washington, D.C.

and

JOHN G. BRADLEY, M.B., CH.B., F.R.C.S.E.
Consultant Orthopaedic Surgeon
Scarborough Hospital, England

FRED CHU, M.D.
Senior Resident in Ophthalmology
Georgetown University Hospital
Washington, D.C.

HARVEY M. PRINCE, M.D.
Washington, D.C.

BETTY HAMILTON, PH.D.
Associate Professor, Department of Anatomy
Georgetown University School of Medicine
Washington, D.C.

DIETER SCHELLINGER, M.D.
Associate Professor, Department of Radiology
Georgetown University School of Medicine
Washington, D.C.

HOMER TWIGG, M.D.
Professor and Chairman
Department of Radiology
Georgetown University School of Medicine
Washington, D.C.

Williams & Wilkins Company
Baltimore

CROSS-SECTIONAL ANATOMY
–an atlas for computerized tomography

ROBERT STEVEN LEDLEY, D.D.S., M.A.

Professor, Department of Radiology,
Department of Physiology and Biophysics
Director, Division of Medical Computing and Biophysics
Department of Physiology and Biophysics
Georgetown University Schools of Medicine and Dentistry
President, National Biomedical Research Foundation
Washington, D.C.

H. K. HUANG, D.Sc.

Assistant Professor, Department of Physiology and Biophysics
Chief of CT Experimental Clinical Laboratory
Division of Medical Computing and Biophysics
Department of Physiology and Biophysics
Georgetown University Schools of Medicine and Dentistry
Washington, D.C.

JOHN C. MAZZIOTTA, M.D., Ph.D.

Postdoctoral Fellow, Division of Medical Computing and Biophysics
Department of Physiology and Biophysics
Georgetown University Schools of Medicine and Dentistry
Washington, D.C.

Copyright © 1977
The Williams & Wilkins Company
428 E. Preston Street
Baltimore, Md. 21202, U.S.A.

Made in the United States of America

Library of Congress Cataloging in Publication Data

Ledley, Robert Steven.
  Cross-sectional anatomy.

  Includes index.
  1. Tomography — Atlases. 2. Anatomy, Human — Atlases. 1. Huang, H. K., 1939– joint author. II. Mazziotta, John C., joint author. III. Title. [DNLM: Anatomy — Atlases. 2. Tomography, Computerized axial — Atlases. QS17 L475c]
  RC78.7.T6L4   616.07′572   77-7099
  ISBN 0-683-04920-8

Composed and printed at the
Waverly Press, Inc.
Mt. Royal and Guilford Aves.
Baltimore, Md. 21202, U.S.A.

to
Terry
Fong and Ling Ling
Bonnie

about the authors

Robert S. Ledley is the inventor of the first whole-body computerized tomograph, which he and his staff first put into clinical operation at the Georgetown University Hospital in 1974. Dr. Ledley is Professor of Radiology and Professor of Physiology and Biophysics in the Schools of Medicine and Dentistry of Georgetown University and has been principal investigator of many National Institutes of Health grants. As the Director of the Medical Computing and Biophysics Division of the Department of Physiology and Biophysics, he leads a group that pioneers in new medical instrumentation. As President of the National Biomedical Research Foundation since 1960, he has been in the forefront of research in the cross-disciplinary field of applications of electronics and computers to medicine. He was formerly Professor of Electrical Engineering at The George Washington University, and is the author of a number of textbooks in the electronic and computer science fields as well as Editor-in-Chief of several scientific journals, including *Computerized Tomography,* published by Pergamon Press.

H. K. Huang is Assistant Professor, Department of Physiology and Biophysics, Georgetown University Schools of Medicine and Dentistry, and Chief of the ACTA Experimental Clinical Laboratory of the Division of Medical Computing and Biophysics. Dr. Huang has pioneered in the development of methods and procedures for the clinical application of computerized tomography. Having earned his D.Sc. degree in Theoretical Mechanics and Applied Mathematics and also having had postdoctoral training in biomedical sciences and anatomy, Dr. Huang has worked extensively in the application of computer science to medical research.

John C. Mazziotta is a Postdoctoral Fellow, Department of Physiology and Biophysics, Georgetown University Schools of Medicine and Dentistry. In addition to his M.D. degree, Dr. Mazziotta received a Ph.D. in Anatomy from Georgetown University and has been working with the anatomical and pathological correlations of computerized tomography.

foreword

The diagnostic radiologist is highly trained and experienced in interpreting complex radiological images composed of many overlapping shadows, scattered radiation and, at times, artifacts. The images are complex owing to the nature and limitations of all of the elements involved in the production of the radiograph, including the X-ray tube, intensifying screens and X-ray film. These images depict body organs as superimposed silhouettes, with the soft tissue structures often not easily distinguishable. Furthermore the critical aspects of these images are frequently subtle, low in contrast and barely discernible, necessitating considerable experience and training to interpret reliably such radiological pictures.

The computerized tomograph represents a new radiological modality with the computerized tomographic scan remarkably different from conventional radiographic images. There are no overlapping shadows in the scan image, and soft tissue structures are depicted with remarkable clarity. Computerized tomographic scanning, however, has limitations, since only a thin slice of tissue may be seen with each CT cross section, and in the present state of the art a three-dimensional organ cannot be visualized in a single scan. Computerized tomographic cross sections are also mainly in the transverse axial (horizontal) plane, and such images are generally unfamiliar to radiologists. Nevertheless, the training of the diagnostic radiologist permits an easy transition into this new art for which new training and experience must be gained.

The purpose of this book is to assist in such training. Since a prerequisite to understanding the pathological is a thorough knowledge of the normal, this volume presents a detailed study of normal cross sections of the body, utilizing line drawings to illustrate in detail the structures seen in actual CT scans. The authors of the book are well-qualified for this project, as the first whole body CT scanner was developed in their laboratory (despite the groundless protestations of other pioneers in this field). Their experience in the field of whole body scanning surpasses that of any others.

ROBERT E. WISE, M.D.
Chairman, Board of Governors
Chief Executive Officer
Chairman, Department of Diagnostic Radiology
Lahey Clinic Foundation
Boston, Massachusetts

acknowledgments

The preparation of a book of this kind is necessarily and completely dependent on the scientific milieu from which it arises. We therefore acknowledge the kind and generous cooperation of our many colleagues and the availability of the specialized equipment provided by the Georgetown University Medical Center and the affiliated National Biomedical Research Foundation.

We are especially indebted to Dr. Lawrence Lilienfield, Chairman of the Department of Physiology and Biophysics, who was responsible for the protocol for scanning normal human volunteers; to Menfai Shiu and Otto Steiner for help in the computer processing of the large volume of scans made, and to Kenneth Franco, who organized the scanning and conventional examination of the volunteer subjects. Domenic DeMichele coordinated both written and graphic materials. We would like to thank Dr. Helen C. Redman of Mount Zion Hospital in San Francisco for her contribution in identifying some of the structures seen in the scans. We also are grateful to Dr. Stephen L. G. Rothman of Yale-New Haven Hospital for contributing many of the ACTA scans of the head. Judith M. Guenther made the final anatomical diagrams, and Dr. Sean Hoare edited and typed the manuscript.

Of course we are especially grateful to the volunteers for allowing their inner selves to be revealed.

introduction

With the advent of the whole-body computerized tomographic scanner (CT scanner) and its important applications in diagnostic radiology, the need arises for a cross-sectional anatomy book that correlates actual CT scans with detailed anatomical structures. This text is intended to fulfill this need by presenting CT scans of normal living humans, together with labeled diagrammatic representations of the structures seen.

The unique property of the CT scan is its ability to distinguish soft-tissue structures, thereby elucidating abnormal features. But a prerequisite to recognizing pathology is a thorough knowledge of the normal. The normal is presented in this volume.

Considerations in the Study of Cross-Sectional Anatomy

In the study of cross-sectional anatomy, it is important to consider two fundamental differences from the more conventional study of anatomy. First, only the structures within the thin two-dimensional slice of the cross section are not seen at all. Conventional anatomical pictures, on the other hand, usually try to present some three-dimensional continuity of overlying and underlying structures. Second, conventional anatomy usually illustrates anterioposterior or lateral views, in which the entire organ, muscle, or bone can most often be seen; while in cross-sectional anatomy, an entire organ, muscle, or bone is rarely visible in one picture.

In the relationship between cross-sectional anatomy and computerized tomography, a number of points should be remembered. First, the appearance of an object can vary in size and shape in different scans. Thus, blood vessels can appear circular when cut axially, or elongated when cut along their longitudinal axis. Furthermore, the arch of the aorta, for example, will be cut axially in its ascending or descending portion, but will be cut lengthwise at the top of the arch in transverse axial sections. Second, structural relations can occasionally vary considerably in the same cross section. For example, cross sections made of the lower cranium can show both cranial structures posteriorly as well as facial structures anteriorly in the same picture. Third, it is not necessarily true that successive sections taken close together will appear the same, e.g., successive sections at the superior part of the thorax will often have greatly different appearances. Fourth, it should not be expected that sections will look symmetrical in areas of the body where right and left symmetries occur. The reason for this is the difficulty in getting the cross-sectional plane precisely axial. Fifth, the injection of contrast-enhancement materials can change the appearance of the picture in a very significant manner. For example, the pelvis of the kidney, which normally appears as a low-density area can appear extremely dense as contrast medium is cleared with the urine. Sixth, it should be noted that some structures, such as the meniscus of the knee or the vertebral discs, are very thin and difficult to cut through. In these cases, care must be taken in interpreting the sections. Finally, some structures, the esophagus, for instance, collapse in the normal state and the lumen may not be visible.

A final consideration in cross-sectional anatomy, especially in its relationship to computerized tomography, is the difference between living anatomy and the anatomy of cadavers. Since living anatomy is seen in computerized tomography, the viewer should visualize the three-dimensional *in vivo* relationships between the structures, of which the cross section being examined is only a small part.

Organization and Features of This Volume

FORMAT. Each two-page layout is devoted to a single cross-sectional study and consists of four presentations. The first of these shows the location of the cross section by means of a diagram and a conventional radiograph. The second shows a drawing of the cross section corresponding to the CT scan, with the anatomical structures labeled in detail. The third and fourth presentations show color and black-and-white versions of the actual CT scan on normal volunteers. (Occasionally we deviate from this format, but in those cases the intent will be clear from the context.)

IMAGE PRESENTATION. The actual CT scans were photographed directly from the black-and-white and color television screens of the ACTA-scanner,* where they are displayed by the scanner's computer; hence, both black-and-white and color renditions of the same scan are shown for each cross section. The radiologist often finds the black-and-white picture a more familiar image; however, color enables more refined discrimination and analysis of the various densities elucidated by the CT scanner. The relation between the two versions of the same scan is straightforward: each of the various grey levels of the black-and-white scan is represented by a corresponding color on the color scan.

The grey level or color of a point on the cross-sectional picture relates to the X-ray linear absorption coefficient of the corresponding point of the patient's body in the cross-sectional plane.

GREY-LEVEL CONVENTION. As a general convention, we use *darker* grey levels to represent lower linear absorption coefficients, such as fat tissue, and lighter grey levels to represent higher linear absorption coefficients, such as muscle tissue. The calcium in bone readily absorbs X-rays, and we represent bone by white; on the other hand, the substance of the lowest linear absorption coefficient is air, as in the sinuses, which we represent by black. The use of contrast media will make tissues appear whiter than normal, owing to the increased X-ray absorption.

USE OF COLOR. In the color television display, the relationship between the color and the linear absorption coefficient is arbitrary and can be chosen at will by the user (this being a unique feature of the ACTA-scanner). In this book, four kinds of color spectra are used: first, the *continuous spectrum*, in which the darker colors represent lower densities, and brighter colors higher densities; second, the *contrasting spectrum*, in which contrasting colors are used to enhance small differences in densities; third, the *highlighting spectrum*, in which a single density range, such as fat tissue, can be made to appear red, while the rest of the picture remains black and white; and fourth, the *multiple-range spectrum*, in which a combination of two (or more) continuous spectra is used simultaneously to show two (or more) density ranges. These *multiple-range spectra* can be used, for example, with hues of orange to show muscle structures and with hues of purple

---

* Trademark Registered, U.S. Patent Office. The ACTA model 0100 was used to make the scans, except for some of the scans of the head for which the ACTA model 0200 FS was used.

to show lung tissue structure on the same picture of the thorax. The selection of a particular spectrum for a scan will be indicated either in each chapter or at the corresponding figure caption.

MULTIPLE WINDOWS. In some areas of the body, tissues of greatly varying linear absorption coefficient occur in the same cross section, such as in the chest where the air in the lungs is of low linear absorption coefficient, and the muscles and bones are of much greater linear absorption coefficients. In order to see details within the lungs and details within the muscles on the same picture, two "windows" can be used in which a distinct range of linear absorption coefficients is spanned by each window. Thus a low linear absorption coefficient range is spanned by one window covering the linear absorption coefficient range of the lungs, and a higher linear absorption coefficient range is spanned by another window covering the muscles. More than two windows can also be used. Grey levels can be used to view multiple-window pictures, but some ambiguity may result if the same levels are used to represent different ranges of linear absorption coefficients. But, as discussed above, using different hues of color for the different window ranges will avoid such ambiguity, while still showing the detailed variations in density within each window range.

When using the ACTA-scanner, each grey level or color is specifically keyed to a range of numerical coefficients, or ACTA-numbers; this key is given in a table which is displayed together with the cross-sectional picture on the television screen. In this ATLAS we have omitted this "color-coded key" because we are only considering normal anatomical features that can be recognized irrespective of the numerical correlations. Hence, the cross sections pictured in this book are typical of CT scans made on any up-to-date computerized tomograph.

OTHER FEATURES. Throughout the book we have selectively taken advantage of other features of the ACTA-scanner, and these have been used for enhancing the presentations. Two of these features are the "enlargement" and the "frontal-plane scan." The enlargement feature presents a selected region of a complete scan as an enlarged picture on the television screen and this enlargement of a portion of a scan can often enable the more subtle details of a scan to be seen with greater clarity. Finally, for the head and for the extremities, it is possible to place the patient in such a position in the CT scanner that a frontal section results. We have illustrated several of these scans.

DIAGRAMS. As mentioned earlier, part of each two-page layout contains a detailed drawing of the structures seen in the cross-sectional scan appearing on the same page. We have correlated as many structures as possible to the scan picture. Often muscle groups and other structures are shown in finer detail on the diagram than in the scan picture; this was done to provide the reader with accurate anatomical references for all structures. Blood vessel lumens are shown in the diagram to facilitate the quick recognition of vascular structures by the reader, even though these lumens may not be well demonstrated in the CT pictures. Similarly, cancellous bone and muscle are depicted by different stippled appearances on the diagram. While we have been careful to position this stippling in anatomically correct areas for cancellous bone, this is not always possible. The stippling therefore serves as a symbol whereby the reader can immediately identify bony structures.

Labeling of structures in the diagrams is designed to give the reader a complete reference for the structures in each tomogram. Some details which have minor clinical significance (e.g., individual muscles found in the anterior neck) have been grouped under one anatomical label (e.g., "Strap muscles") in order to facilitate the uncluttered access to important clinical structures by the reader. Structures which are truly bilaterally symmetric are labeled on only one side of the diagram, while all asymmetric structures are labeled individually.

TEN PARTS. In this ATLAS we have organized the body into 10 parts, namely: (1) the cranium, (2) the orbit, (3) the lower face and neck, (4) the chest, (5) the upper abdomen, (6) the lower abdomen, (7) the male pelvis, (8) the female pelvis, (9) the upper extremity, and (10) the lower extremity. These 10 divisions were chosen for convenience in presentation. We have, therefore,rather arbitrarily defined each of the 10 parts as follows (see *Anatomical Structure Index* (on inside covers):

(1) *Cranium* — vertex to foramen magnum in plane sections at $-25°$ to orbital-meatal line
(2) *Orbit* — orbital roof to orbital floor in plane sections at $+15°$ to orbital-meatal line
(3) *Lower face and neck* — inferior orbital rim to first thoracic vertebra (T_1)
(4) *Chest* — lung apex to costodiaphragmatic recess (T_2 to T_{11})
(5) *Upper abdomen* — diaphragmatic crus to iliac crest (T_{12} to L_4)
(6) *Lower abdomen* — iliac crest to pelvic brim (L_4 to sacrum)
(7) *Male pelvis* — pelvic brim to upper thigh
(8) *Female pelvis* — pelvic brim to upper thigh
(9) *Upper extremity* — excluding shoulder joint
(10) *Lower extremity* — excluding hip joint

It should be pointed out that many of the CT scans are made in planes having various angles to the axial line. These angles are defined at the beginning of each section and in the figure legends. Also, we use several systems to adequately describe the location of a scan, depending on the part of the body on which the scan was made. These *location nomenclatures* are also described at the beginning of each part and in the figure legends.

CONVENTIONS USED. The computerized tomographic scans were made on normal volunteers, who were first screened with physical examinations and conventional radiographs. All patients were scanned supine unless otherwise noted. No volunteer under the age of 50 was used for a pelvic scan. Occasionally, small discontinuities exist in the series because of the necessity of using many different volunteers; nonetheless, care was taken to standardize, as much as possible, the stature and build of the volunteers. *In all of the scans the left side of the patient appears on the right side of the page.* Thus, since the patient is supine, we are viewing the section from below. The reason for this convention is that the computerized tomography scans will thereby be comparable with the viewing of routine radiographs. This convention has been adopted because this text is primarily intended for use by the clinical radiologist.

ANATOMICAL STRUCTURE INDEX. A scan-level dictionary is provided in chart form on the inside covers of the book. This chart provides a cross-reference for many structures, relating the extent of organs in the sagittal plane to vertebral level and to appropriate page numbers. This chart can be used as a convenient reference for the location of structures when studying this volume and also as a means for locating specific structures in a patient who is to undergo CT scan examination. The use of this chart can thus facilitate the location of structures during clinical studies, thereby reducing the number of "base line" scans required for organ localization.

CONTENTS

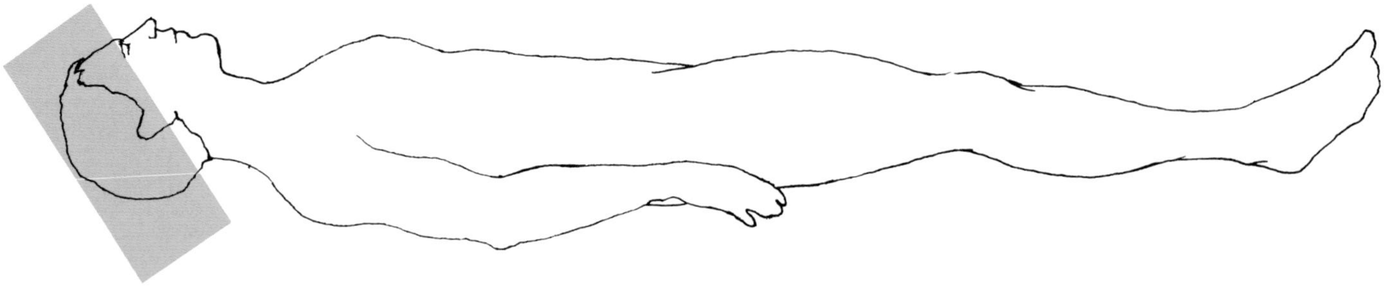

chapter one

Cranium

This section of the ATLAS includes all structures within the cranial cavity, and the scans comprising this section therefore range from the vertex of the head to the foramen magnum.

One of the most important medical applications of CT scanning is in the examination of the cranium and its contents. CT scanning has, for the first time, allowed for the direct and accurate soft tissue imaging of the brain and the ventricular system. It can demonstrate pathology directly, while at the same time delineating the distorting effects of the pathological process on normal structures. With CT scanning, areas of increased or decreased density within the brain substance (e.g., tumors, cysts, infarcts, hematomas, etc.) and the size and shape of cerebrospinal fluid spaces can be evaluated.

Other radiologic methods which delineate details of the intracranial structures include angiography and pneumoencephalography, Even though both of these methods are well established in neuroradiological diagnostics, they are attended by risk and discomfort to the patient. In addition, these methods often demonstrate pathology only indirectly, owing to the displacement of normal structures (e.g., blood vessels or ventricular contours). On the other hand, while CT scanning of the intracranial contents does not eliminate the need for angiography and pneumoencephalography in selected cases, it is truly a new and powerful tool for the direct visualization of many brain structures in neuroradiological diagnosis.

The use of intravenous contrast materials has further extended the use and accuracy of intracranial CT diagnoses. Areas of the brain that are undergoing specific types of pathological alterations may be enhanced by the use of these agents. A recent technique involves the introduction of water-soluble contrast material into the subarachnoid spaces. Such techniques allow for the imaging of cerebrospinal fluid-containing spaces and have promising future applications.

It is customary to scan the brain at an angle of $-25°$ to the orbital-meatal line (refer to the schematic drawing provided with each cross-sectional level). In this chapter we present normal CT scans made parallel to this base line. Cross-sectional imaging at this angle has the advantage of encompassing structures of all of the cranial fossae (in the lower levels) simultaneously, a useful survey feature. Cross-sections of the brain at other angles are included in the sections on the orbits and face. All scans were obtained at the above specified angle with the subjects in the supine position, using a 7.5-mm section thickness and a 1-cm scan interval.

In addition to the normal cross sections, we are including several CT scans representing cerebral atrophy. These were added with the intention of demonstrating ventricular and cerebral surface anatomy in exaggerated form.

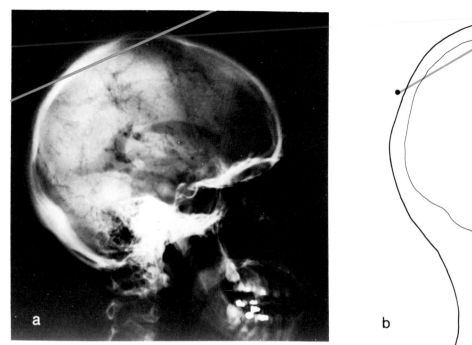

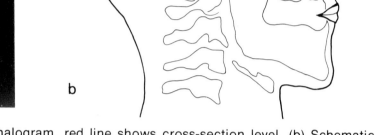

1.1 Scan level. (a) Normal lateral pneumoencephalogram, red line shows cross-section level. (b) Schematic drawing of scan level, angle of approximately −25° to the orbital-meatal line (*dashed line*).

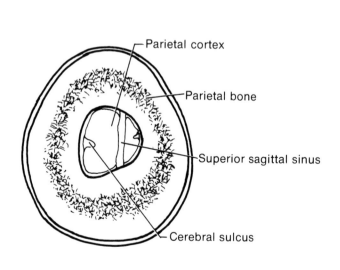

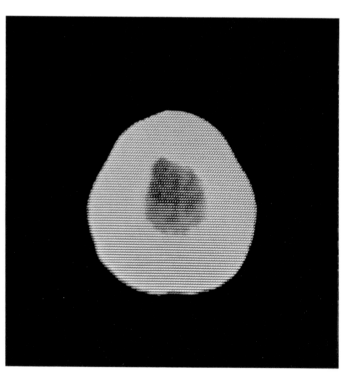

1.2

1.3

1.2 Anatomical diagram at the level of the vertex of the skull.
1.3 CT scan illustrating the presence of the superior parietal cortex.

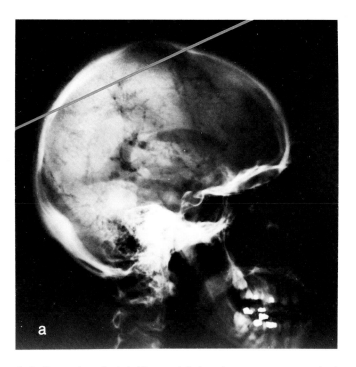

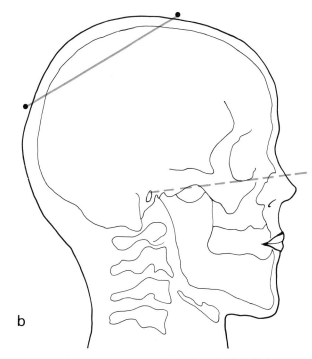

a

b

1.4 Scan level. (a) Normal lateral pneumoencephalogram, red line shows cross-section level. (b) Schematic drawing of scan level, angle of approximately −25° to the orbital-meatal line (*dashed line*).

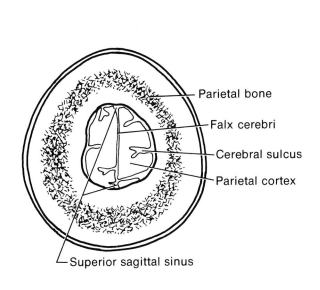

Parietal bone

Falx cerebri

Cerebral sulcus

Parietal cortex

Superior sagittal sinus

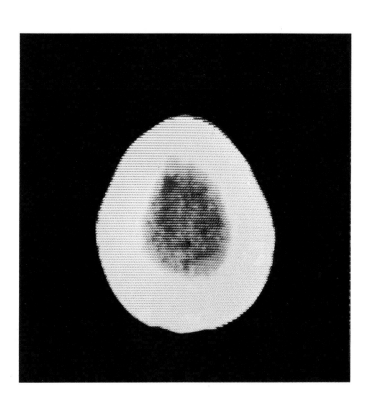

1.5

1.6

1.5 Anatomical diagram through the superior parietal lobe.
1.6 CT scan. Note the presence of the interhemispheric fissure and the cortical sulci.

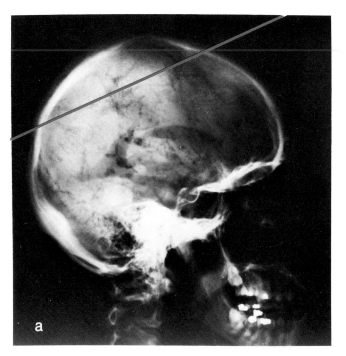
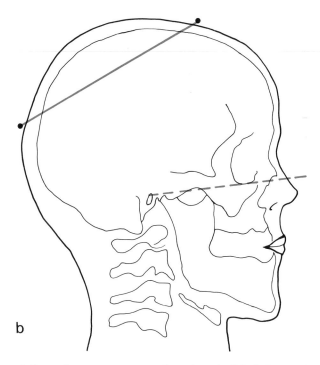

1.7 Scan level. (a) Normal lateral pneumoencephalogram, red line shows cross-section level. (b) Schematic drawing of scan level, angle of approximately −25° to the orbital-meatal line (*dashed line*).

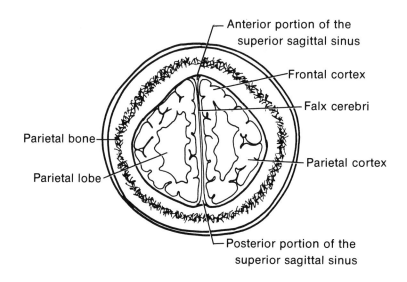

1.8 Anatomical diagram through the superior portion of the cerebral hemispheres.

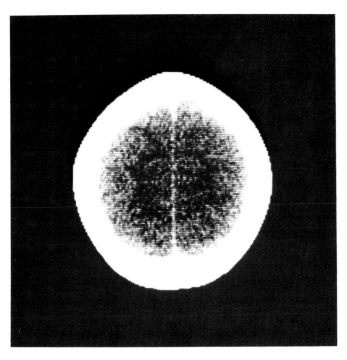

1.9 CT scan at a somewhat different angle from the anatomical diagram and demonstrating the appearance of the superior sagittal sinus and the falx cerebri with intravenous contrast material.

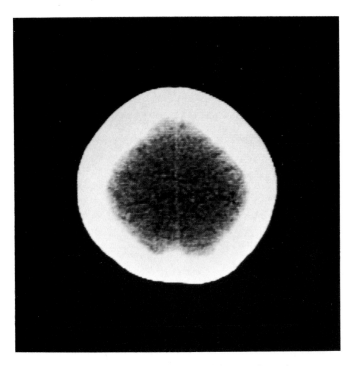

1.10 CT scan corresponding to the diagram in Figure 1.8 and illustrating the presence of the falx cerebri and the parietal lobe.

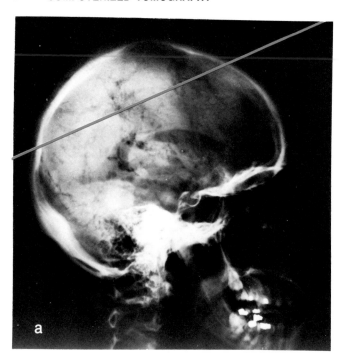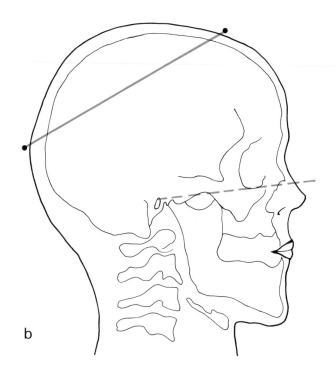

1.11 Scan level. (a) Normal lateral pneumoencephalogram, red line shows cross-section level. (b) Schematic drawing of scan level, angle of approximately −25° to the orbital-meatal line (*dashed line*).

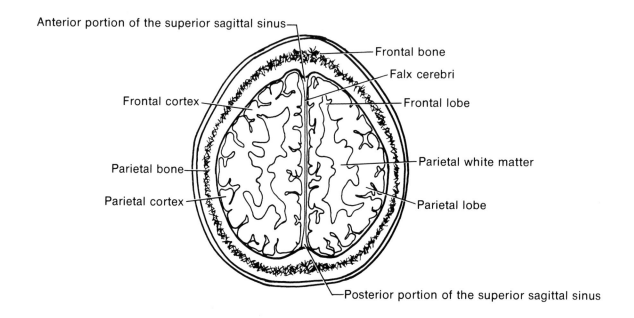

1.12 Anatomical diagram through the superior portion of the cerebral hemispheres.

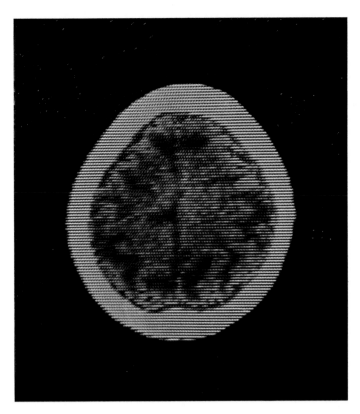

1.13 ABNORMAL color CT scan illustrating widened cortical sulci at approximately the same scan level.

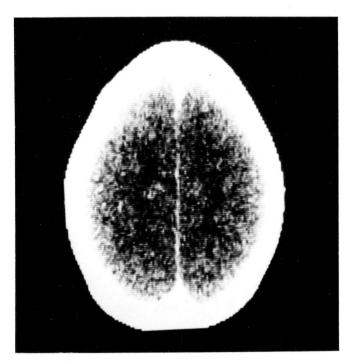

1.14 Black and white CT scan corresponding to the diagram in Figure 1.12 and demonstrating the appearance of the falx cerebri and superior sagittal sinus with intravenous contrast infusion.

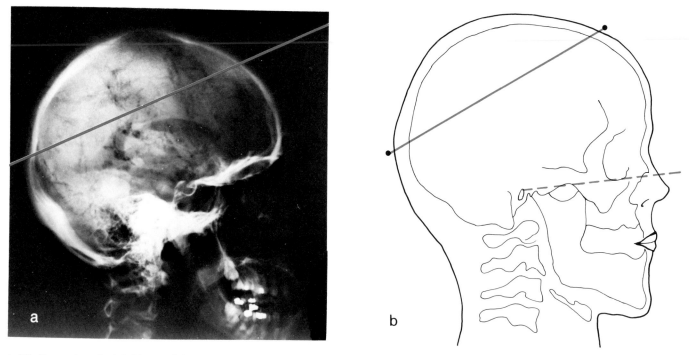

1.15 Scan level. (a) Normal lateral pneumoencephalogram, red line shows cross-section level. (b) Schematic drawing of scan level, angle of approximately −25° to the orbital-meatal line (*dashed line*).

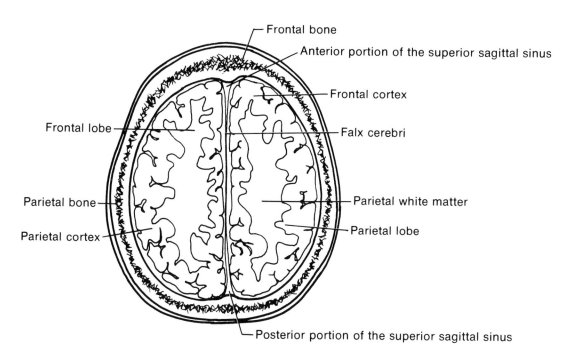

1.16 Anatomical diagram through the cerebral hemispheres.

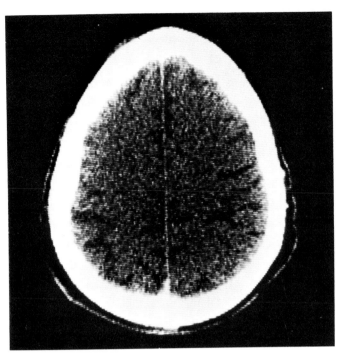

1.17 ABNORMAL CT scan at a corresponding level illustrating widened cortical sulci and a somewhat enlarged anterior portion of the interhemispheric fissure (cortical atrophy).

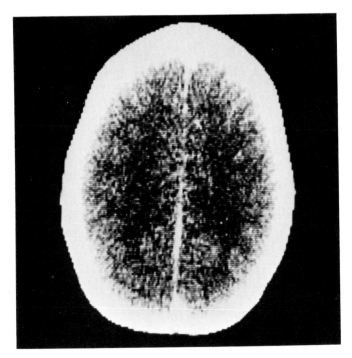

1.18 CT scan corresponding to the diagram in Figure 1.16 and demonstrating grey and white matter. Note again the appearance of the superior sagittal sinus and falx cerebri with intravenous contrast infusion.

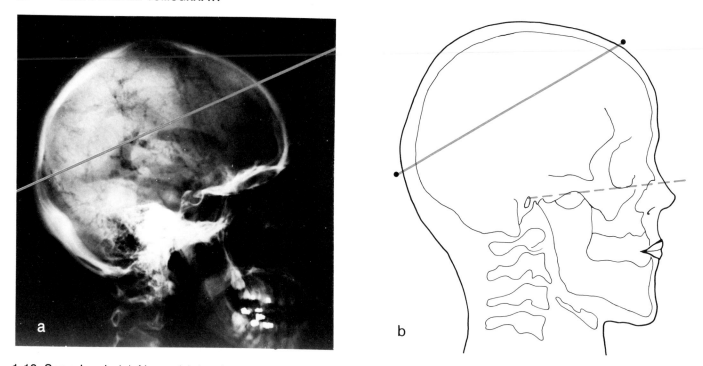

1.19 Scan level. (a) Normal lateral pneumoencephalogram, red line shows cross-section level. (b) Schematic drawing of scan level, angle of approximately −25° to the orbital-meatal line (*dashed line*).

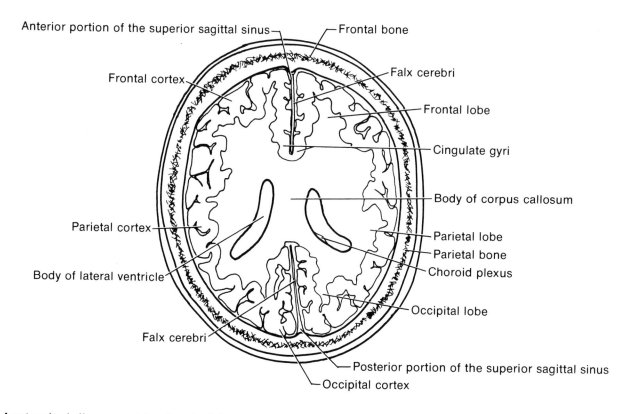

1.20 Anatomical diagram at the level of the roofs of the lateral ventricles.

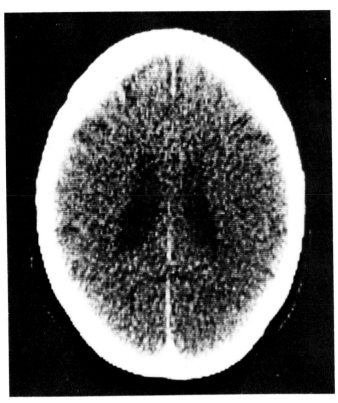

1.21 ABNORMAL CT scan at approximately the same level with slightly increased size of the ventricles and cortical sulci (atrophy).

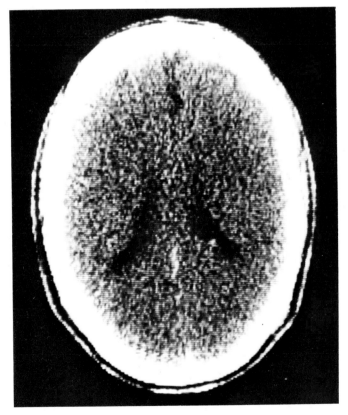

1.22 CT scan corresponding to the diagram in Figure 1.20 and demonstrating the lateral ventricles.

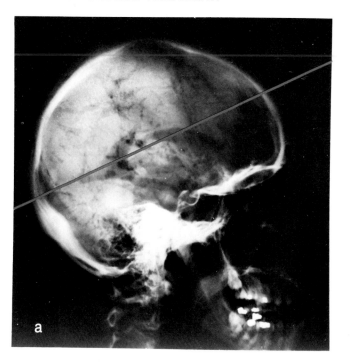
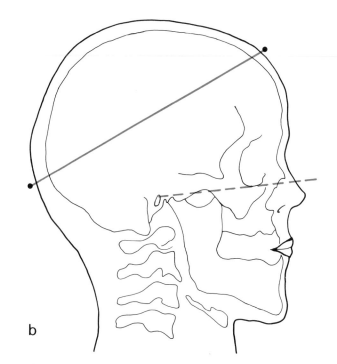

1.23 Scan level. (a) Normal lateral pneumoencephalogram, red line shows cross-section level. (b) Schematic drawing of scan level, angle of approximately −25° to the orbital-meatal line (*dashed line*).

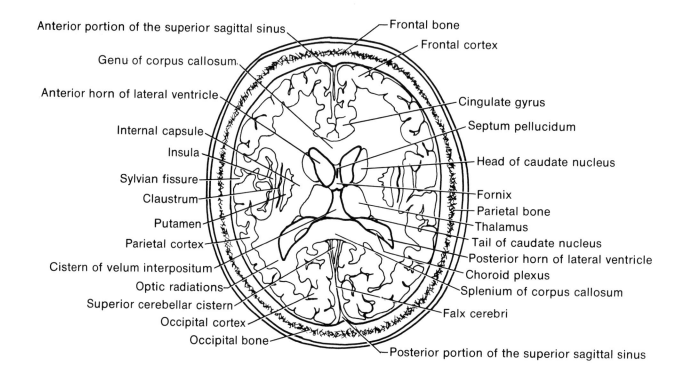

1.24 Anatomical digaram through the superior portion of the thalamus.

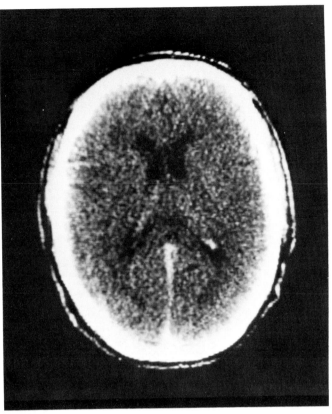

1.25 CT scan at a slightly higher level and showing the appearance of the choroid plexi of the lateral ventricles as they appear with intravenous contrast enhancement.

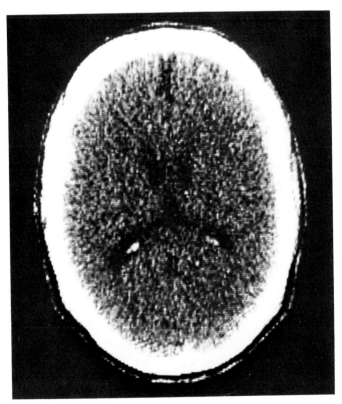

1.26 CT scan corresponding to the diagram in Figure 1.24 and demonstrating the appearance of the anterior and posterior horns of the lateral ventricles.

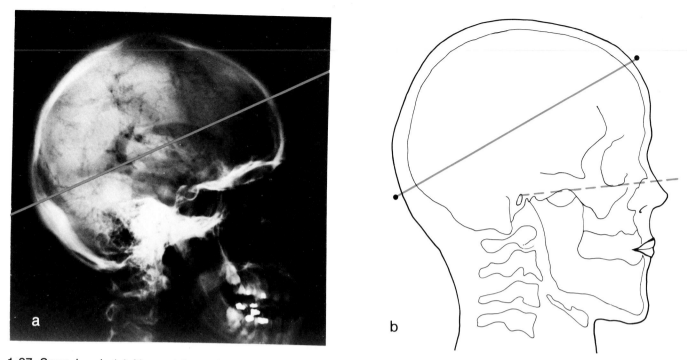

1.27 Scan level. (a) Normal lateral pneumoencephalogram, red line shows cross-section level. (b) Schematic drawing of scan level, angle of approximately −25° to the orbital-meatal line (*dashed line*).

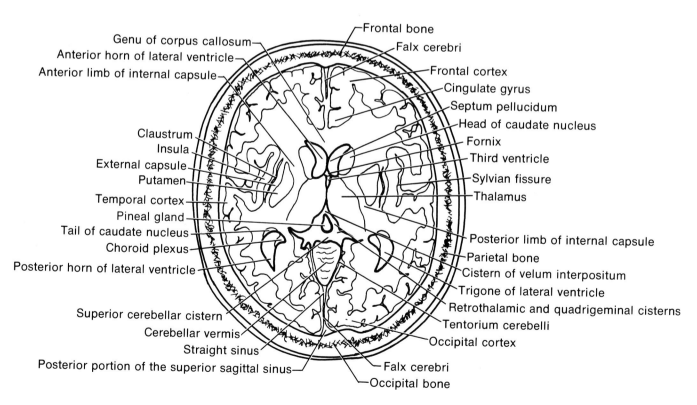

1.28 Anatomical diagram at the level of the pineal gland.

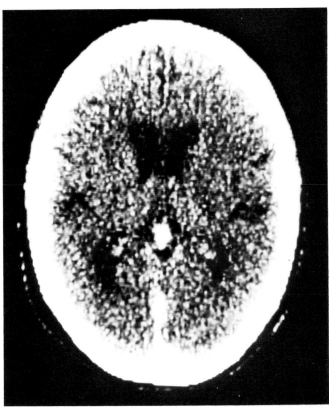

1.29 ABNORMAL CT scan at a slightly different angle and demonstrating brain atrophy. Note the pineal gland, the anterior and posterior horns of the lateral ventricles, as well as the widening of the cortical sulci and Sylvian fissures.

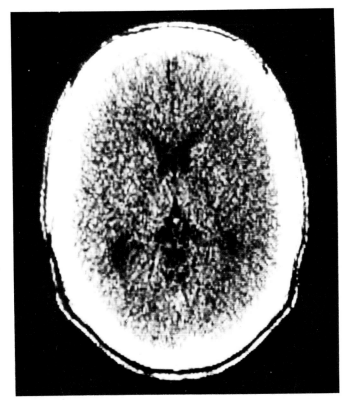

1.30 CT scan corresponding to the diagram in Figure 1.28 and demonstrating the appearance of the anterior and posterior horns of the lateral ventricles and the pineal gland. Also note the quadrigeminal and superior cerebellar cisterns. The heads of the caudate nuclei are seen lateral to the frontal horns of the lateral ventricles.

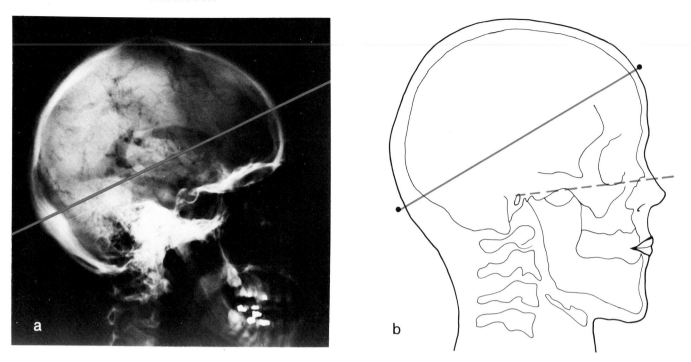

1.31 Scan level. (a) Normal lateral pneumoencephalogram, red line shows cross-section level. (b) Schematic drawing of scan level, angle of approximately −25° to the orbital-meatal line (*dashed line*).

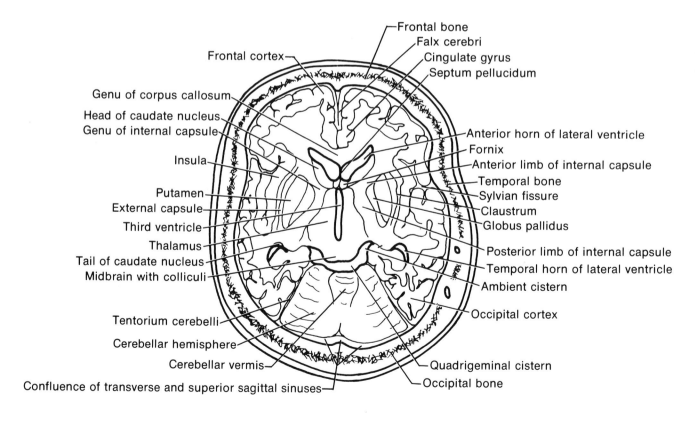

1.32 Anatomical diagram through the superior portion of the third ventricle.

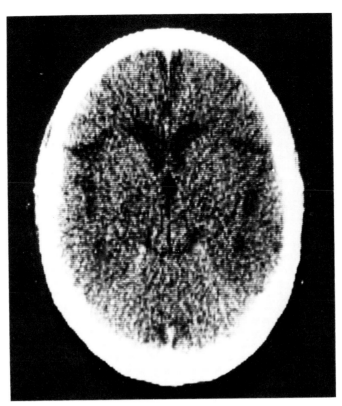

1.33 ABNORMAL CT scan demonstrating slightly widened anterior horns of the lateral ventricles, third ventricle and Sylvian fissures (atrophy).

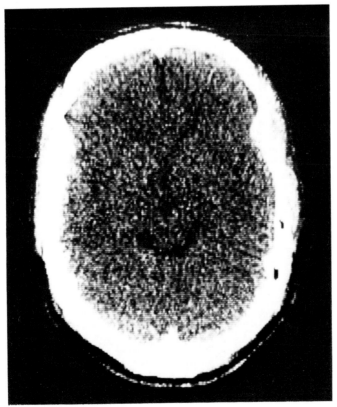

1.34 CT scan corresponding to the diagram in Figure 1.32. Note the appearance of the anterior horns of the lateral ventricles as well as the third ventricle and Sylvian fissures. At this level, the quadrigeminal cistern and the ambient cisterns can be seen.

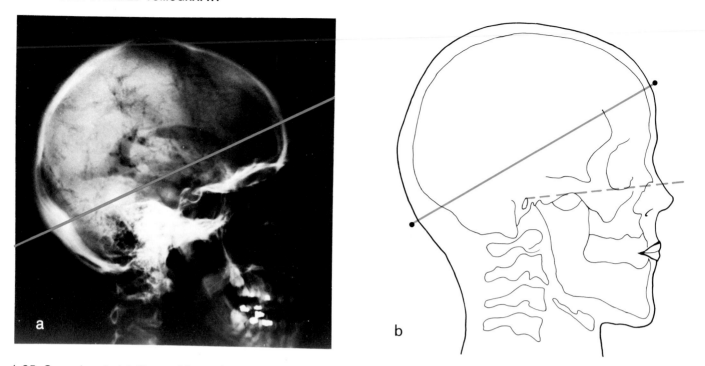

1.35 Scan level. (a) Normal lateral pneumoencephalogram, red line shows cross-section level. (b) Schematic drawing of scan level, angle of approximately −25° to the orbital-meatal line (*dashed line*).

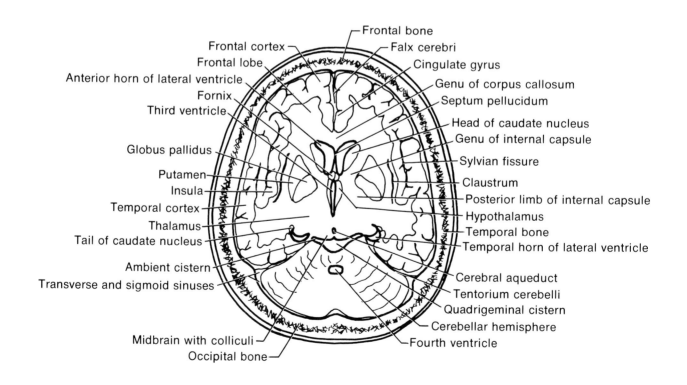

1.36 Anatomical diagram through the inferior portion of the third ventricle.

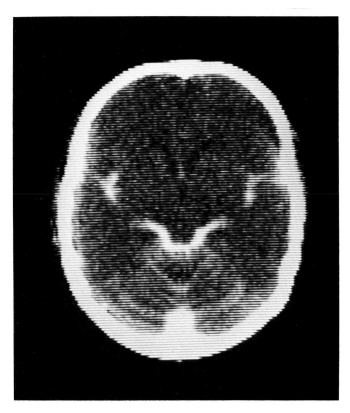

1.37 CT scan following introduction of a water-soluble contrast material (metrizamide) into the subarachnoid space and demonstrating the Sylvian fissures, the ambient and quadrigeminal cisterns, as well as the cisterna magna and the cerebellar sulci, all seen in white.

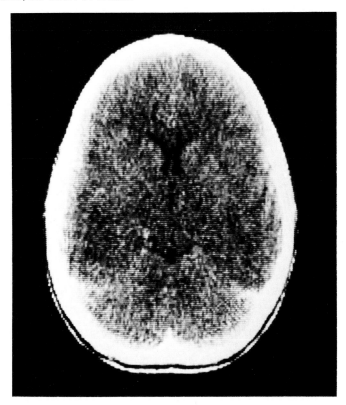

1.38 CT scan corresponding to the diagram in Figure 1.36 and demonstrating the appearance of the anterior horns of the lateral ventricles, the inferior portion of the third ventricle, and the quadrigeminal and ambient cisterns.

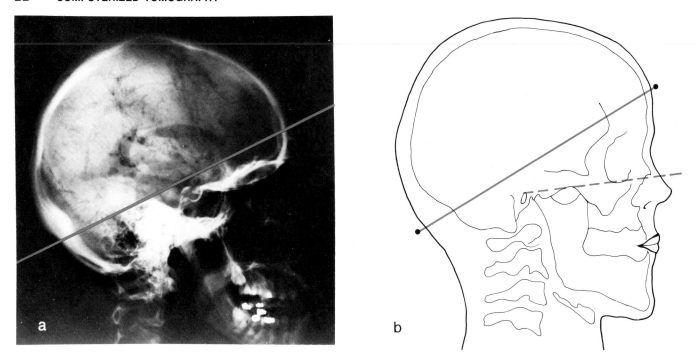

1.39 Scan level. (a) Normal lateral pneumoencephalogram, red line shows cross-section level. (b) Schematic drawing of scan level, angle of approximately −25° to the orbital-meatal line (*dashed line*).

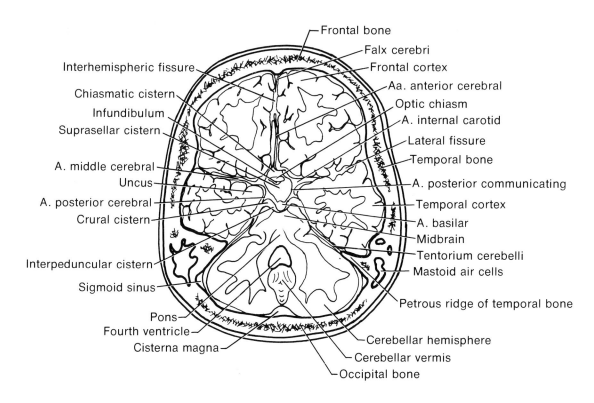

1.40 Anatomical diagram at the level of the suprasellar cistern.

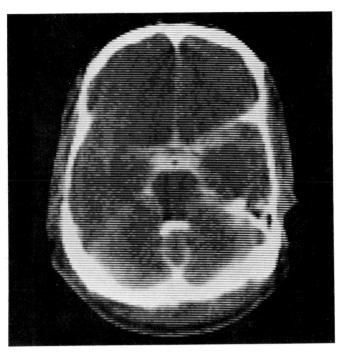

1.41 CT scan following introduction of a water-soluble contrast medium (metrizamide) into the subarachnoid space. It demonstrates the continuity of the suprasellar, interpeduncular, crural and ambient cisterns; the central filling defect represents the tip of the basilar artery. Note the fourth ventricle and the subarachnoid space surrounding the anterior and middle cerebral arteries.

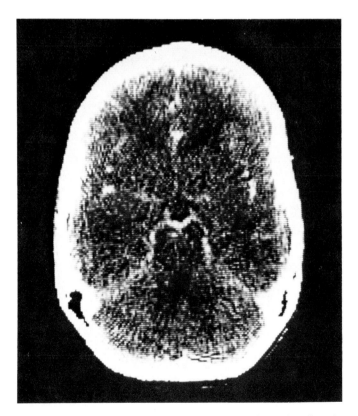

1.42 CT scan corresponding to the diagram in Figure 1.40 and produced using intravenous contrast enhancement. Note the elements of the circle of Willis including the internal carotid, anterior and middle cerebral arteries as well as the basilar and posterior cerebral arteries. The fourth ventricle can be seen, as well as the mastoid cells and the cisterna magna.

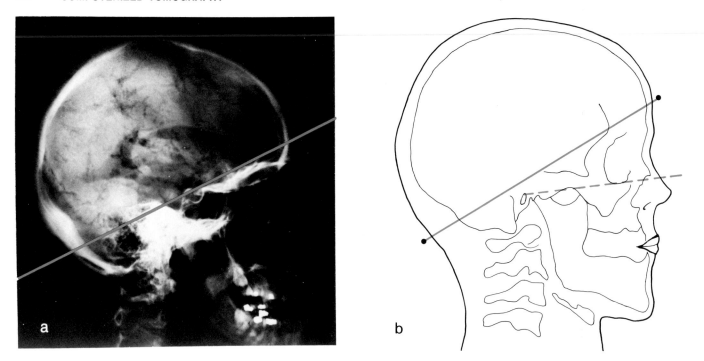

1.43 Scan level. (a) Normal lateral pneumoencephalogram, red line shows cross-section level. (b) Schematic drawing of scan level, angle of approximately −25° to the orbital-meatal line (*dashed line*).

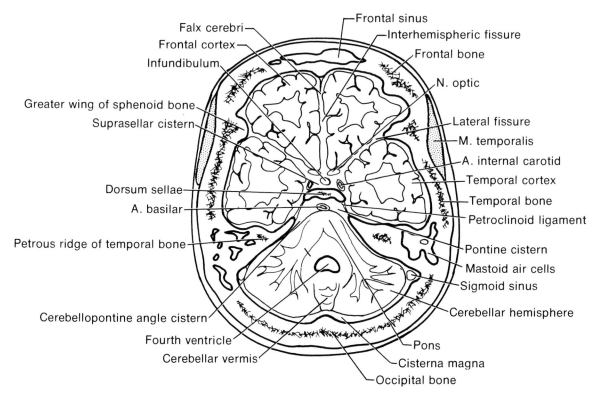

1.44 Anatomical diagram at the level of the dorsum sellae.

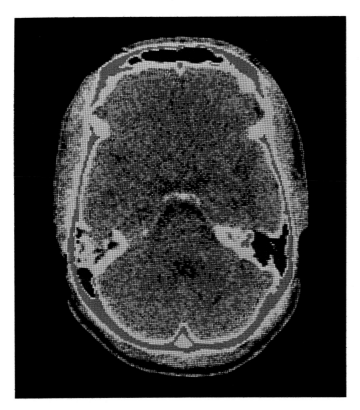

1.45 Color CT scan corresponding to the diagram in Figure 1.44.

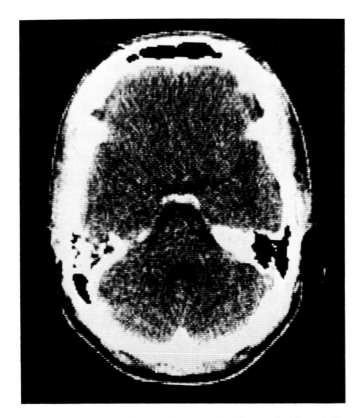

1.46 Black and white CT scan corresponding to the diagram in Figure 1.44 and demonstrating the petrous ridge of the temporal bones, mastoid air cells and the greater wings of the sphenoid bone as well as the frontal sinus. The pontine, cerebellopontine angle and the suprasellar cisterns are visible. Note also the appearance of the fourth ventricle.

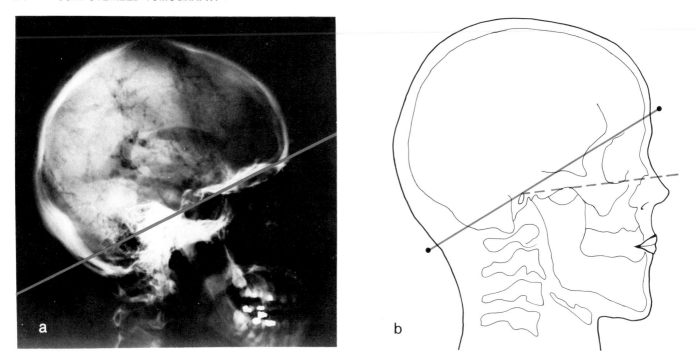

1.47 Scan level. (a) Normal lateral pneumoencephalogram, red line shows cross-section level. (b) Schematic drawing of scan level, angle of approximately −25° to the orbital-meatal line (*dashed line*).

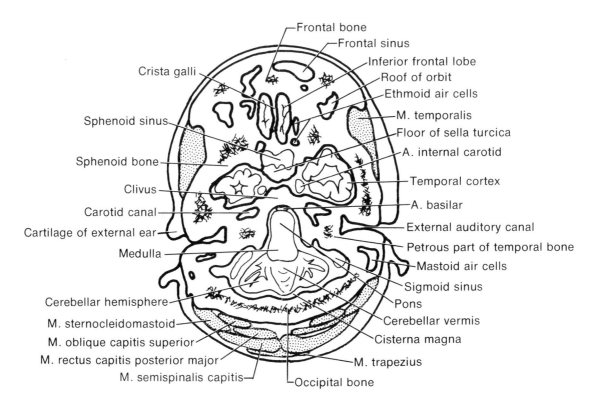

1.48 Anatomical diagram at the level of the orbital roofs.

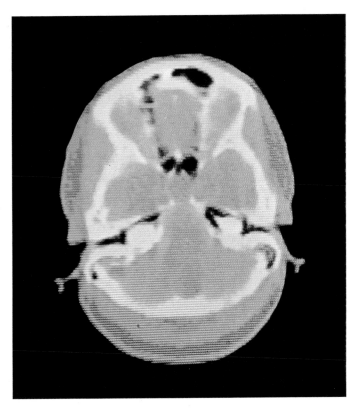

1.49 Color CT scan demonstrating the following bony structures: external auditory canal, mastoid air cells and sphenoid and frontal sinuses.

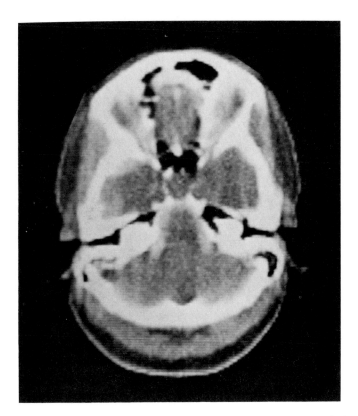

1.50 Black and white CT scan corresponding to the diagram in Figure 1.48 and demonstrating the cerebellar hemispheres and the inferior portions of the temporal and frontal lobes.

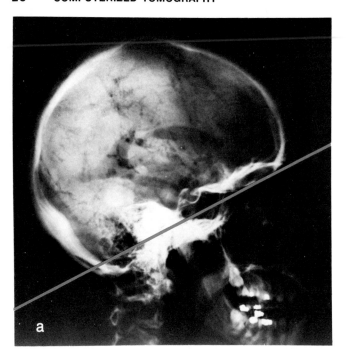

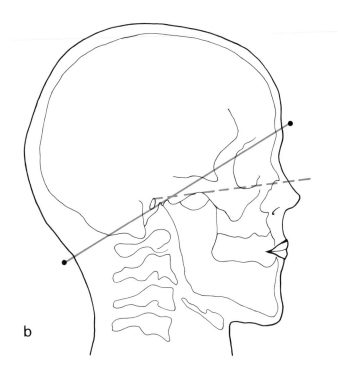

1.51 Scan level. (a) Normal lateral pneumoencephalogram, red line shows cross-section level. (b) Schematic drawing of scan level, angle of approximately −25° to the orbital-meatal line (*dashed line*).

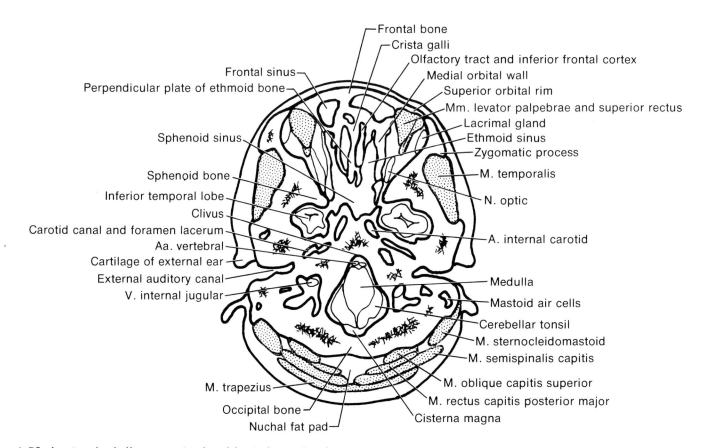

1.52 Anatomical diagram at a level just above the foramen magnum.

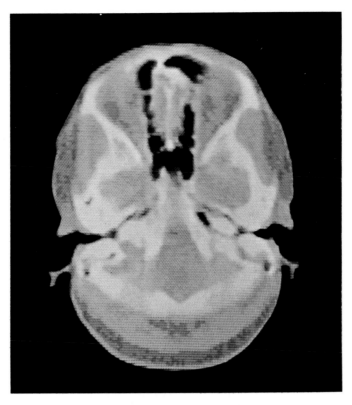

1.53 Color CT scan demonstrating the superior portion of the orbits and the frontal, ethmoid and sphenoid sinuses.

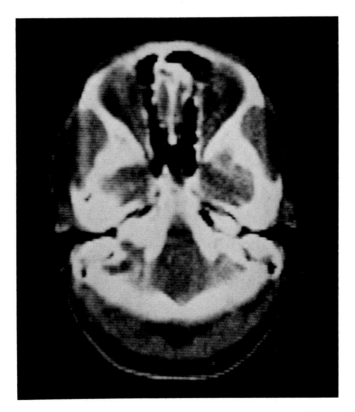

1.54 Black and white CT scan corresponding to the diagram in Figure 1.52 and demonstrating the inferior portions of the cerebellum, the medulla and the inferior portions of the temporal and frontal lobes.

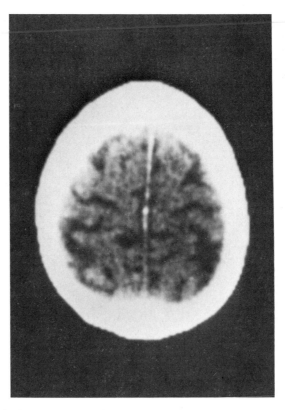

1.55 ABNORMAL CT scan through the upper cerebrum produced using intravenous contrast enhancement and demonstrating the falx cerebri. This scan demonstrates increased size of the interhemispheric fissure as well as the widened cortical sulci (atrophy).

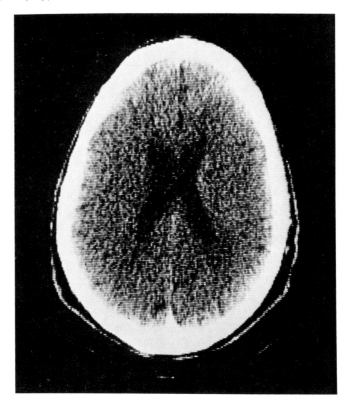

1.56 ABNORMAL CT scan through the upper portion of the lateral ventricles and demonstrating slight ventricular enlargement and minimal dilation of the cortical sulci (borderline atrophy).

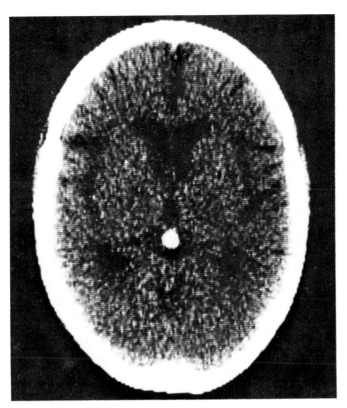

1.57 ABNORMAL CT scan at the level of the pineal gland. This scan illustrates an increase in the dimensions of the anterior and temporal horns of the lateral ventricles, as well as the cortical sulci, the interhemispheric fissure and the Sylvian fissures (atrophy).

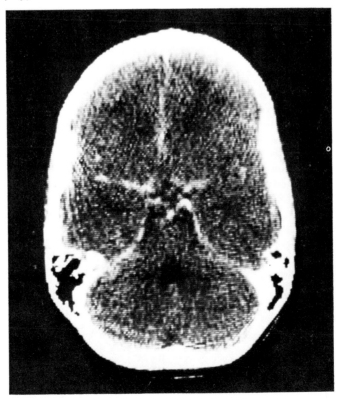

1.58 NORMAL CT scan produced using intravenous contrast enhancement and demonstrating the circle of Willis including the basilar, posterior cerebral and posterior communicating arteries as well as the middle and anterior cerebral arteries.

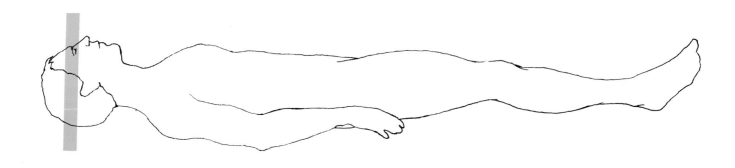

chapter two

Orbit

In this section of the ATLAS, the orbits and their contents are examined. This region extends from the orbital roof to the floor and includes the globes, optic nerves, extraocular muscles, and lacrimal glands.

CT scanning of the orbit provides accurate anatomical imaging of soft tissue structures within the bony confines of the orbit as well as within the globe itself. The fact that images are not superimposed on one another, as is the case with conventional radiographic studies, makes CT scanning of the orbit a precise tool for the three-dimensional localization of lesions within this region. The presence of low density orbital fat makes imaging of the individual extraocular muscles and the optic nerve routinely possible. Using CT scanning, the globe itself can be radiographically subdivided into its component parts, the anterior segment, the lens, and the posterior cavity containing the vitreous.

Tumors within the globe, along the optic nerve, and involving the orbital walls are readily visualized using CT methods. Thickening of the extraocular muscles in hyperthyroidism has been documented by CT scanning. In addition, pathological enlargement of the lacrimal gland and tumor extension through the orbital walls can be delineated by CT scans without the need for the more invasive procedures of orbital arteriography and venography or orbitography, all of which involve infusion of contrast material into orbital structures. The potential for precise three-dimensional localization of nonmetallic foreign bodies within the globe is a further use for CT techniques.

In this section are presented transverse views of the orbit, which were obtained with the subject in the supine position and using as a reference the canthomeatal line (i.e., a line drawn from the lateral canthus of the eye to the center of the external auditory meatus). Because most information in the orbit can be obtained by scanning in a plane parallel to the optic nerve, all transverse scans were collected at an angle of +15° to the canthomeatal line (i.e., the meatal end of the transverse plane rotated superiorly) and using a section thickness of 4 mm. A coronal scan was made with the patient in the prone position, with the neck hyperextended using a section thickness of 7.5 mm.

Although grey-level coding systems are useful in delineating adjacent structures, it is occasionally difficult to rely entirely on this feature, particularly if the absorption coefficients for adjacent structures are similar. Assigning a color to a specific grey level can be particularly useful in the orbit. For example, orbital fat can be made red in order to distinguish the outline of the optic nerve or the extraocular muscles from the surrounding tissues. Similarly, the lens can be made to stand out in color against the grey-level background. The color assignment is explained in more detail in the figure captions of each color image.

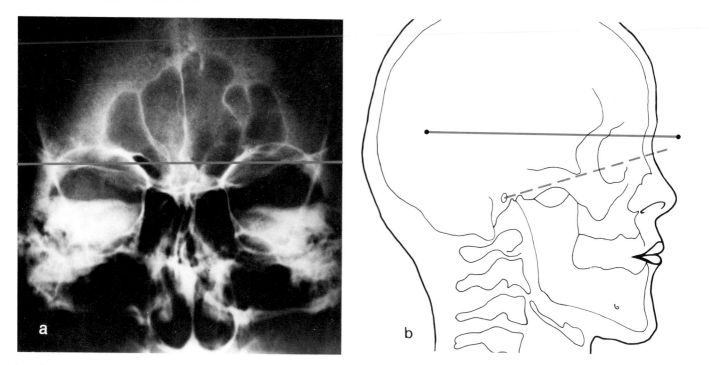

2.1 Scan level. (a) Normal skull roentgenogram; red line shows cross-section level. (b) Schematic drawing of scan level approximately 26 mm above the lateral canthus of the eye at an angle of +15° to the canthomeatal line (*dashed line*).

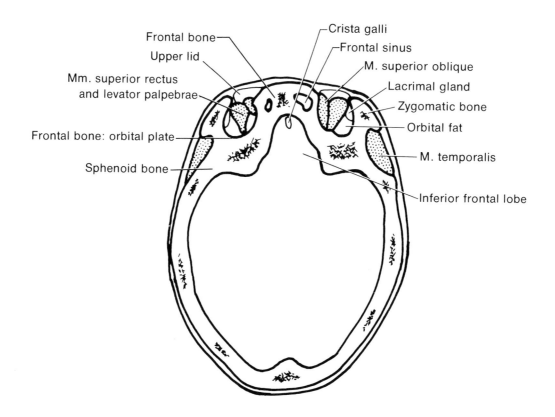

2.2 Anatomical diagram showing the superior extraocular muscles.

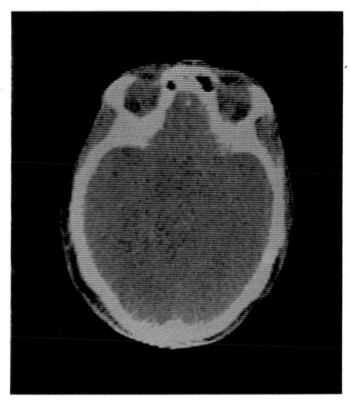

2.3 Color CT scan showing the superior extraocular muscles in yellow-green color.

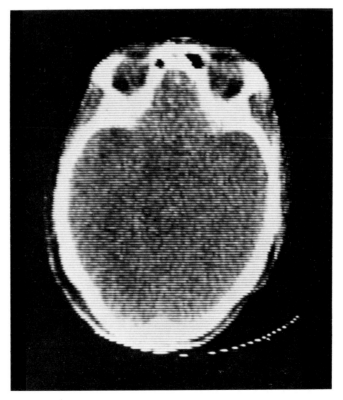

2.4 Black and white CT scan.

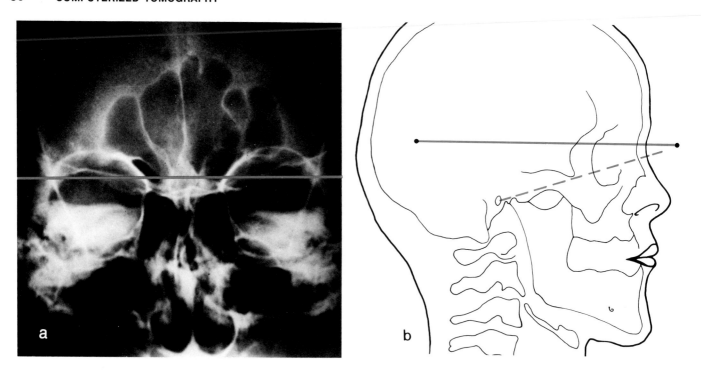

2.5 Scan level. (a) Normal skull roentgenogram; red line shows cross-section level. (b) Schematic drawing of scan level approximately 21 mm above the lateral canthus of the eye at an angle of +15° to the canthomeatal line (*dashed line*).

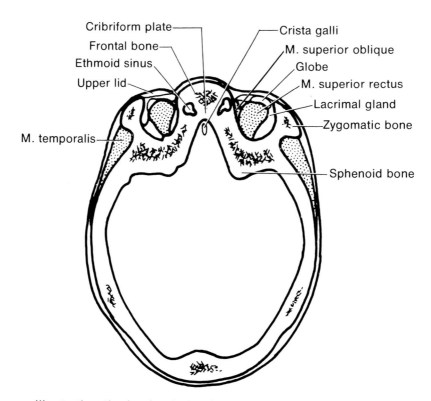

2.6 Anatomical diagram illustrating the lacrimal gland.

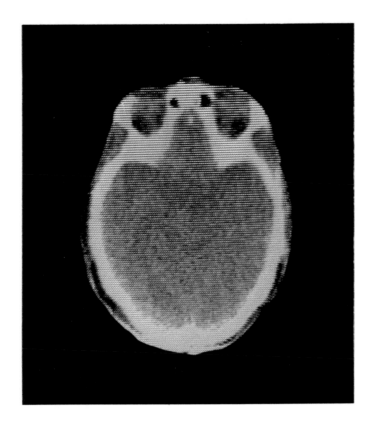

2.7 Color CT scan.

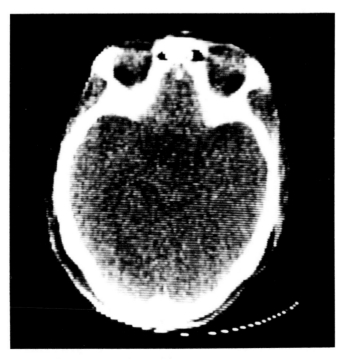

2.8 Black and white CT scan through the superior orbit.

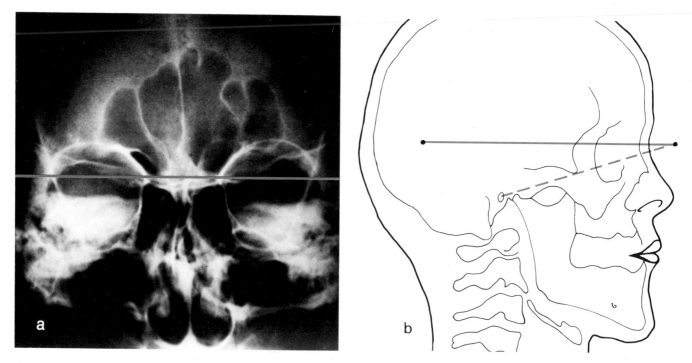

2.9 Scan level. (a) Normal skull roentgenogram; red line shows cross-section level. (b) Schematic drawing of scan level approximately 18 mm above the lateral canthus of the eye at an angle of +15° to the canthomeatal line (*dashed line*).

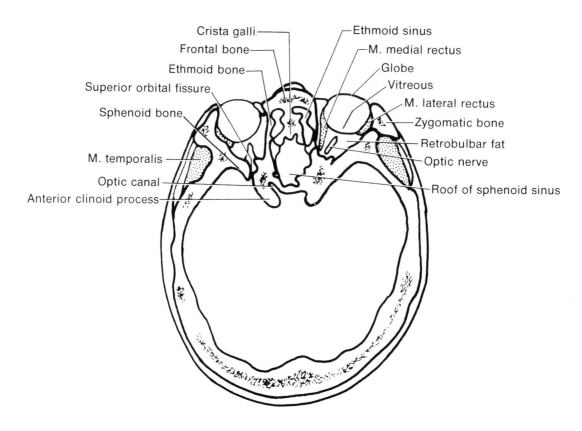

2.10 Anatomical diagram at a level through the superior hemisphere of the globe.

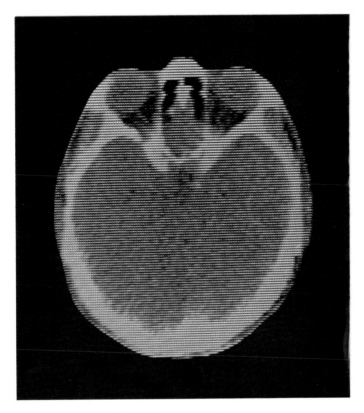

2.11 Color CT scan showing the optic nerve in light green color.

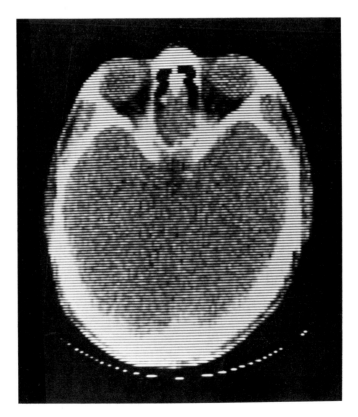

2.12 Black and white CT scan.

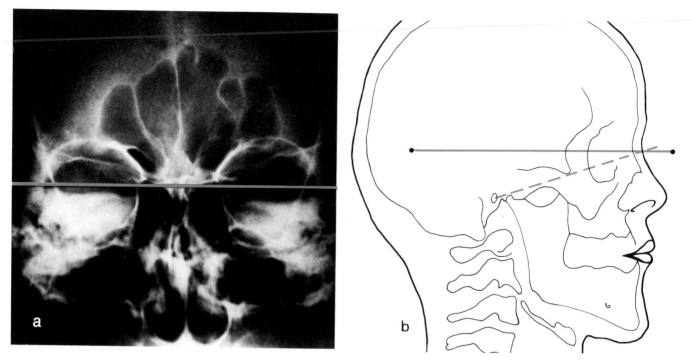

2.13 Scan level. (a) Normal skull roentgenogram; red line shows cross-section level. (b) Schematic drawing of scan level approximately 13 mm above the lateral canthus of the eye at an angle of +15° to the canthomeatal line (*dashed line*).

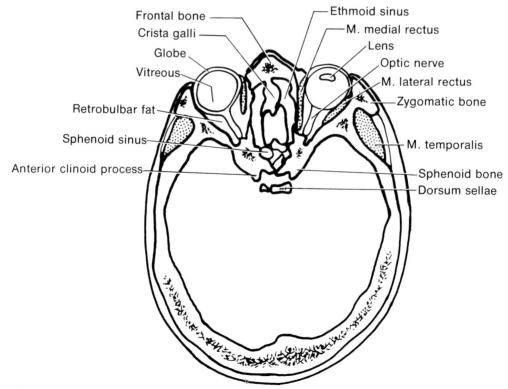

2.14 Anatomical diagram at the level of the dorsum sellae.

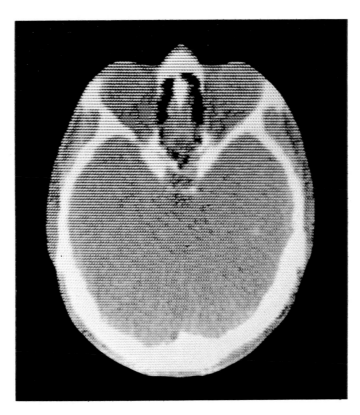

2.15 Color CT scan. Note the retrobulbar fat colored red, thereby allowing for the easy visualization of the optic nerve and extraocular muscles also seen in this section.

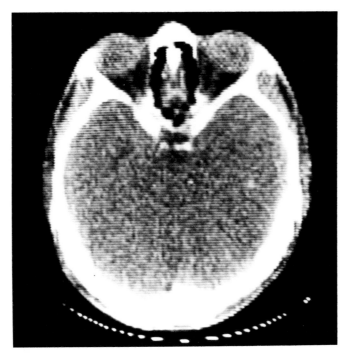

2.16 Black and white CT scan.

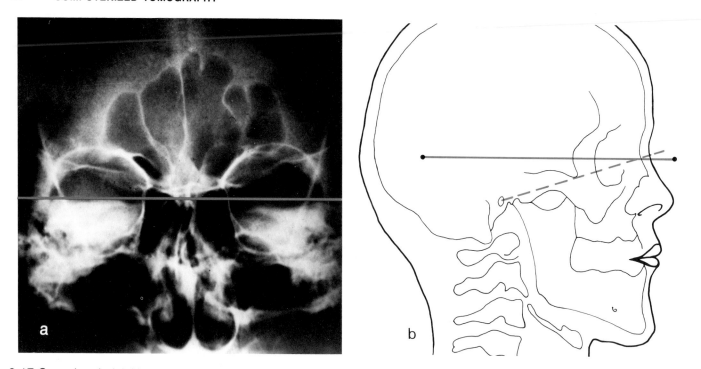

2.17 Scan level. (a) Normal skull roentgenogram; red line shows cross-section level. (b) Schematic drawing of scan level approximately 10 mm above the lateral canthus of the eye at an angle of +15° to the canthomeatal line (*dashed line*).

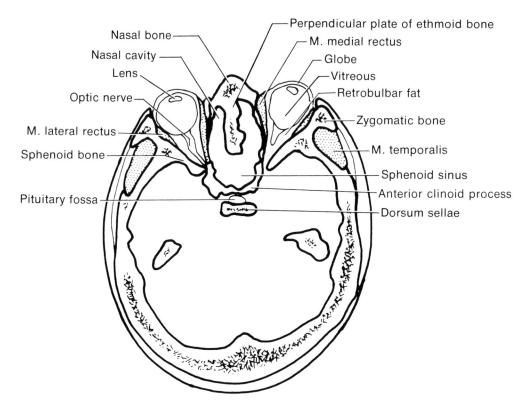

2.18 Anatomical diagram through the center of the globe.

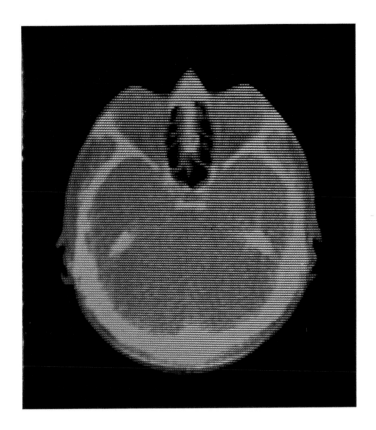

2.19 Color CT scan.

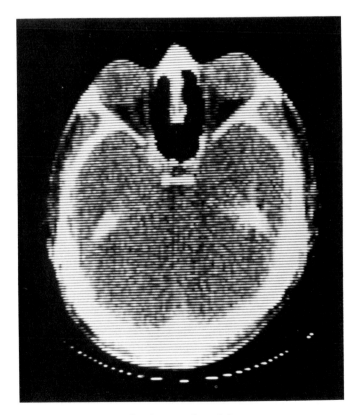

2.20 Black and white CT scan demonstrating the lenses in white.

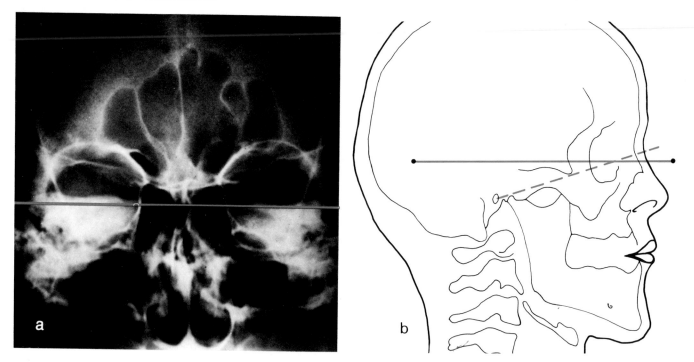

2.21 Scan level. (a) Normal skull roentgenogram; red line shows cross-section level. (b) Schematic drawing of scan level approximately 5 mm above the lateral canthus of the eye at an angle of +15° to the canthomeatal line (*dashed line*).

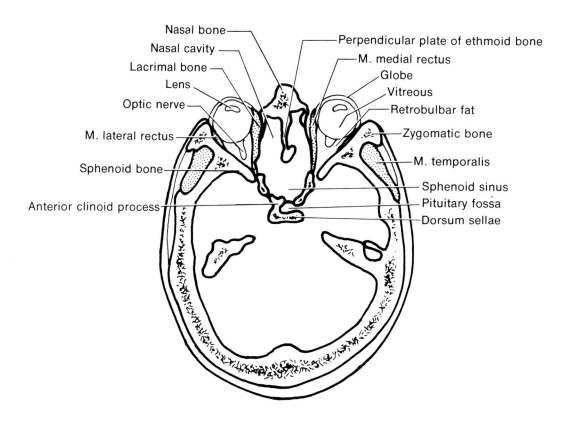

2.22 Anatomical diagram.

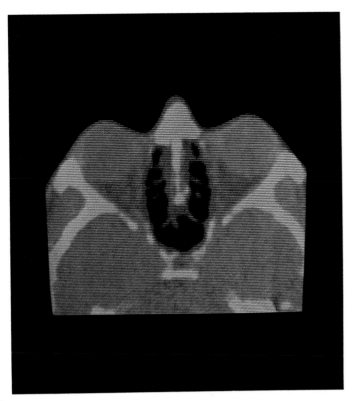 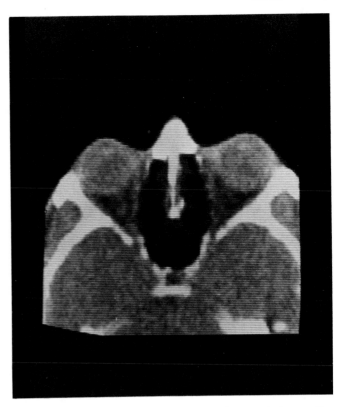

2.23 Enlarged CT scans. (*Left*) Color scan demonstrating the medial and lateral rectus muscles and the optic nerves in orange. (*Right*) Black and white scan illustrating the lenses.

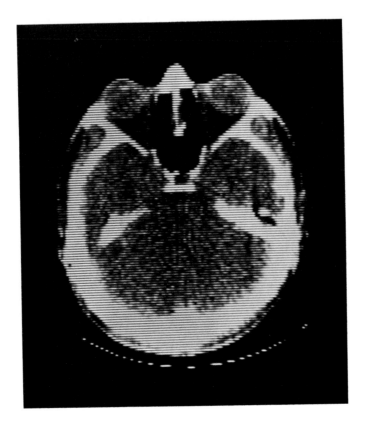

2.24 Black and white CT scan.

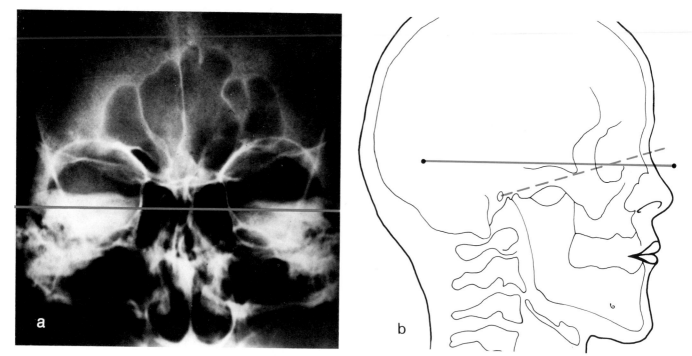

2.25 Scan level. (a) Normal skull roentgenogram, red line shows cross-section level. (b) Schematic drawing of scan level approximately 2 mm above the lateral canthus of the eye at an angle of +15° to the canthomeatal line (*dashed line*).

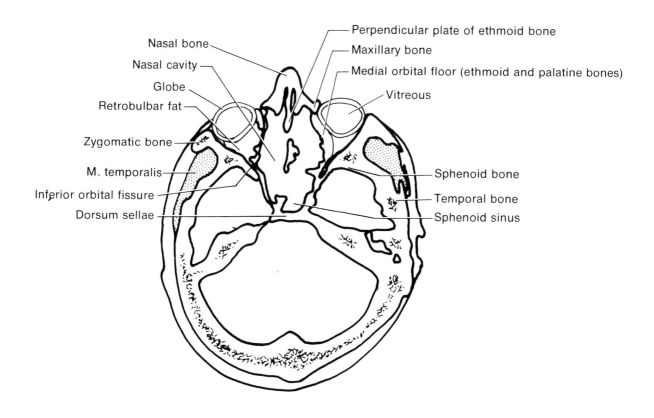

2.26 Anatomical diagram.

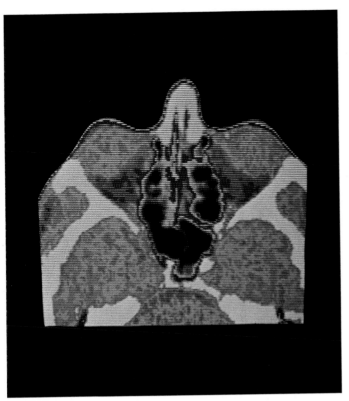 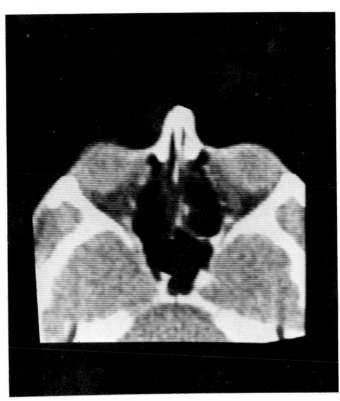

2.27 Enlarged CT scans. (*Left*) Color scan demonstrating the nasal concha within the nasal cavity. (*Right*) Black and white scan.

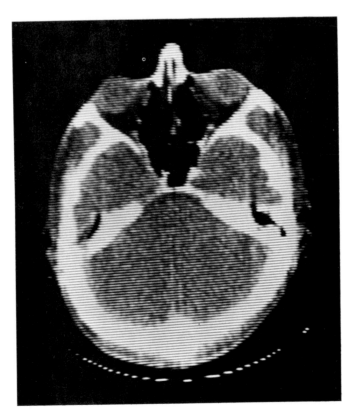

2.28 Black and white CT scan.

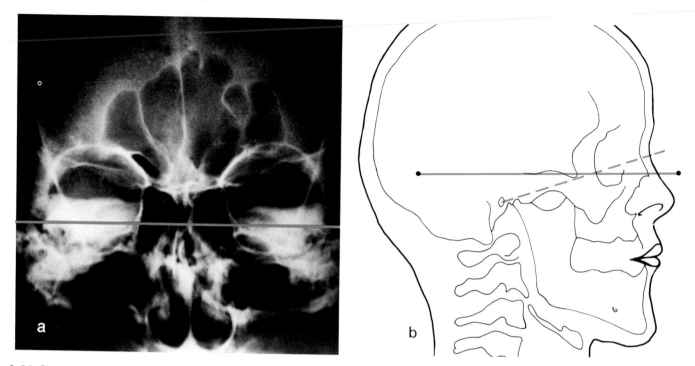

2.29 Scan level. (a) Normal skull roentgenogram; red line shows cross-section level. (b) Schematic drawing of scan level approximately 1 mm below the lateral canthus of the eye at an angle of +15° to the canthomeatal line (*dashed line*).

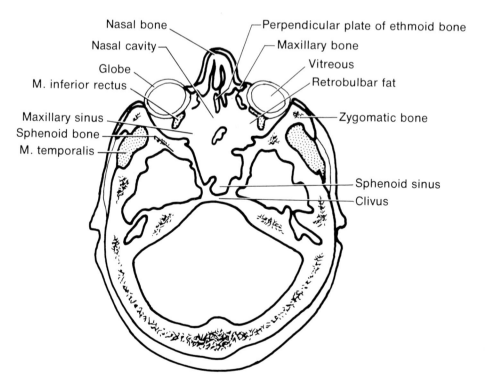

2.30 Anatomical diagram.

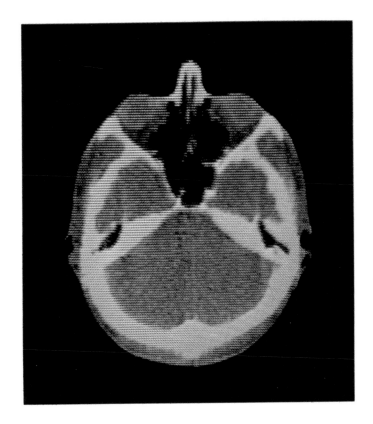

2.31 Color CT scan.

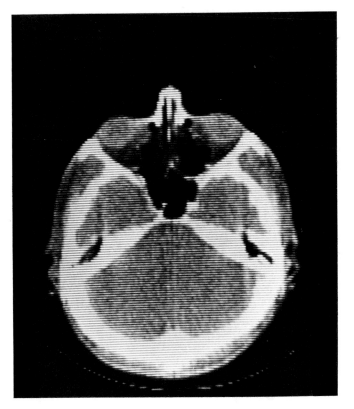

2.32 Black and white CT scan.

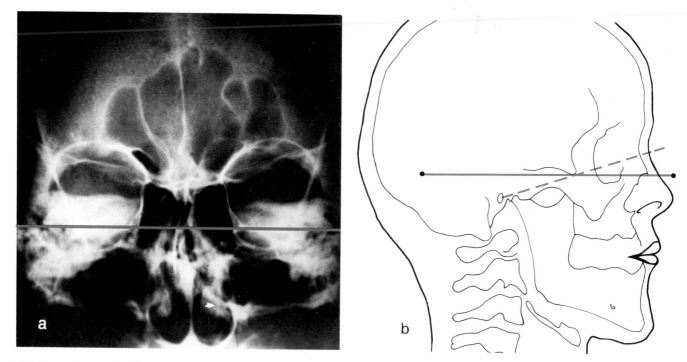

2.33 Scan level. (a) Normal skull roentgenogram; red line shows cross-section level. (b) Schematic drawing of scan level approximately 6 mm below the lateral canthus of the eye at an angle of +15° to the canthomeatal line (*dashed line*).

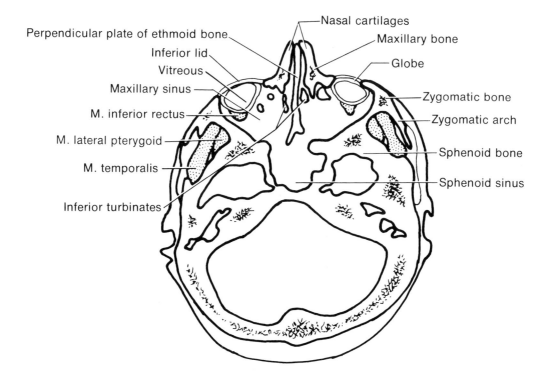

Perpendicular plate of ethmoid bone

Inferior lid

Vitreous

Maxillary sinus

M. inferior rectus

M. lateral pterygoid

M. temporalis

Inferior turbinates

Nasal cartilages

Maxillary bone

Globe

Zygomatic bone

Zygomatic arch

Sphenoid bone

Sphenoid sinus

2.34 Anatomical diagram at the upper border of the zygomatic arch.

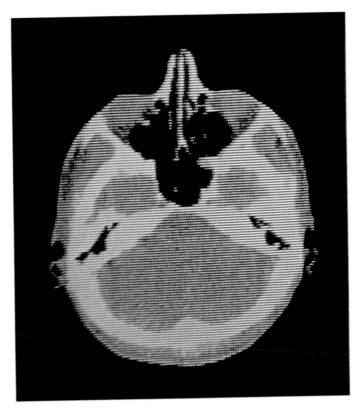

2.35 Color CT scan. Note the appearance of the muscles of the infratemporal fossa colored yellow.

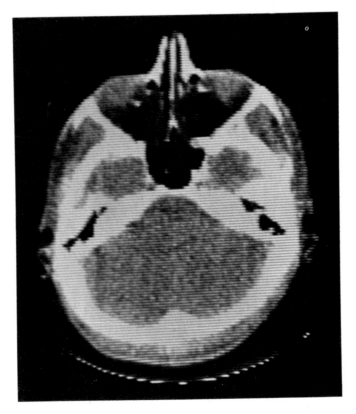

2.36 Black and white CT scan.

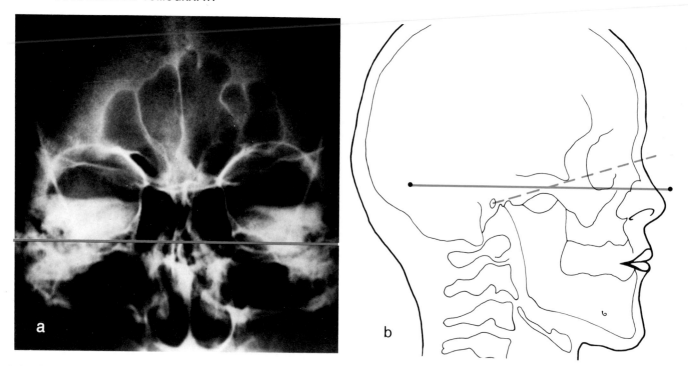

2.37 Scan level. (a) Normal skull roentgenogram; red line shows cross-section level. (b) Schematic drawing of scan level approximately 10 mm below the lateral canthus of the eye at an angle of +15° to the canthomeatal line (*dashed line*).

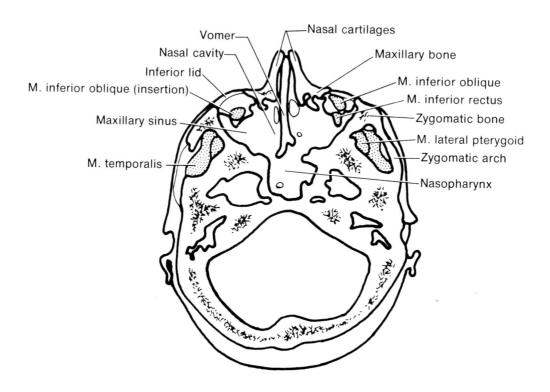

2.38 Anatomical diagram through the inferior portion of the orbit.

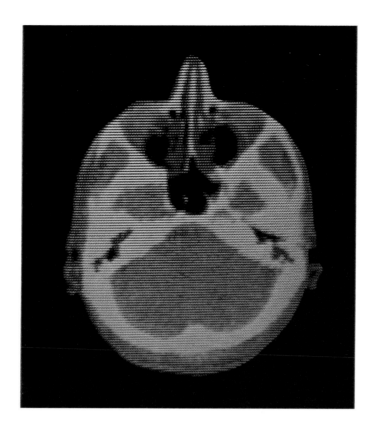

2.39 Color CT scan.

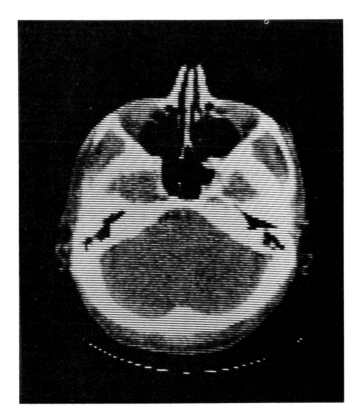

2.40 Black and white CT scan.

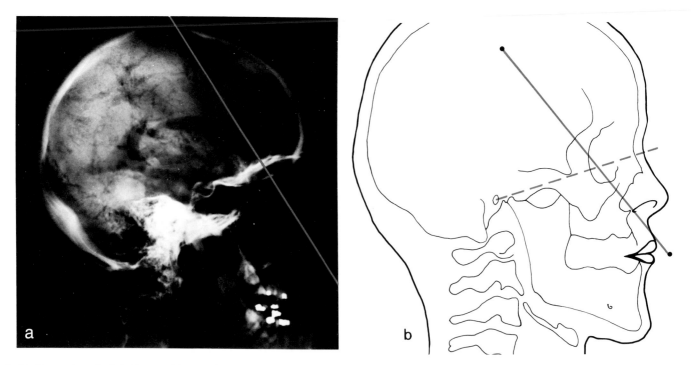

2.41 Scan level. (a) Normal lateral pneumoencephalogram; red line shows cross-section level. (b) Schematic drawing of scan level.

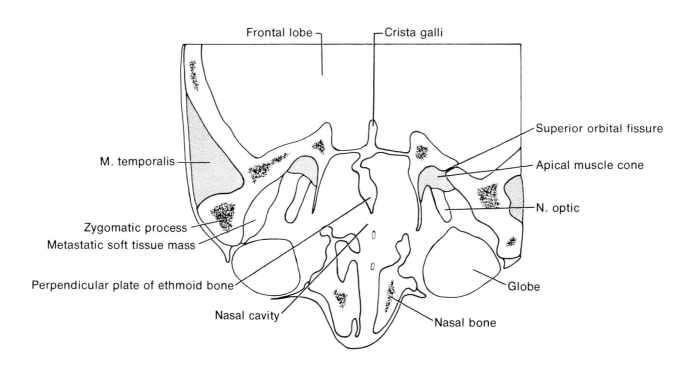

2.42 Anatomical diagram of ABNORMAL coronal section through the orbit.

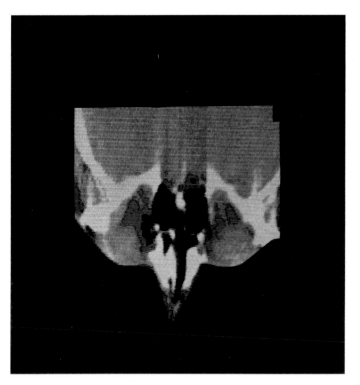 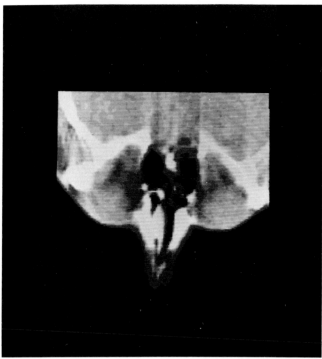

2.43 ABNORMAL enlarged coronal CT scans. (*Left*) Color scan with retrobulbar fat in red, optic nerve in green and a metastatic tumor in yellow; seen on the lateral wall of the orbit. (*Right*) Corresponding black and white scan showing nasal concha and the outline of the nose.

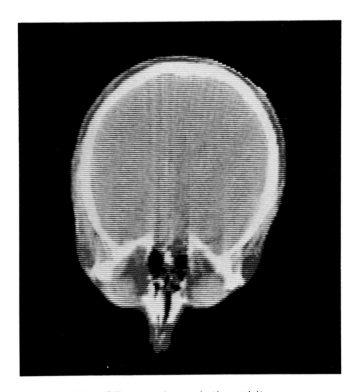

2.44 ABNORMAL coronal black and white CT scan through the orbit.

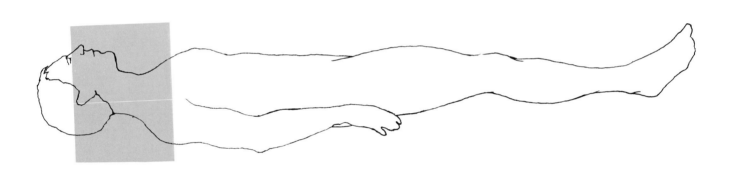

chapter three

Lower Face and Neck

This section of the ATLAS includes all structures from the floor of the orbit down to the level of T_1, a region which encompasses all the structures of the face, nasal cavity, mouth, pharynx, larynx, and neck.

Some of the first clinical uses of CT scanning in the face and neck were in the examination of the paranasal sinuses. Scanning these structures has given reliable studies for the detection of neoplasms arising from the mucosal linings of the facial sinuses. CT scanning in such cases delineates not only the location of a tumor mass but also its regional extension, and could permit nonsurgical staging of such lesions. In addition to neoplastic diseases of the head and neck, fluid collections, abscesses in the sinuses and prevertebral spaces, and pathology of the infratemporal and pterygopalatine fossae can be evaluated.

The structures of the hypopharynx, larynx, and epiglottis are well visualized with CT scans, and lesions of these structures may be examined by scanning at the appropriate level. The thyroid gland can be seen in its entirety; enlargements, cysts, and tumor masses have already been described using CT. The carotid system can be imaged by CT techniques and in addition contrast material enables the visualization of other major vessels in the head and neck. Finally, changes in the cervical spinal cord, such as occur in syringomyelia, may be studied using CT techniques.

All subjects studied for this section were lying supine with their arms at their sides. The subjects were scanned with their mouths closed using a 7.5-mm section thickness at 0° gantry tilt and a 1-cm scan interval. The presence of dental amalgams, gold crowns, and other metallic restorations cause significant artifacts when the scan level passes through these objects. For this reason, subjects with few such amalgams were used for the scans demonstrating the mouth region. If neck structures in the mouth region are needed for study, various positions (e.g., open mouth, hyperextension of the head) may be used to eliminate the teeth from the scan plane.

As in other sections, reference lines are provided on a standard A-P X-ray film of the cervical spine and on a patient profile. The following colors in the scans of this section represent those tissues listed below:

White .Compact bone
Light blue, orange . . . . .Bone marrow, ligament, and tendon
Light purple . . . . .Muscle
Dark purple . . . . .Fat
Black . . . . .Air

The following landmarks are provided to correlate patient positioning with the figures in this ATLAS:

External auditory meatus Figures 3.1–3.4
Angle of mandible . . . . . . .Figures 3.25–3.28
Top of thyroid cartilage . .Figures 3.41–3.44
Acromioclavicular joint . .Figures 3.53–3.56

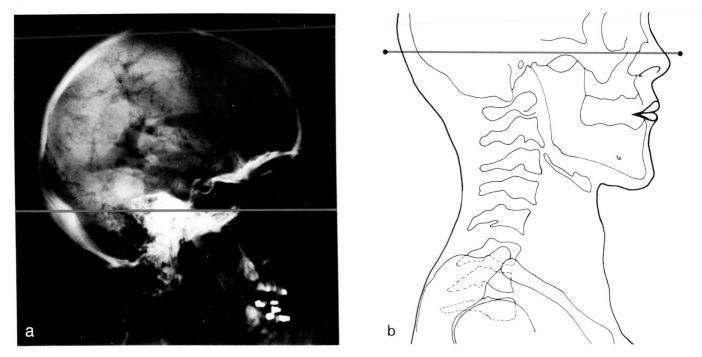

3.1 Scan level. (a) Normal lateral pneumoencephalogram; red line shows cross-section level. (b) Schematic drawing of scan level.

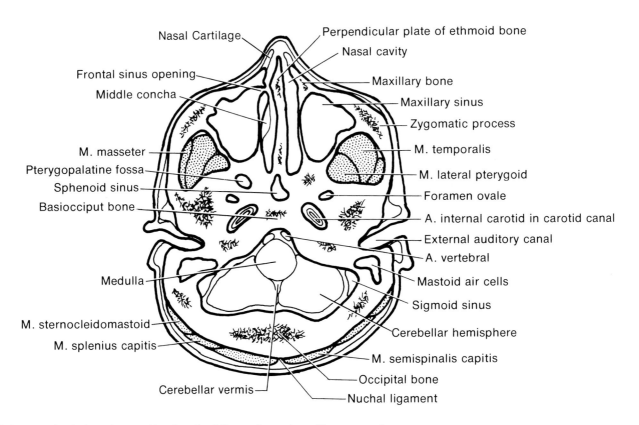

3.2 Anatomical drawing at the level of the external auditory canal.

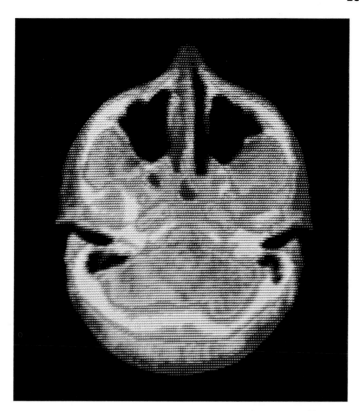

3.3 Color CT scan. Note the appearance of the carotid artery in the carotid canal and the muscles of the infratemporal fossa.

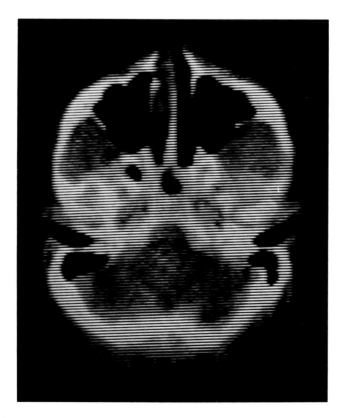

3.4 Black and white CT scan.

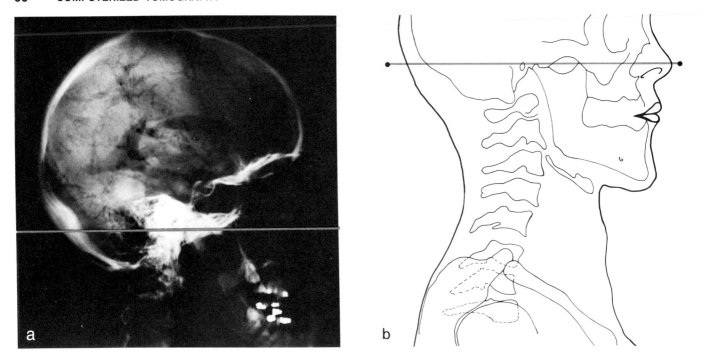

3.5 Scan level. (a) Normal lateral pneumoencephalogram; red line shows cross-section level. (b) Schematic drawing of scan level.

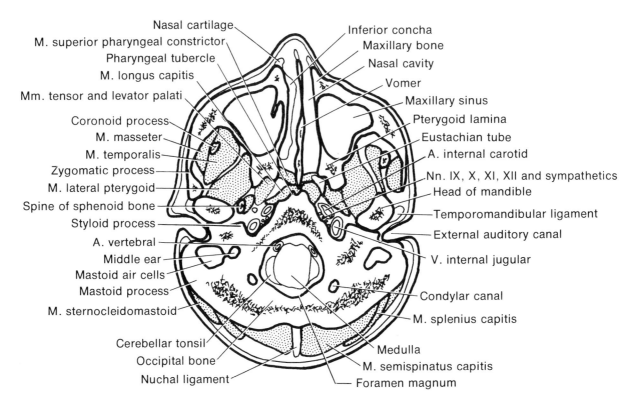

3.6 Anatomical drawing at the level of the base of the skull.

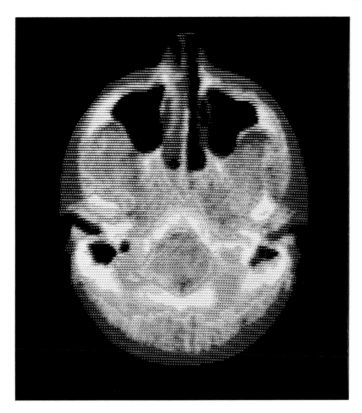

3.7 Color CT scan illustrating the temporomandibular joint.

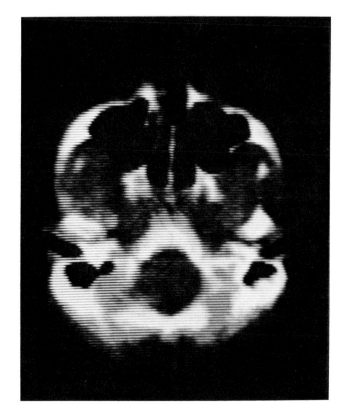

3.8 Black and white CT scan.

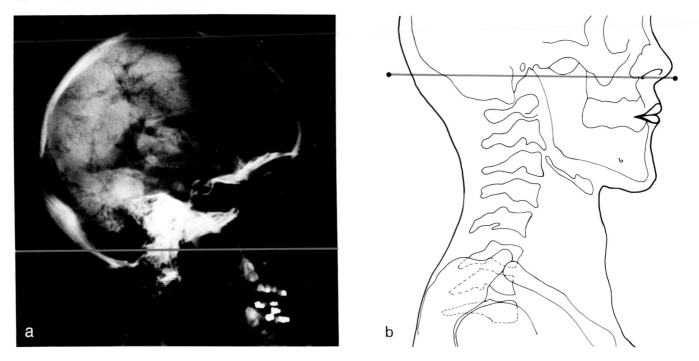

3.9 Scan level. (a) Normal lateral pneumoencephalogram; red line shows cross-section level. (b) Schematic drawing of scan level.

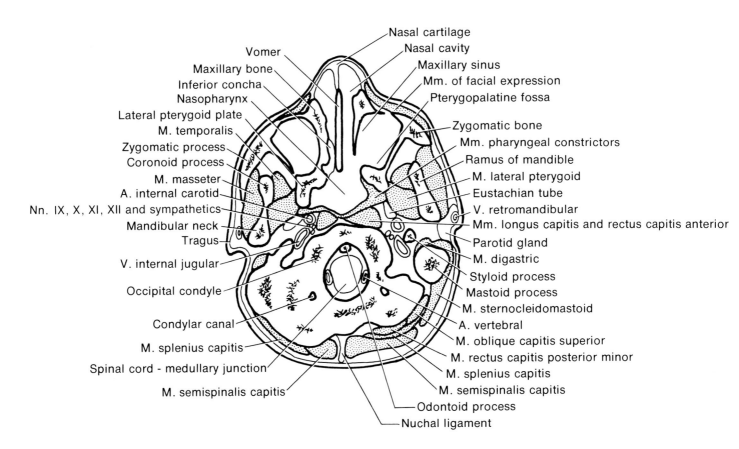

3.10 Anatomical diagram at the level of the foramen magnum.

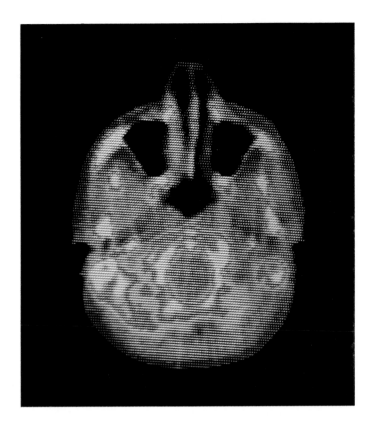

3.11 Color CT scan.

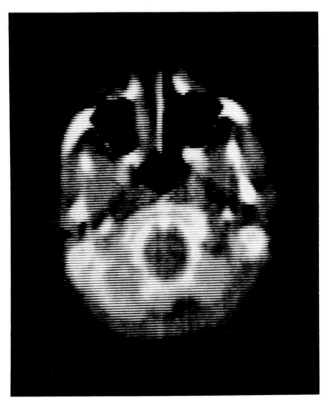

3.12 Black and white CT scan. Note the musculature of the infratemporal fossa and in the prevertebral region.

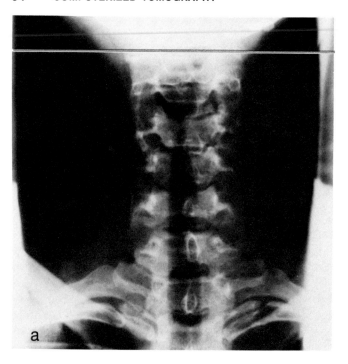
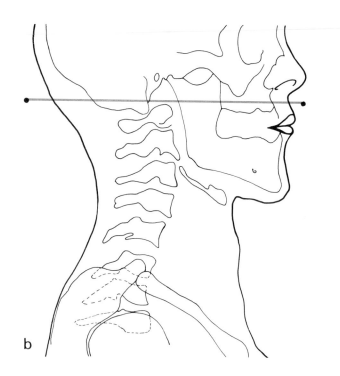

3.13 Scan level. (a) Normal A-P cervical spine roentgenogram; red line shows cross-section level. (b) Schematic drawing of scan level.

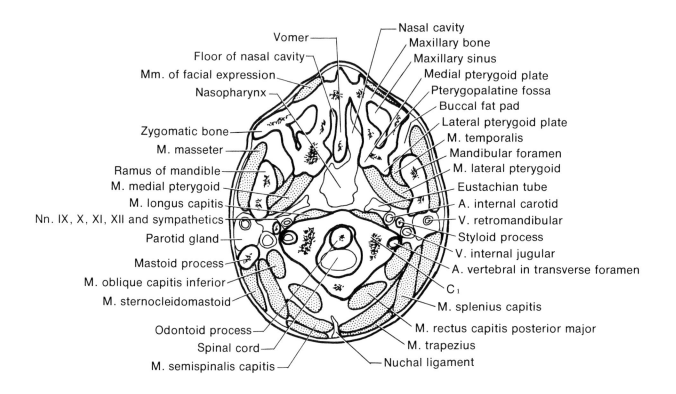

3.14 Anatomical diagram at the level of the nasopharynx and C_1.

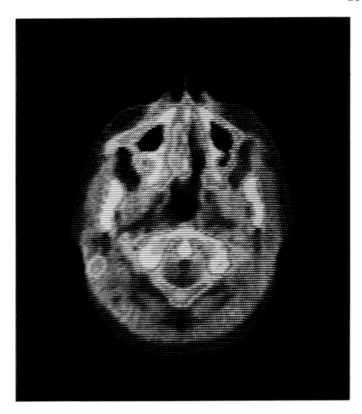

3.15 Color CT scan.

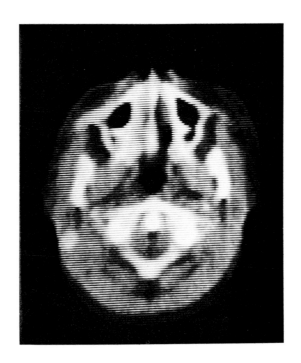

3.16 Black and white CT scan illustrating the odontoid process and the lower facial sinuses.

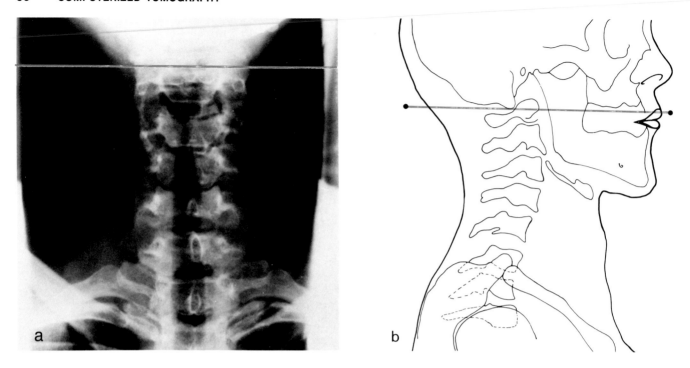

3.17 Scan level. (a) Normal A-P cervical spine roentgenogram; red line shows cross-section level. (b) Schematic drawing of scan level.

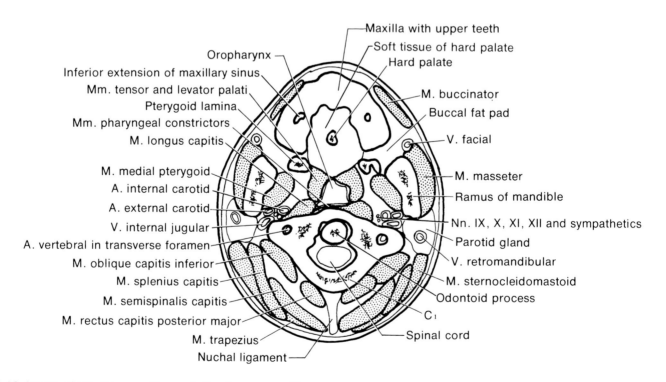

3.18 Anatomical diagram through the lower maxilla.

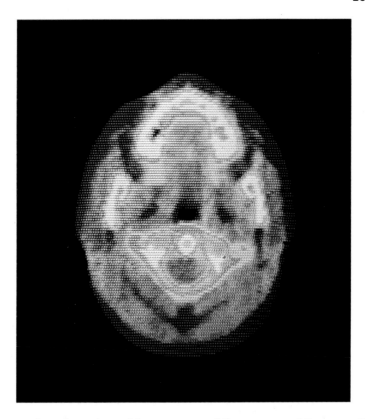

3.19 Color CT scan demonstrating the odontoid process and the ramus of the mandible.

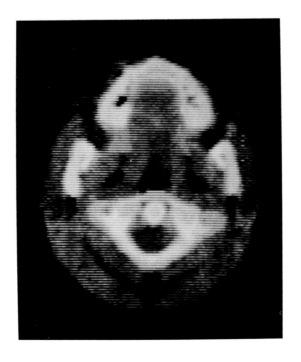

3.20 Black and white CT scan.

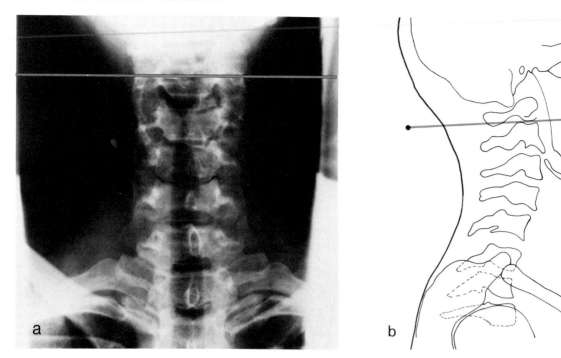

3.21 Scan level. (a) Normal A-P cervical spine roentgenogram; red line shows cross-section level. (b) Schematic drawing of scan level.

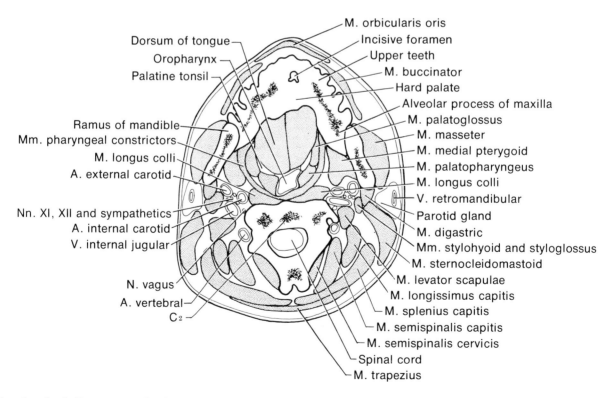

3.22 Anatomical diagram at the level of the oropharynx.

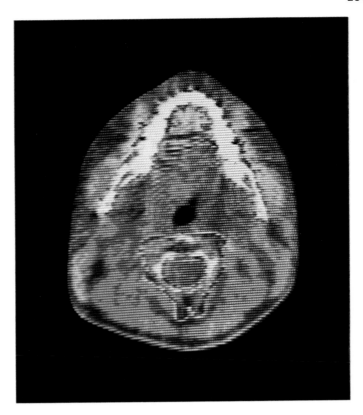

3.23 Color CT scan demonstrating the suboccipital musculature in light purple.

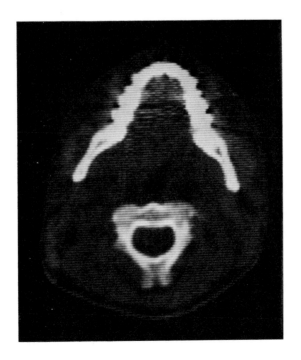

3.24 Black and white CT scan.

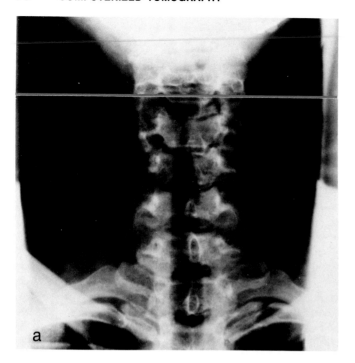 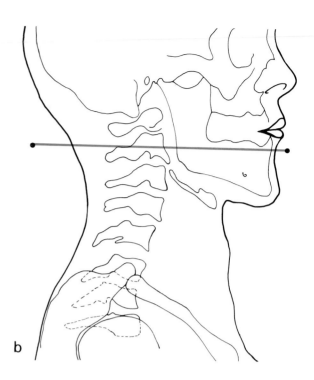

3.25 Scan level. (a) Normal A-P cervical spine roentgenogram; red line shows cross-section level. (b) Schematic drawing of scan level.

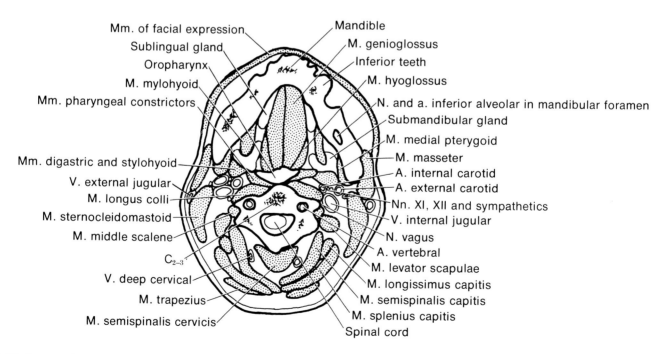

3.26 Anatomical diagram at the level of the oropharynx and tongue.

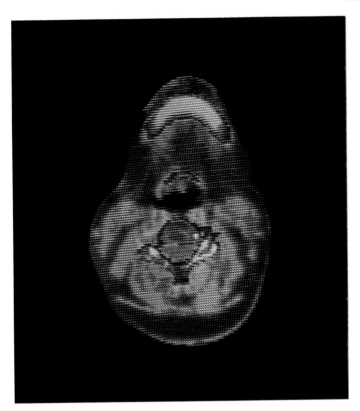

3.27 Color CT scan.

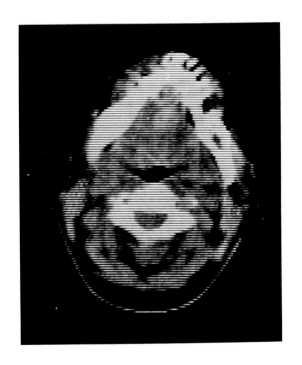

3.28 Black and white CT scan.

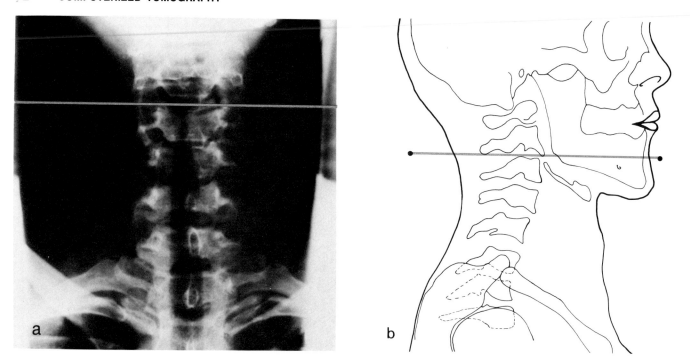

3.29 Scan level. (a) Normal A-P cervical spine roentgenogram; red line shows cross-section level. (b) Schematic drawing of scan level.

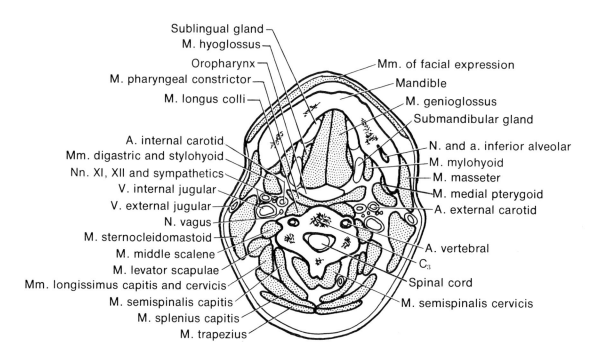

Sublingual gland
M. hyoglossus
Oropharynx
M. pharyngeal constrictor
M. longus colli

Mm. of facial expression
Mandible
M. genioglossus
Submandibular gland

A. internal carotid
Mm. digastric and stylohyoid
Nn. XI, XII and sympathetics
V. internal jugular
V. external jugular
N. vagus
M. sternocleidomastoid
M. middle scalene
M. levator scapulae
Mm. longissimus capitis and cervicis
M. semispinalis capitis
M. splenius capitis
M. trapezius

N. and a. inferior alveolar
M. mylohyoid
M. masseter
M. medial pterygoid
A. external carotid

A. vertebral
C₃
Spinal cord
M. semispinalis cervicis

3.30 Anatomical diagram.

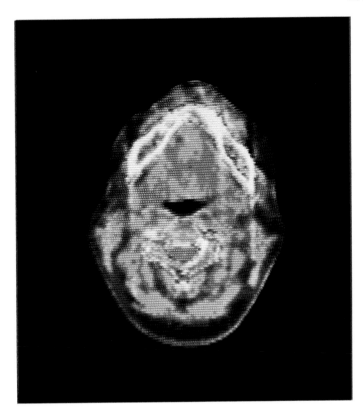

3.31 Color CT scan with the cervical musculature colored light purple.

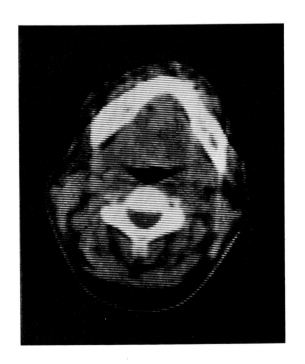

3.32 Black and white CT scan.

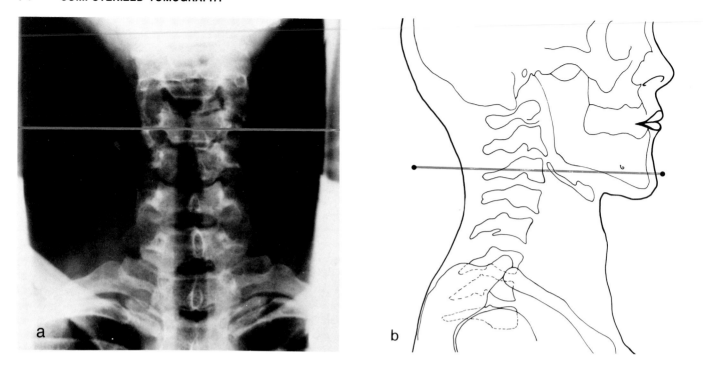

3.33 Scan level. (a) Normal A-P cervical spine roentgenogram; red line shows cross-section level. (b) Schematic drawing of scan level.

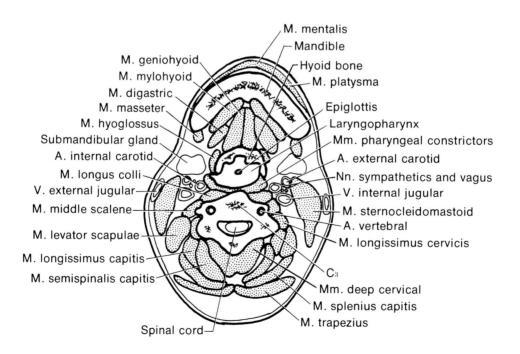

3.34 Anatomical diagram at the level of the hyoid bone.

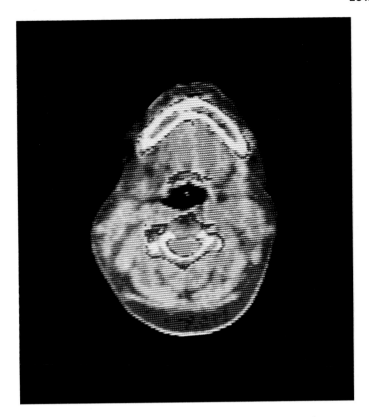

3.35 Color CT scan. Note the presence of the epiglottis within the laryngopharynx.

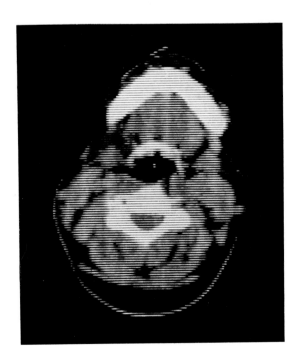

3.36 Black and white CT scan.

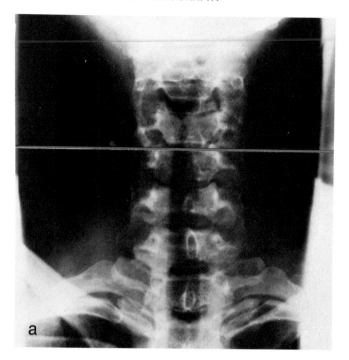
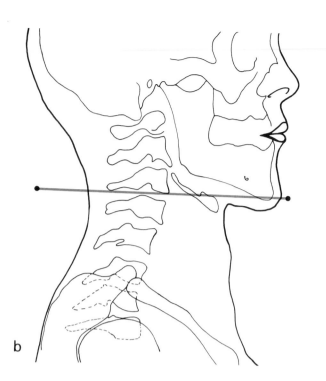

3.37 Scan level. (a) Normal A-P cervical spine roentgenogram; red line shows cross-section level. (b) Schematic drawing of scan level.

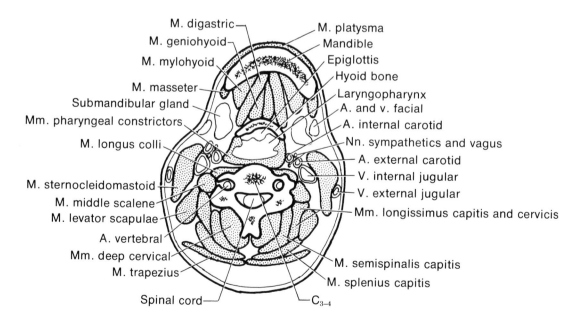

3.38 Anatomical diagram at the level of the hyoid bone.

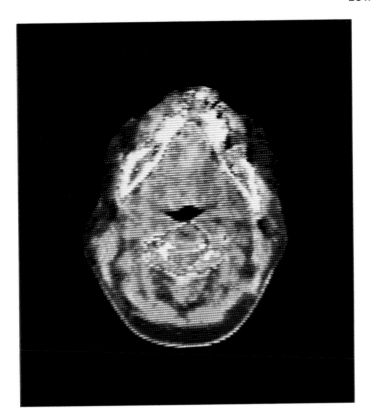

3.39 Color CT scan.

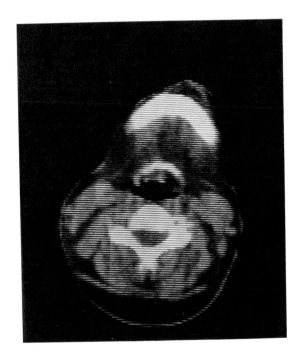

3.40 Black and white CT scan.

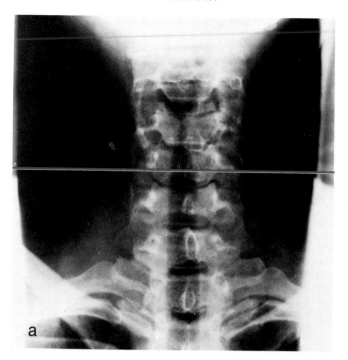

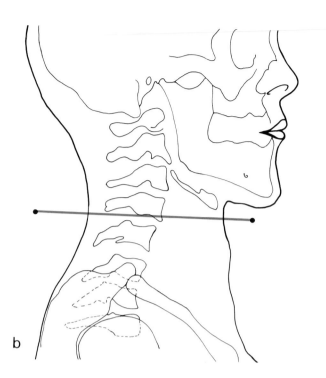

3.41 Scan level. (a) Normal A-P cervical spine roentgenogram; red line shows cross-section level. (b) Schematic drawing of scan level.

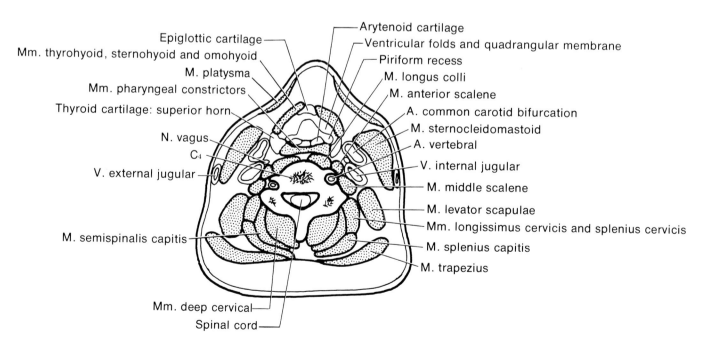

3.42 Anatomical diagram through the superior portion of the thyroid cartilage.

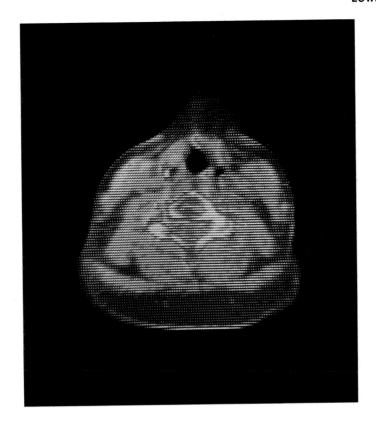

3.43 Color CT scan.

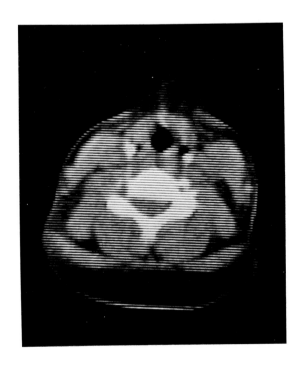

3.44 Black and white CT scan.

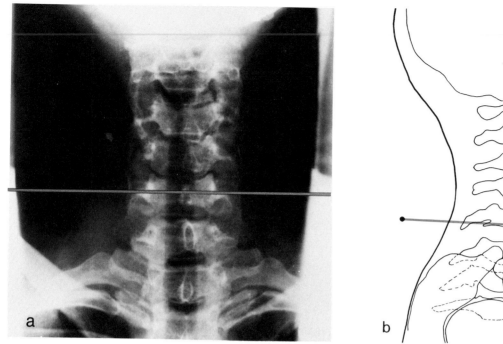

3.45 Scan level. (a) Normal A-P cervical spine roentgenogram; red line shows cross-section level. (b) Schematic drawing of scan level.

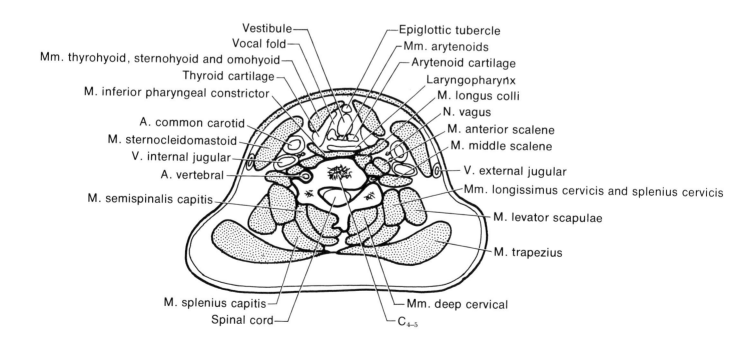

3.46 Anatomical drawing at the level of the larynx.

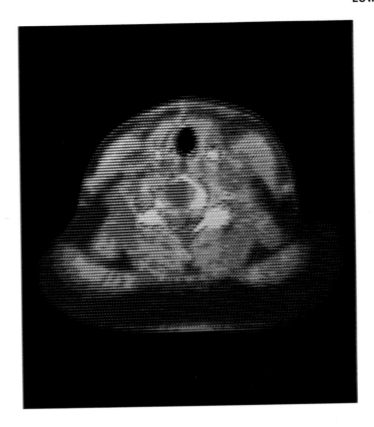

3.47 Color CT scan.

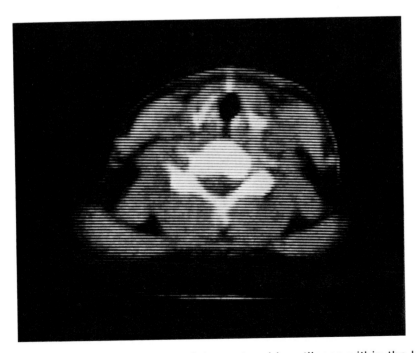

3.48 Black and white CT scan. Note the presence of the arytenoid cartilages within the larynx.

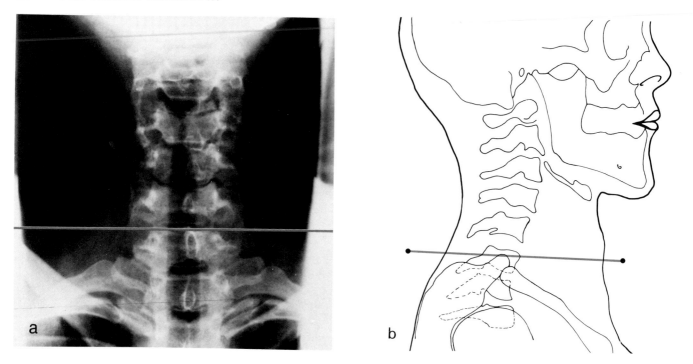

3.49 Scan level. (a) Normal A-P cervical spine roentgenogram; red line shows cross-section level. (b) Schematic drawing of scan level.

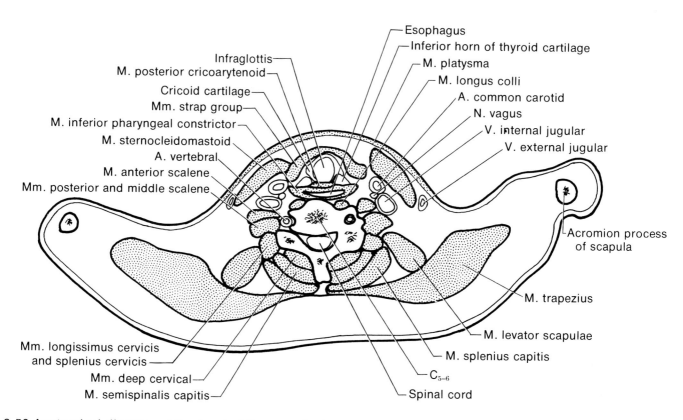

3.50 Anatomical diagram at the level of the superior border of the cricoid cartilage.

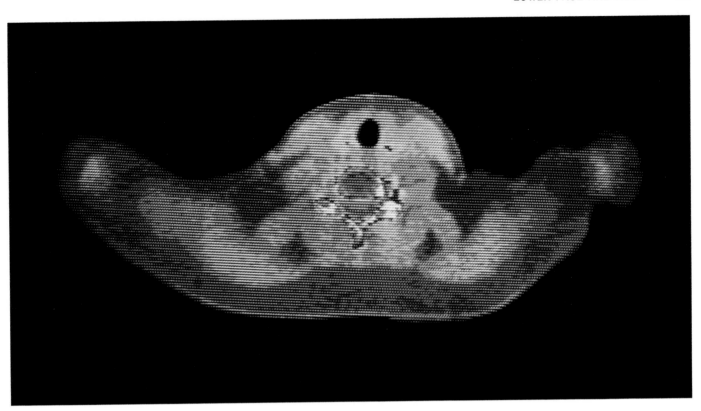

3.51 Color CT scan showing the superior border of the acromion process of the scapula.

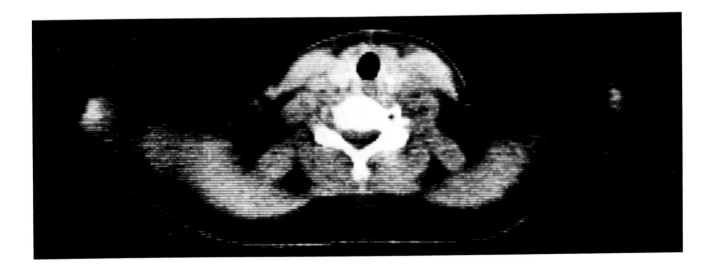

3.52 Black and white CT scan.

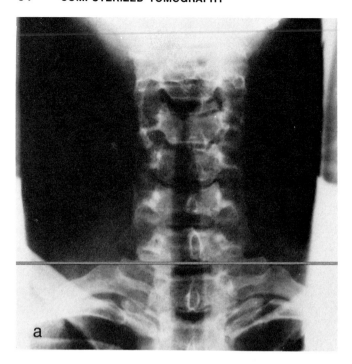 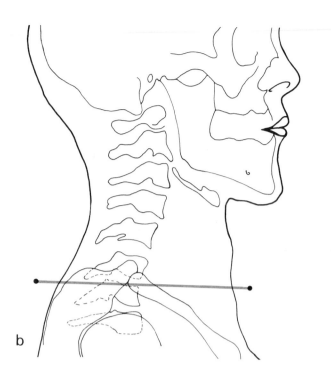

3.53 Scan level. (a) Normal A-P cervical spine roentgenogram; red line shows cross-section level. (b) Schematic drawing of scan level.

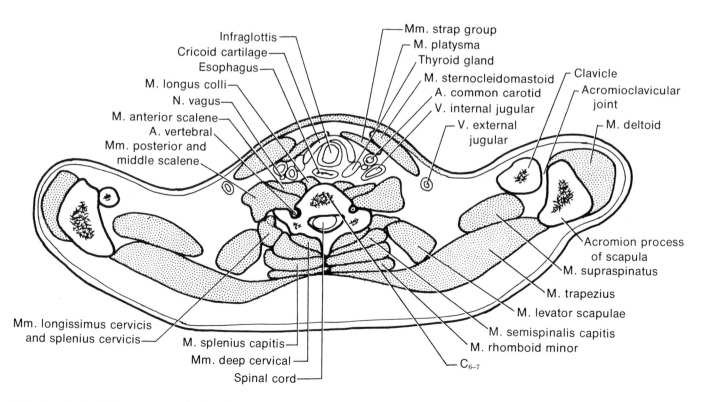

3.54 Anatomical diagram at the level of the lower portion of the cricoid cartilage.

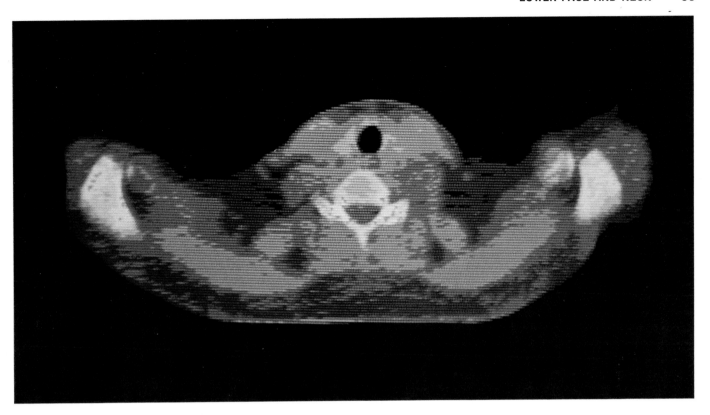

3.55 Color CT scan demonstrating the acromioclavicular joint.

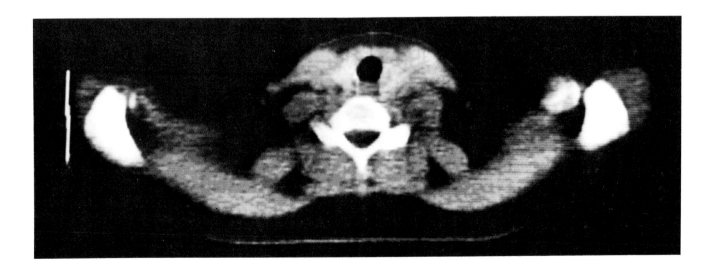

3.56 Black and white CT scan.

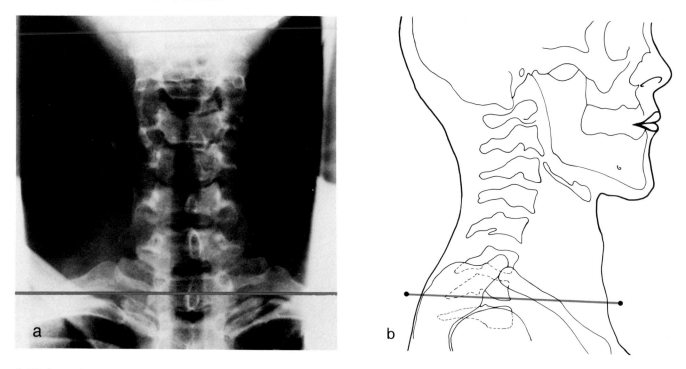

3.57 Scan level. (a) Normal A-P cervical spine roentgenogram; red line shows cross-section level. (b) Schematic drawing of scan level.

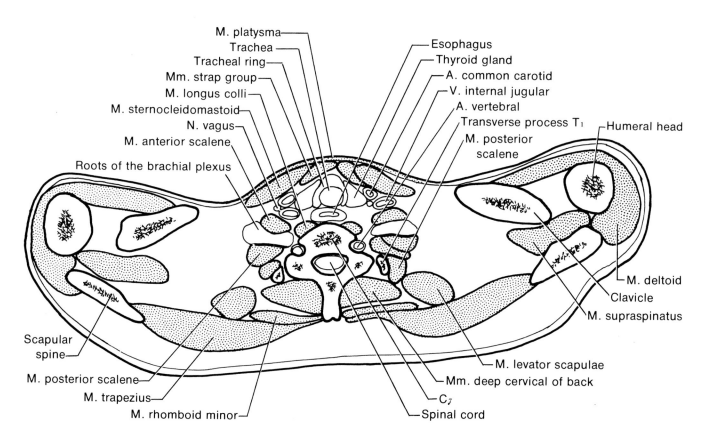

3.58 Anatomical drawing at the level of the upper trachea and C_7.

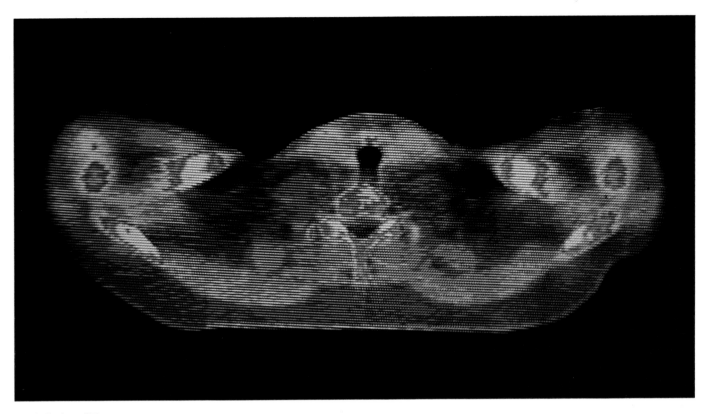

3.59 Color CT scan.

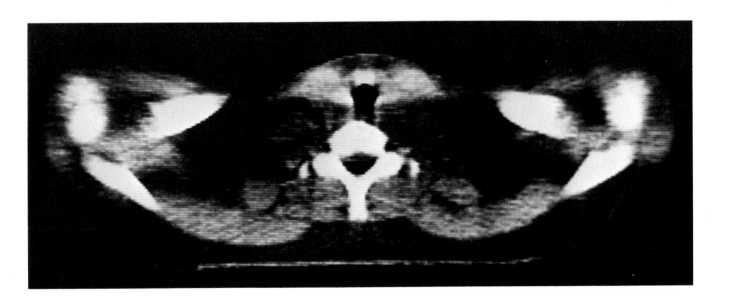

3.60 Black and white CT scan. Notice the appearance of the radiodense thyroid gland.

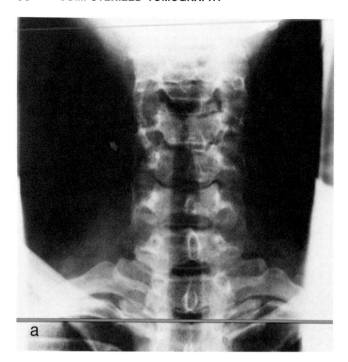

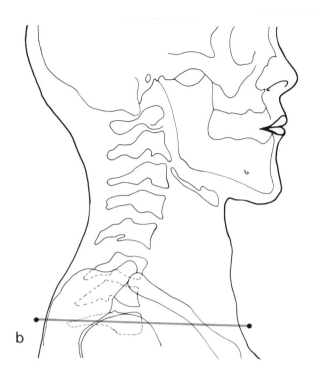

a

b

3.61 Scan level. (a) Normal A-P cervical spine roentgenogram; red line shows cross-section level. (b) Schematic drawing of scan level.

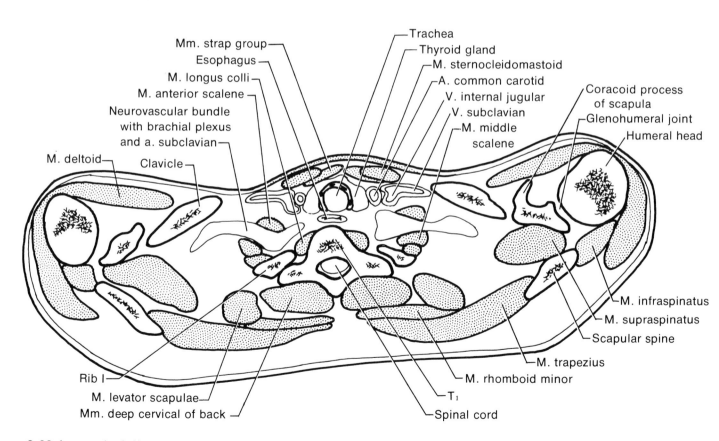

Mm. strap group
Esophagus
M. longus colli
M. anterior scalene
Neurovascular bundle
with brachial plexus
and a. subclavian
M. deltoid
Clavicle
Trachea
Thyroid gland
M. sternocleidomastoid
A. common carotid
V. internal jugular
V. subclavian
M. middle
scalene
Coracoid process
of scapula
Glenohumeral joint
Humeral head
M. infraspinatus
M. supraspinatus
Scapular spine
M. trapezius
M. rhomboid minor
T_1
Spinal cord
Rib I
M. levator scapulae
Mm. deep cervical of back

3.62 Anatomical diagram at the level of T_1.

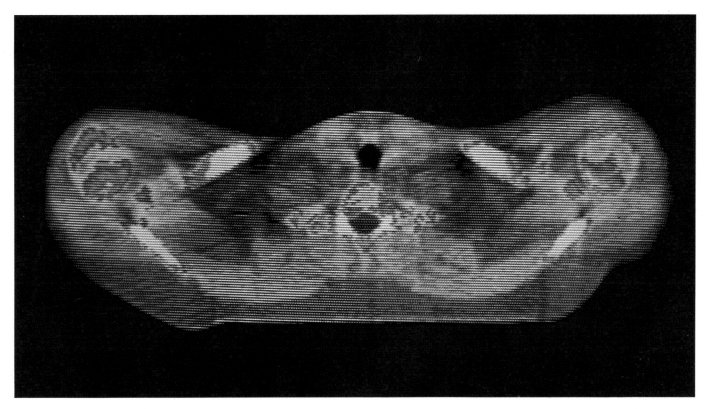

3.63 Color CT scan.

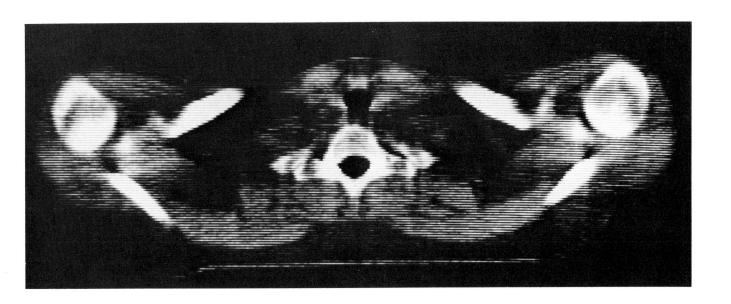

3.64 Black and white CT scan. Note the glenohumeral joint and the musculature of the shoulder.

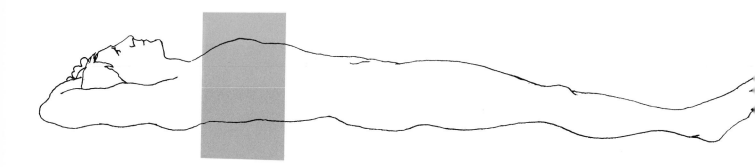

chapter four

Chest

This section of the ATLAS includes all structures from the lung apices to the costodiaphragmatic recesses, which in CT scanning can cover an area that extends from the second to the eleventh thoracic vertebra.

As is the case with other regions of the body, serial two-dimensional CT scans provide the clinician with an exact three-dimensional localization of abnormalities within the chest, a feature useful for percutaneous biopsy, for preoperative evaluation, and especially for radiation therapy planning and evaluation. Diseases involving the pleura and pericardium may be studied quite feasibly using CT methods. Conventional radiological methods are of great value in the study of chest pathology because of the marked differences in the radioabsorption of the structures within the thoracic cage. CT scanning, however, constitutes an additional potential for diagnostic formation because it provides a precisely localized image throughout the region. For example, imaging of the mediastinum, as well as the hilar and peritracheal lymph nodes, for enlargement secondary to occult malignancy and local or systemic inflammatory processes is an important diagnostic radiographic finding. CT scans are particularly effective for just such mediastinal and hilar structures, the constituents of which are of similar radioabsorption and often overlap in conventional radiographic imaging.

All subjects were scanned in the supine position with their arms extended above the head. A section thickness of 7.5 mm was used at a 0° gantry tilt with a scan interval of 1 cm. The conventional X-ray image displayed along with each CT scan was obtained with the subject in the same supine position and at mid-expiration in the respiratory cycle. A reference line has been drawn on each conventional X-ray image to correspond as closely as possible to the level shown on the CT scan and diagram.

The colors used in the CT image correspond to the following tissue densities:

White . . . . .Bone
Yellow-orange . . . . .Muscle
Purple . . . . .Lung parenchyma
with air

Double windows (as explained in the Introduction) were utilized in the CT scans in this section in order to provide increased detail in the areas of both high and low radioabsorption.

In two instances, muscles (the strap muscles of the neck and the paravertebral muscles of the deep back) are named collectively in groups rather than individually, to allow for clearer, more detailed labeling of structures of greater clinical importance.

In order to facilitate patient positioning, we have included the following list of bony landmarks to correlate surface anatomy with their corresponding figure numbers:

Jugular notch . . . . . . .Figures 4.9–4.12
Xiphoid . . . . .Figures 4.77–4.80

Because the distance between landmarks varies from one individual to the next (in this ATLAS the distance from the jugular notch to the xiphoid was 16 cm), it is necessary to adjust scanning levels proportionally to this difference in distances, in order to compare scans which correspond to the figures in the ATLAS.

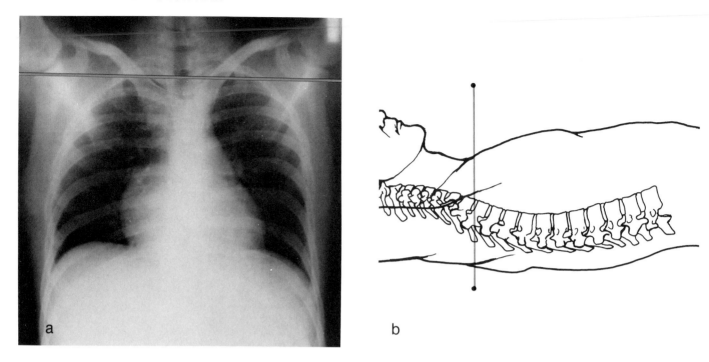

4.1 Scan level. (a) Normal mid-expiration chest roentgenogram; red line shows cross-section level. Note the glenohumeral joint is slightly elevated relative to the scan level. (b) Schematic drawing of scan level.

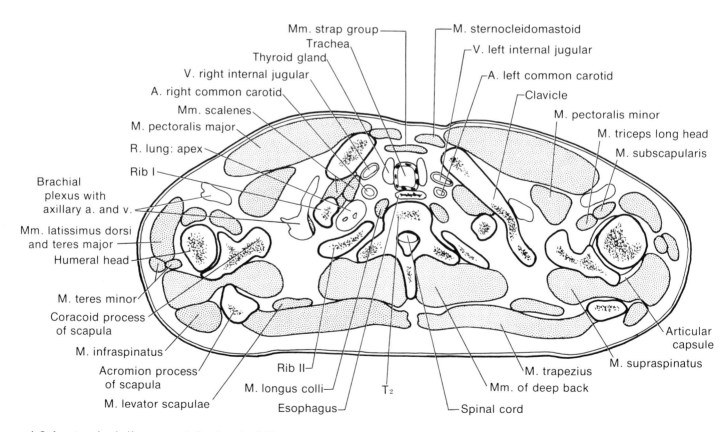

4.2 Anatomical diagram at the level of T_2.

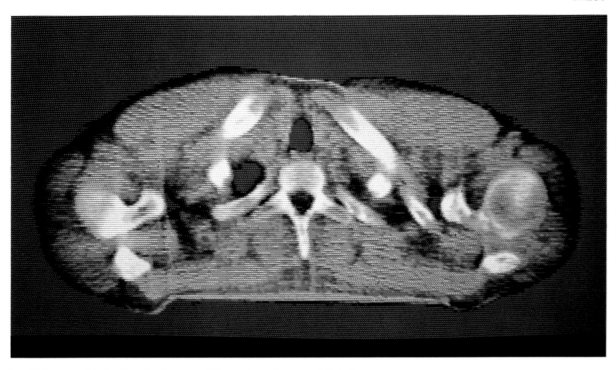

4.3 Color CT scan. Note the features of the glenohumeral joint.

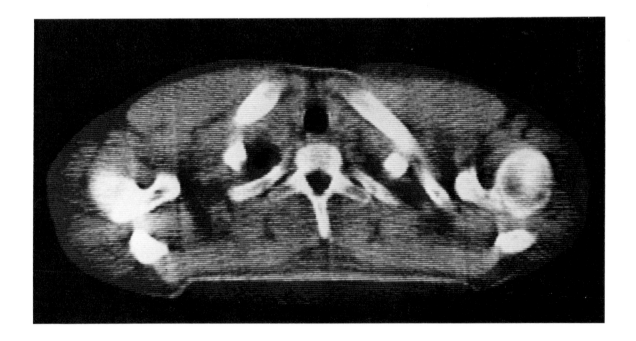

4.4 Black and white CT scan.

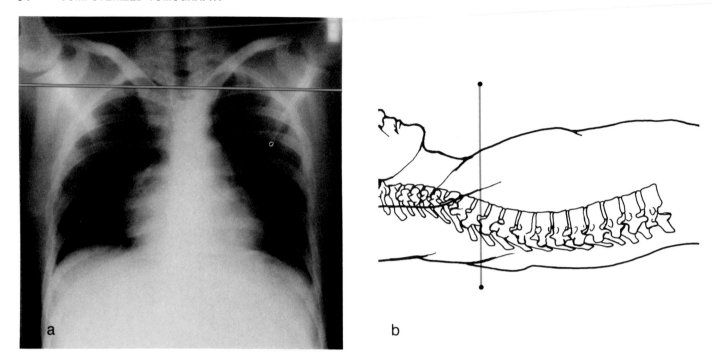

4.5 Scan level. (a) Normal mid-expiration chest roentgenogram; red line shows cross-section level. Note the glenohumeral joint is slightly elevated relative to the scan level. (b) Schematic drawing of scan level.

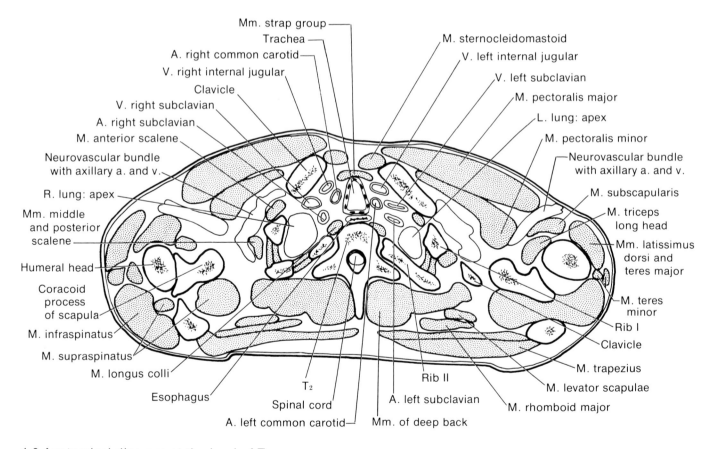

4.6 Anatomical diagram at the level of T_2.

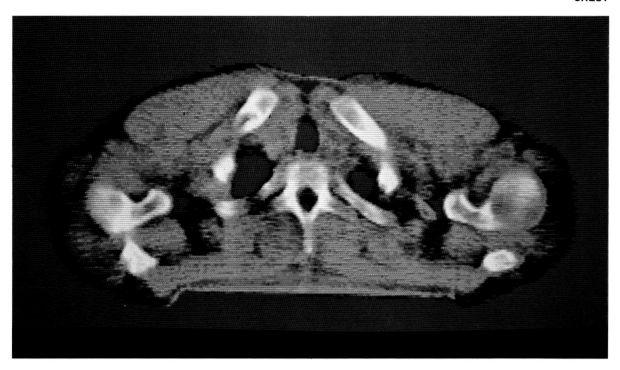

4.7 Color CT scan.

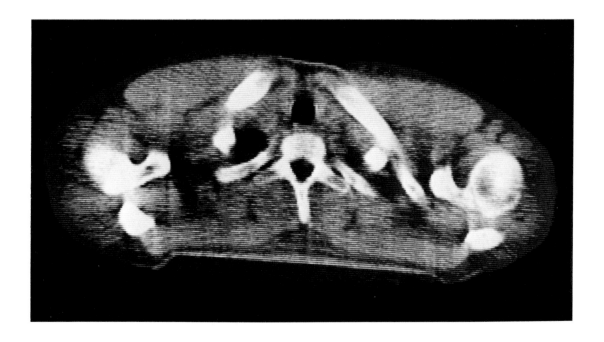

4.8 Black and white CT scan.

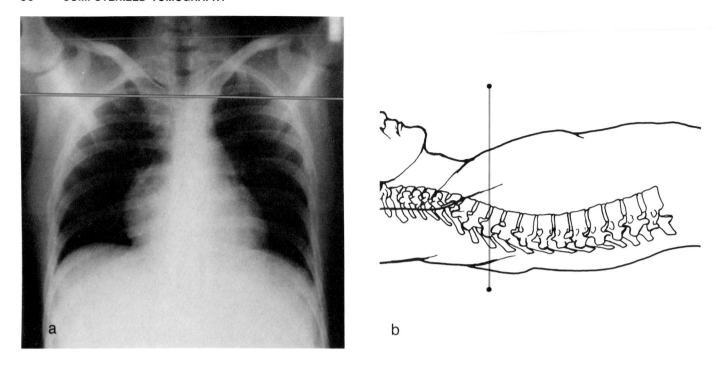

4.9 Scan level. (a) Normal mid-expiration chest roentgenogram; red line shows cross-section level. Note the glenohumeral joint is slightly elevated relative to the scan level. (b) Schematic drawing of scan level.

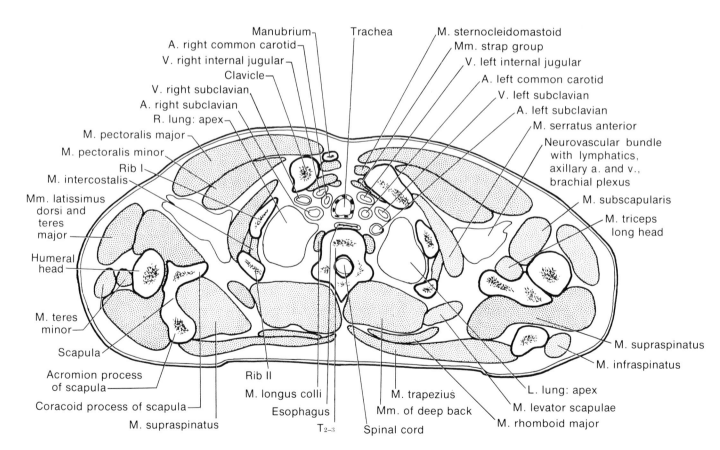

4.10 Anatomical diagram at the T_{2-3} level.

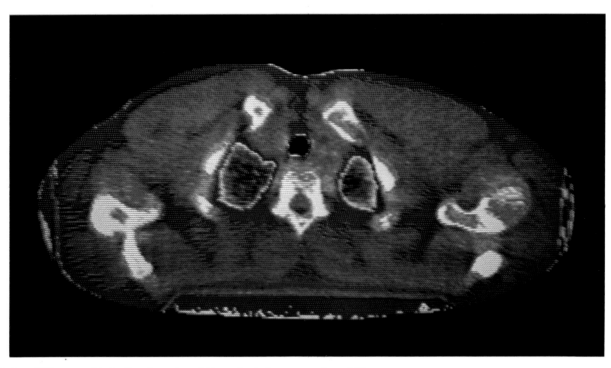

4.11 Color CT scan. Note the heads of the clavicles seen in white.

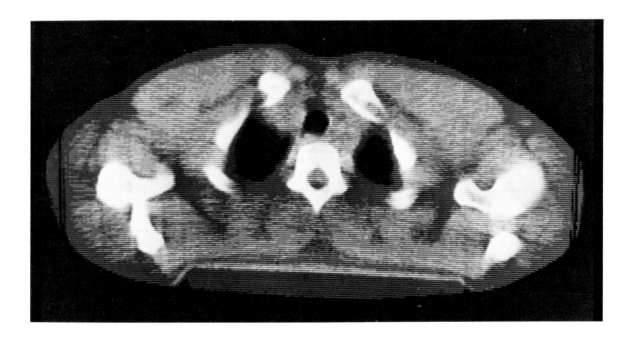

4.12 Black and white CT scan.

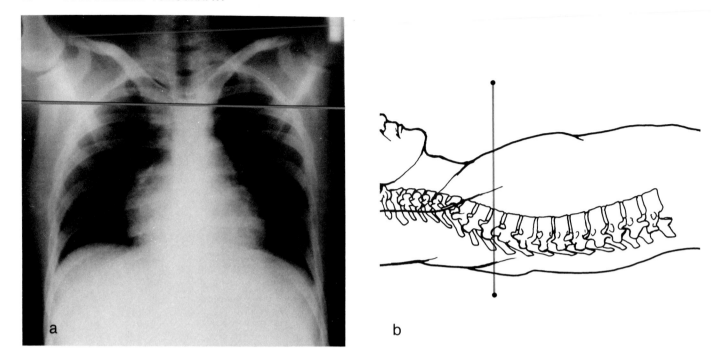

4.13 Scan level. (a) Normal mid-expiration chest roentgenogram; red line shows cross-section level. (b) Schematic drawing of scan level.

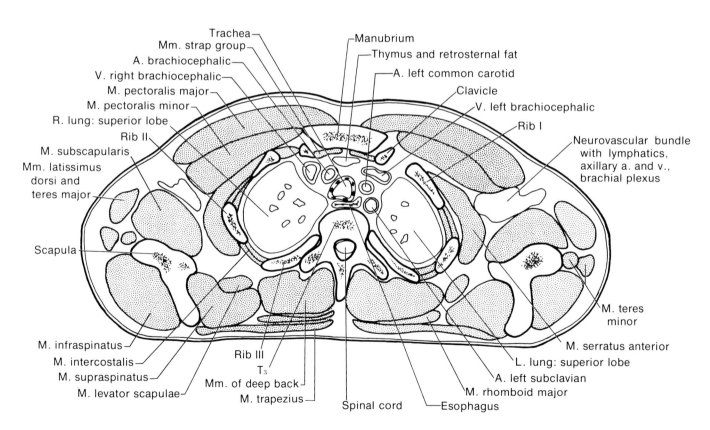

4.14 Anatomical diagram at the level of T₃.

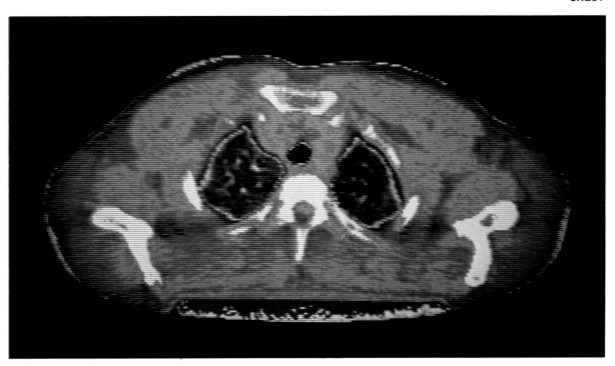

4.15 Color CT scan. Note the upper border of the manubrium and the details of the lung parenchyma using this double window display.

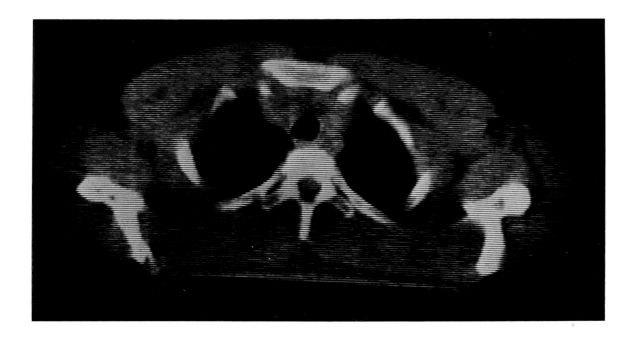

4.16 Black and white CT scan.

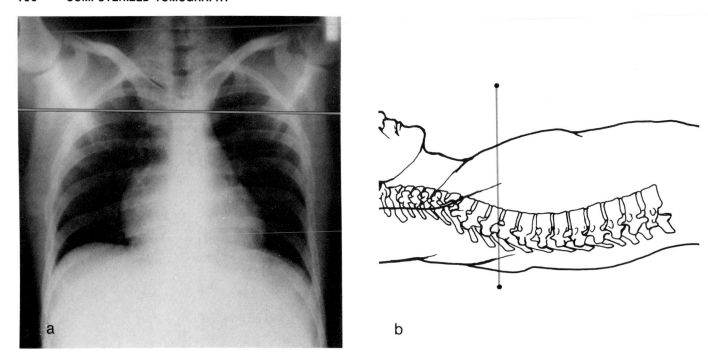

4.17 Scan level. (a) Normal mid-expiration chest roentgenogram; red line shows cross-section level. (b) Schematic drawing of scan level.

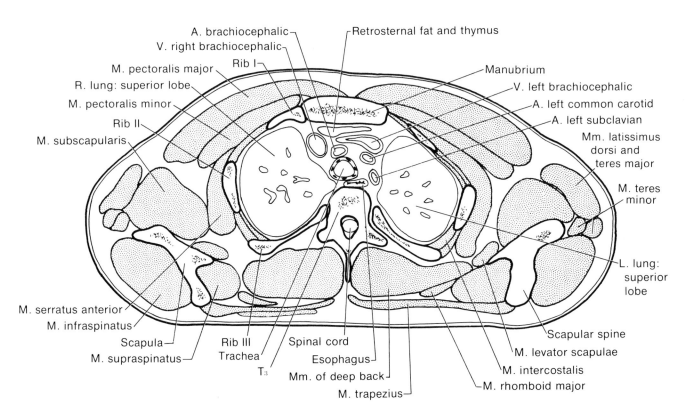

4.18 Anatomical diagram at the level of T₃.

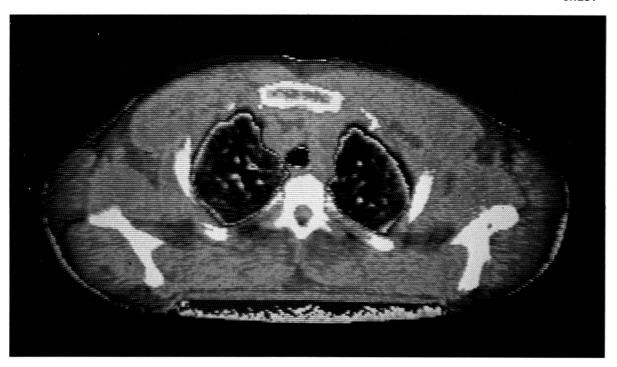

4.19 Color CT scan.

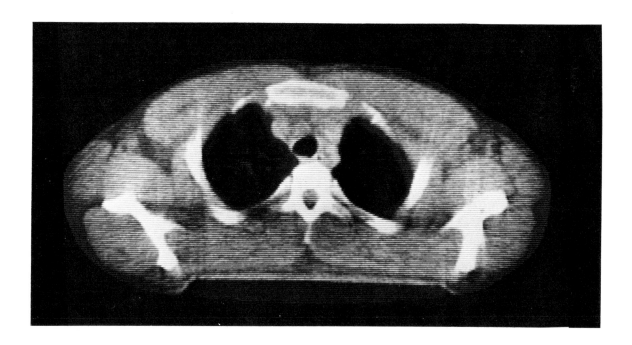

4.20 Black and white CT scan.

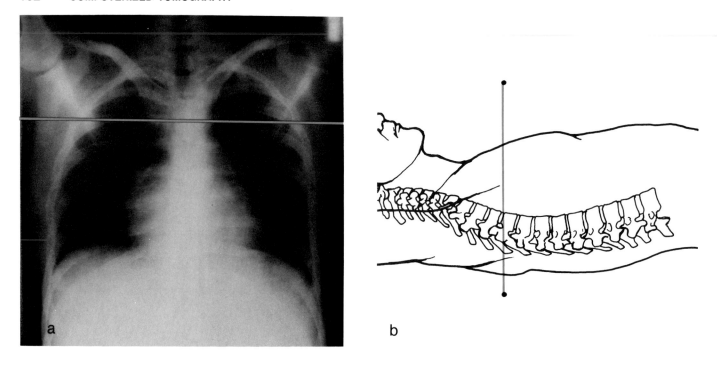

4.21 Scan level. (a) Normal mid-expiration chest roentgenogram; red line shows cross-section level. (b) Schematic drawing of scan level.

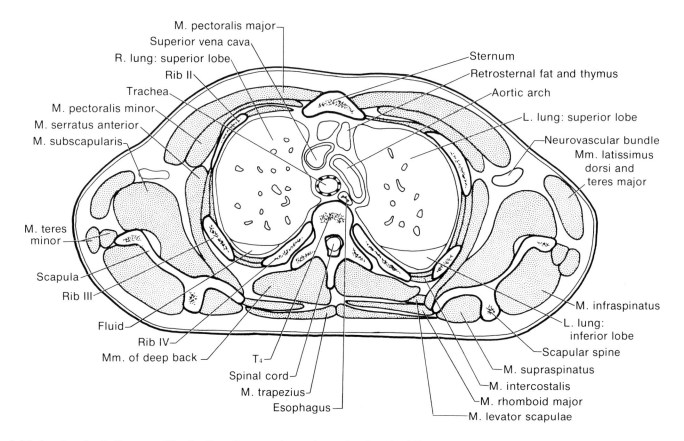

4.22 Anatomical diagram illustrating the aortic arch at the level of T$_4$.

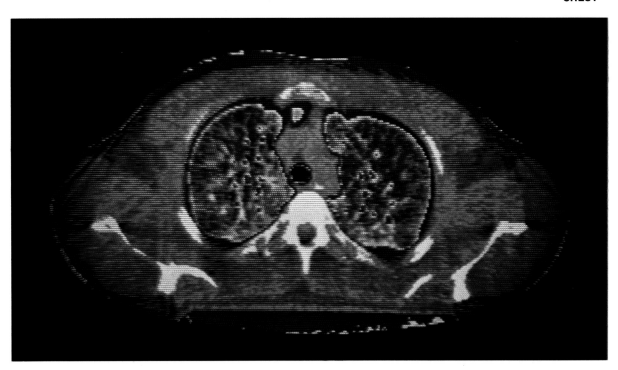

4.23 Color CT scan. Note the presence of segmental pulmonary bronchi and pulmonary vasculature which appear lighter than the purple-shaded lung parenchyma.

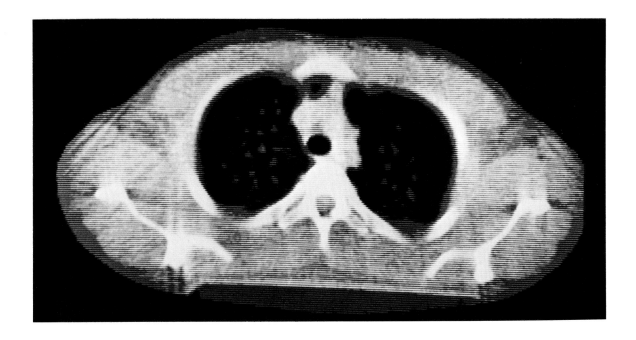

4.24 Black and white CT scan.

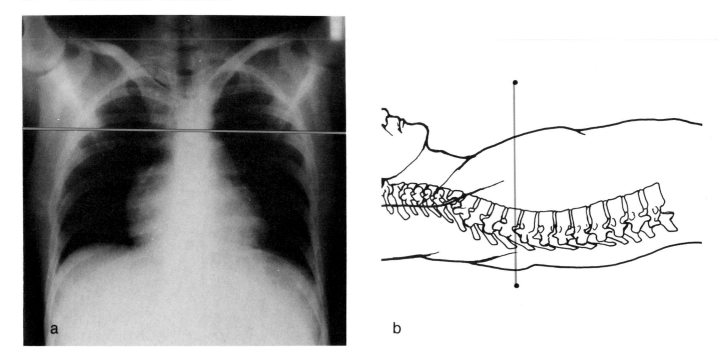

4.25 Scan level. (a) Normal mid-expiration chest roentgenogram; red line shows cross-section level. (b) Schematic drawing of scan level.

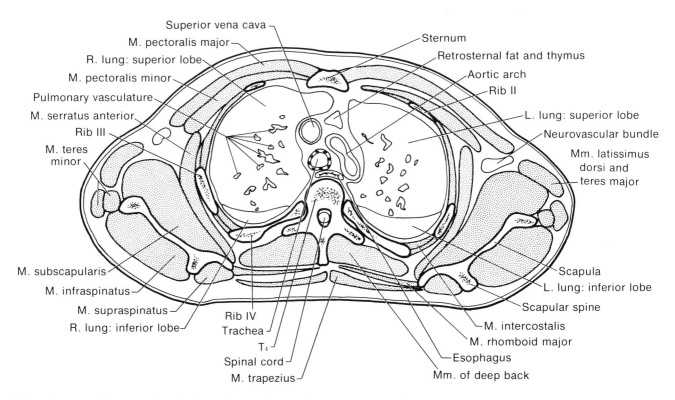

4.26 Anatomical diagram illustrating the aortic arch at the level of T_4.

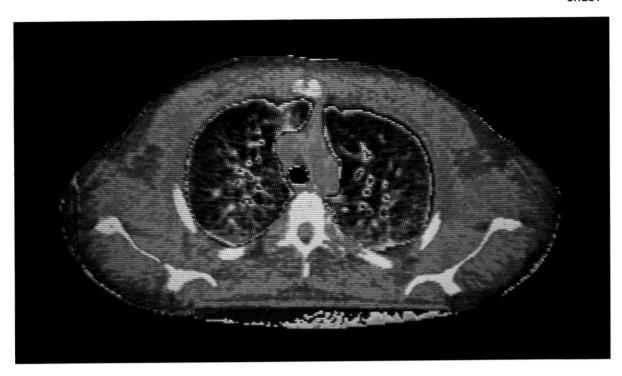

4.27 Color CT scan.

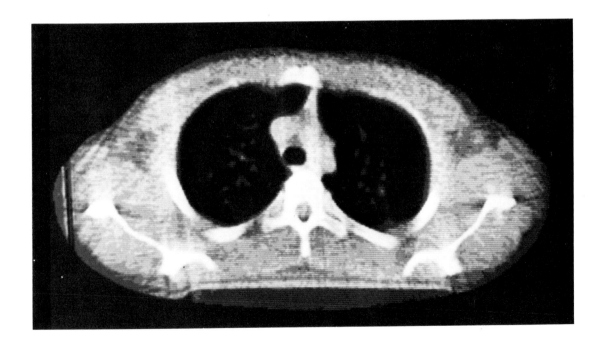

4.28 Black and white CT scan.

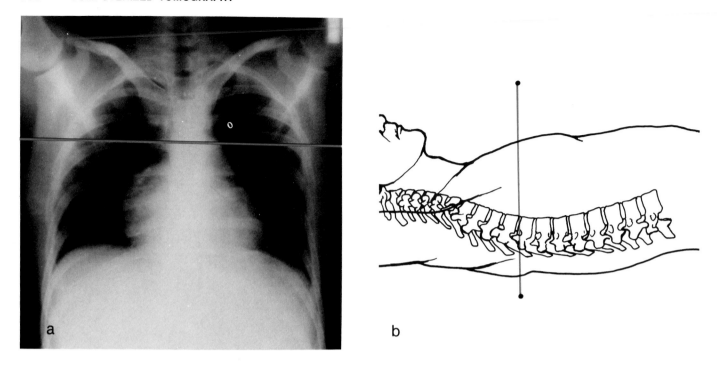

4.29 Scan level. (a) Normal mid-expiration chest roentgenogram; red line shows cross-section level. (b) Schematic drawing of scan level.

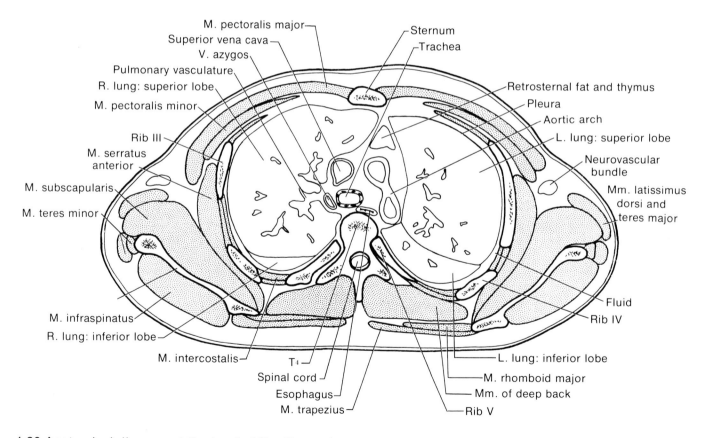

4.30 Anatomical diagram at the level of T_{4-5} illustrating the aortic arch and azygos vein.

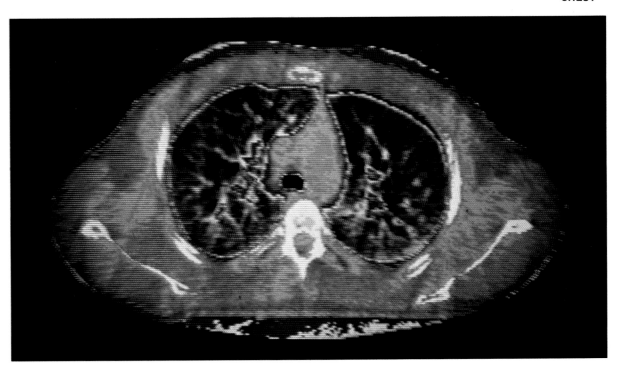

4.31 Color CT scan. Note the more oval shape of the trachea at this level and the prominence of the pulmonary vasculature.

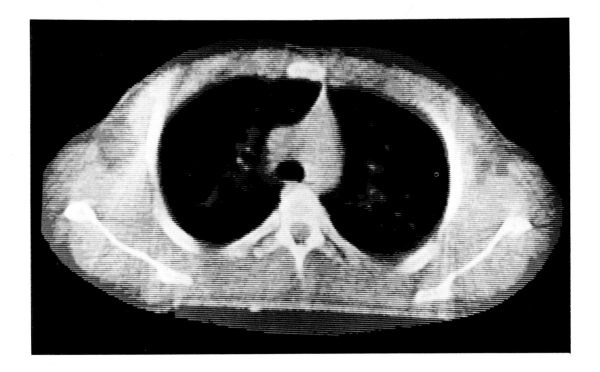

4.32 Black and white CT scan. Note the contour of the mediastinum at this level caused by the aortic arch, superior vena cava and the azygos vein.

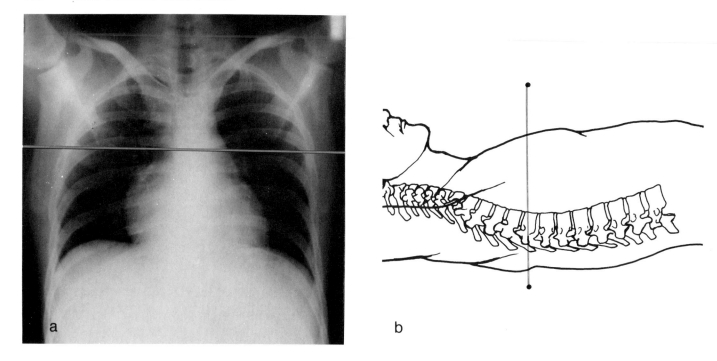

4.33 Scan level. (a) Normal mid-expiration chest roentgenogram; red line shows cross-section level. (b) Schematic drawing of scan level.

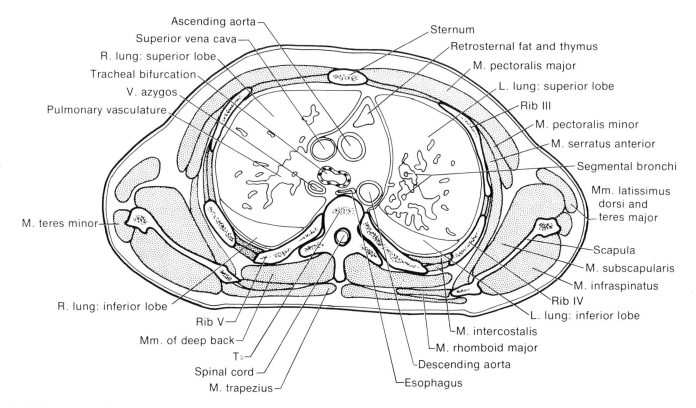

4.34 Anatomical diagram at the tracheal bifurcation at the level of T₅.

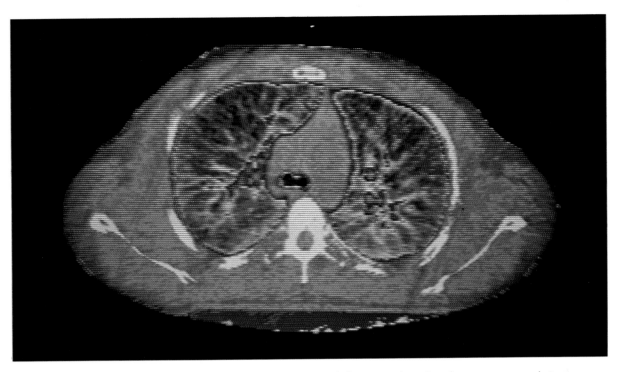

4.35 Color CT scan. Note the bifurcation of the trachea and the prominent pulmonary vasculature.

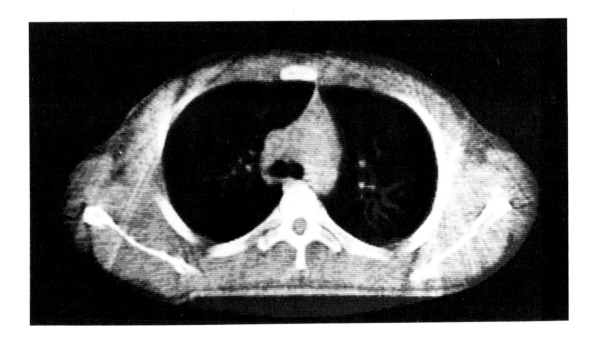

4.36 Black and white CT scan.

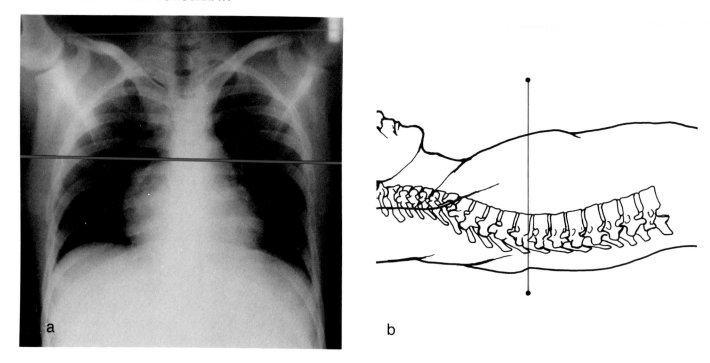

4.37 Scan level. (a) Normal mid-expiration chest roentgenogram; red line shows cross-section level. (b) Schematic drawing of scan level.

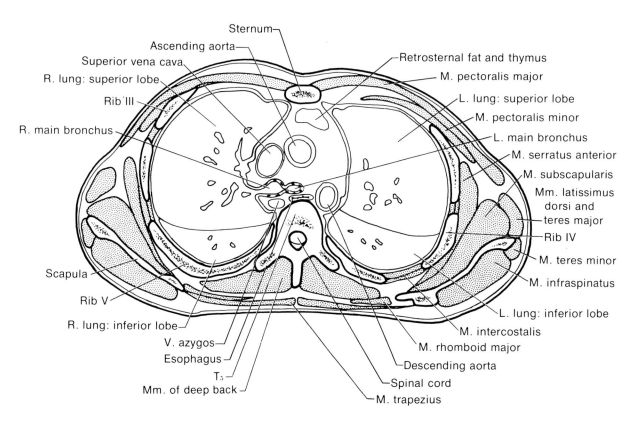

4.38 Anatomical diagram at the level of T_5.

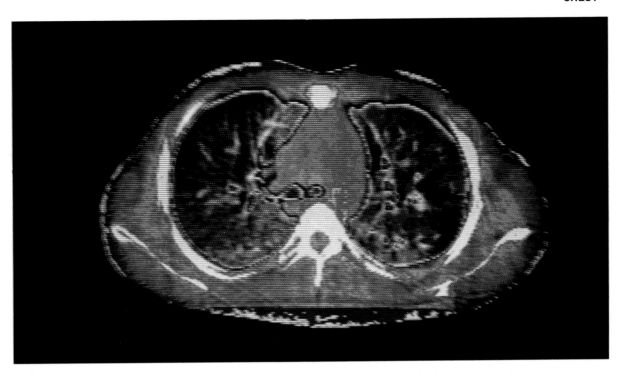

4.39 Color CT scan illustrating the carina between the cartilage-surrounded main bronchi.

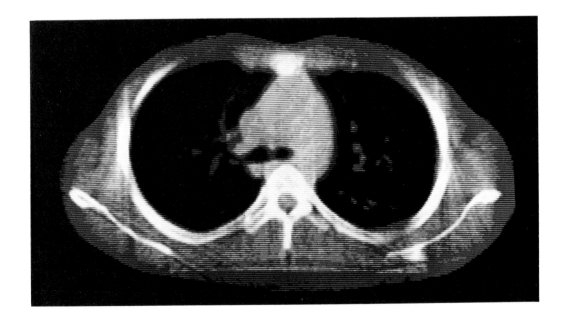

4.40 Black and white CT scan.

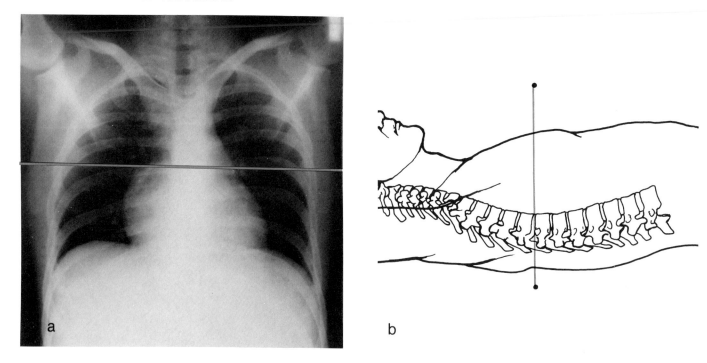

4.41 Scan level. (a) Normal mid-expiration chest roentgenogram; red line shows cross-section level. (b) Schematic drawing of scan level.

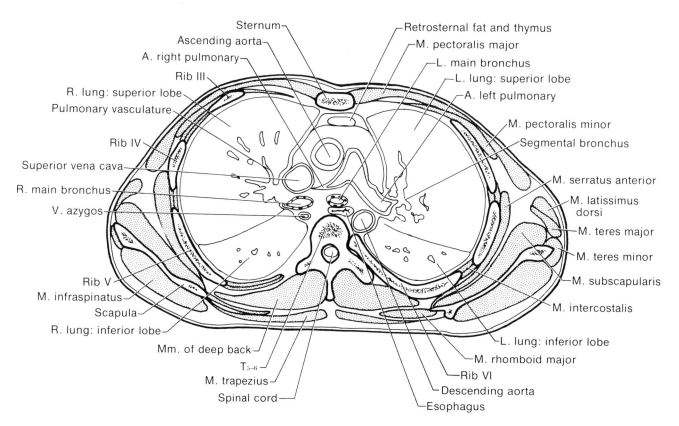

4.42 Anatomical diagram illustrating the course of the pulmonary artery at the level of T_{5-6}.

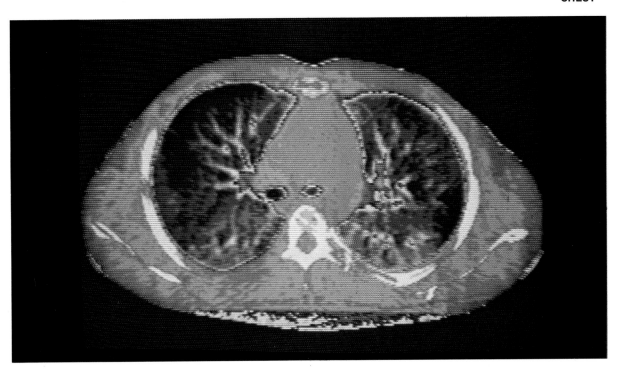

4.43 Color CT scan.

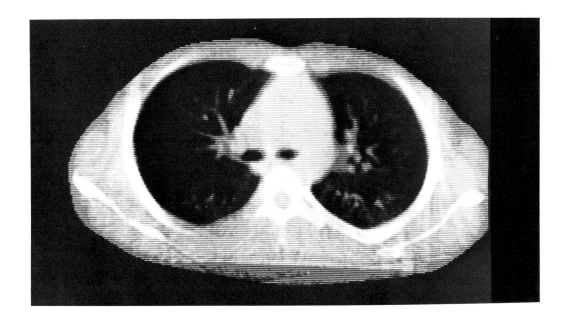

4.44 Black and white CT scan.

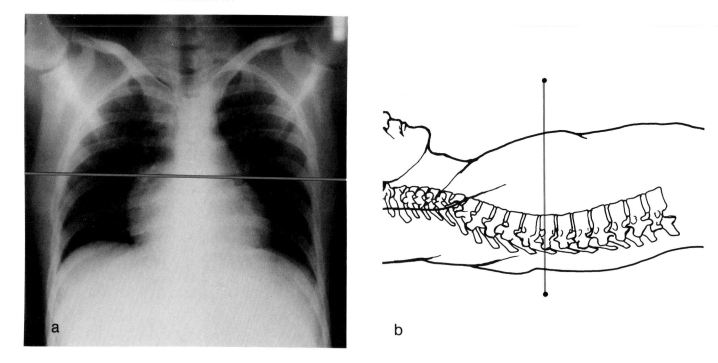

4.45 Scan level. (a) Normal mid-expiration chest roentgenogram; red line shows cross-section level. (b) Schematic drawing of scan level.

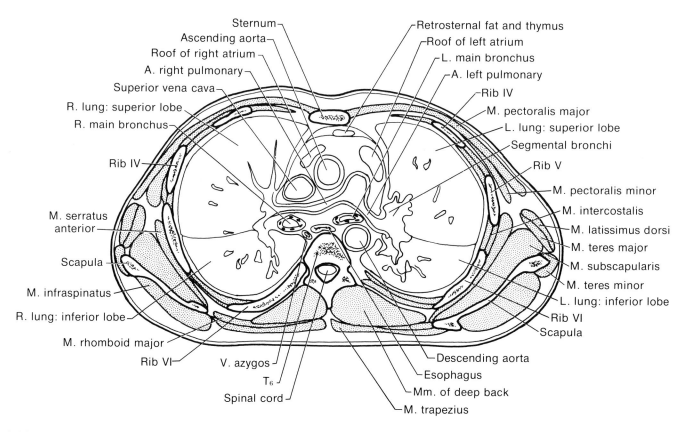

4.46 Anatomical diagram at the level of T_6.

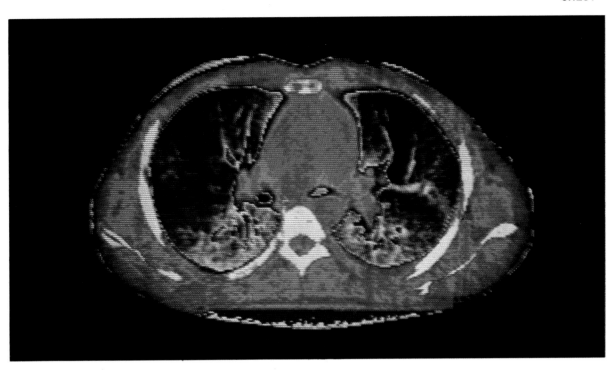

4.47 Color CT scan. Note the lighter shaded higher density lung parenchyma in the dependent portion of the lung seen in the posterior quarter of the lung field.

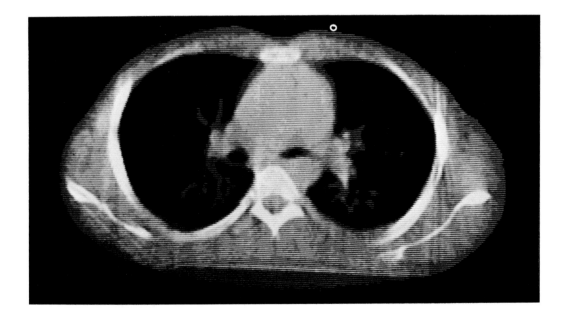

4.48 Black and white CT scan.

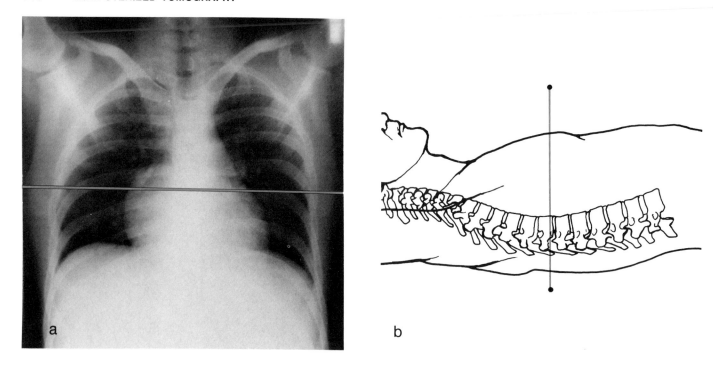

4.49 Scan level. (a) Normal mid-expiration chest roentgenogram; red line shows cross-section level. (b) Schematic drawing of scan level.

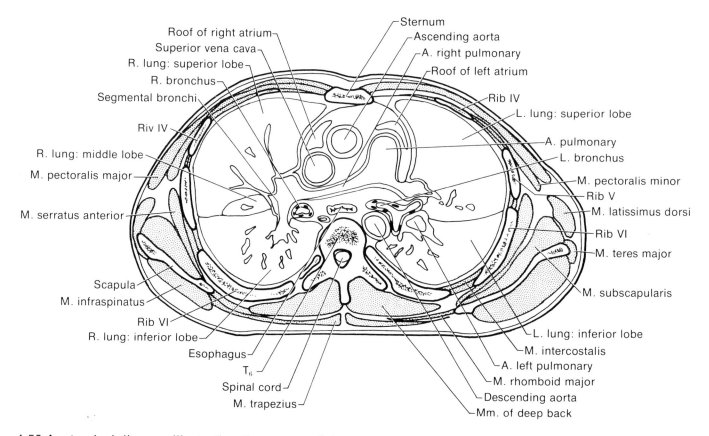

4.50 Anatomical diagram illustrating the course of the pulmonary artery at spinal level T$_6$.

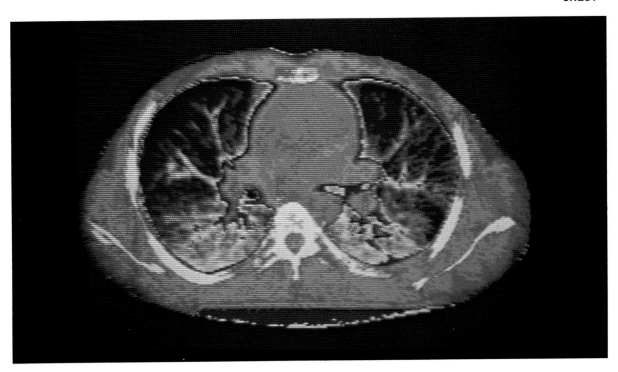

4.51 Color CT scan demonstrating the radiation of pulmonary vasculature and bronchi from the hilum of the lungs.

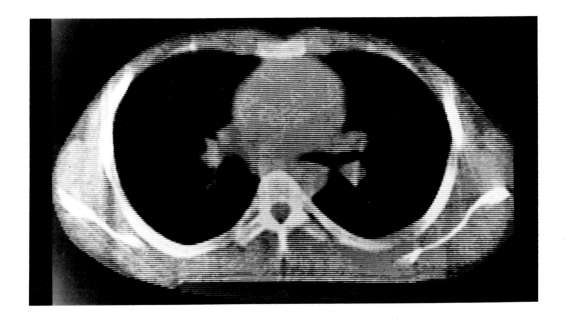

4.52 Black and white CT scan.

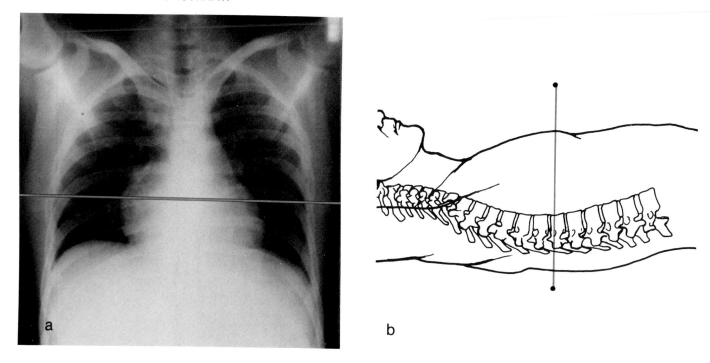

4.53 Scan level. (a) Normal mid-expiration chest roentgenogram; red line shows cross-section level. (b) Schematic drawing of scan level.

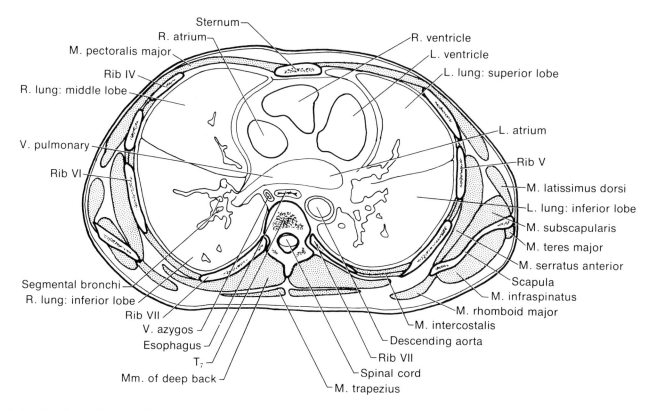

4.54 Anatomical diagram illustrating the course of the pulmonary vein at the level of T₇.

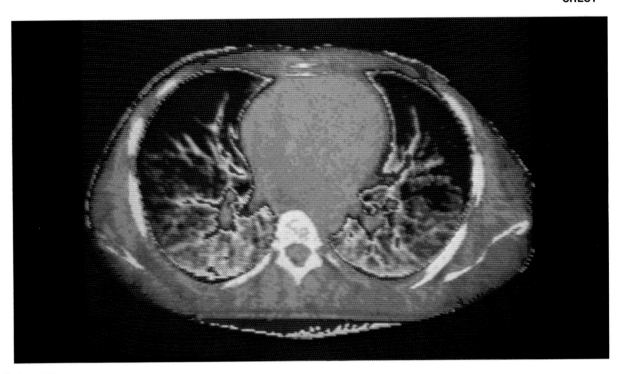

4.55 Color CT scan.

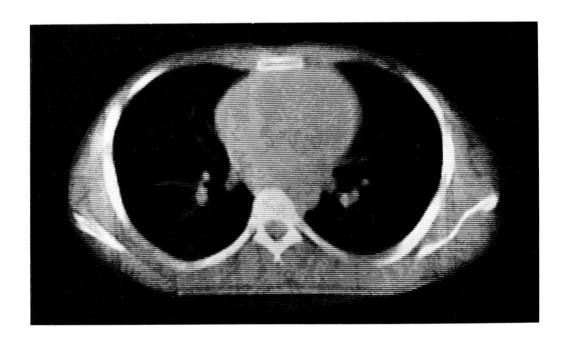

4.56 Black and white CT scan.

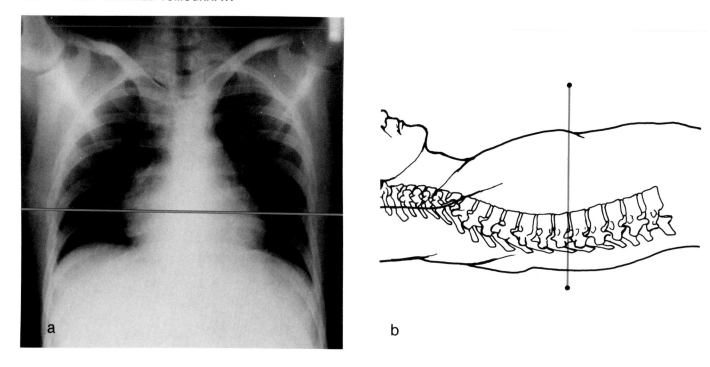

4.57 Scan level. (a) Normal mid-expiration chest roentgenogram; red line shows cross-section level. (b) Schematic drawing of scan level.

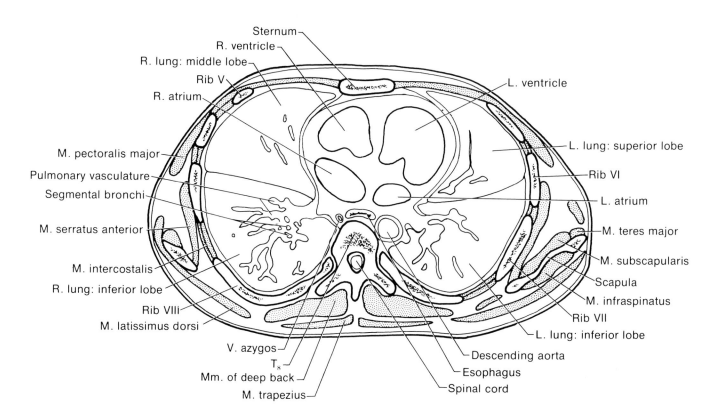

4.58 Anatomical diagram depicting the chambers of the heart at the level of T$_8$.

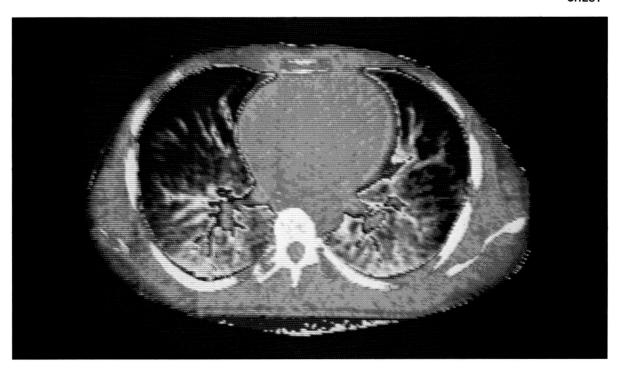

4.59 Color CT scan.

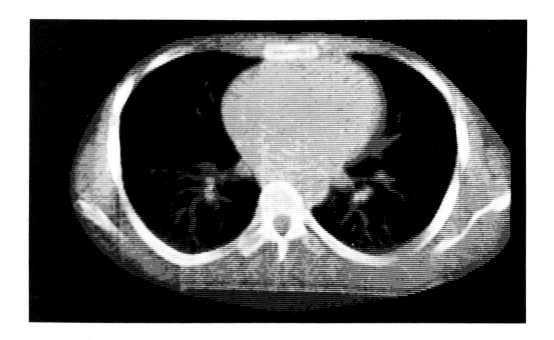

4.60 Black and white CT scan.

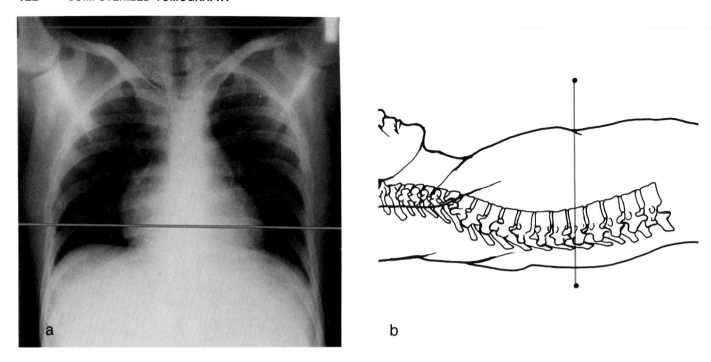

4.61 Scan level. (a) Normal mid-expiration chest roentgenogram; red line shows cross-section level. (b) Schematic drawing of scan level.

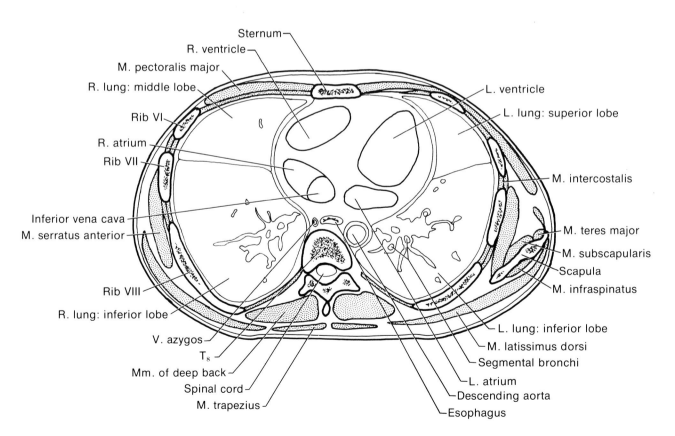

4.62 Anatomical diagram illustrating the appearance of the inferior vena cava in the right atrium at the level of T_8.

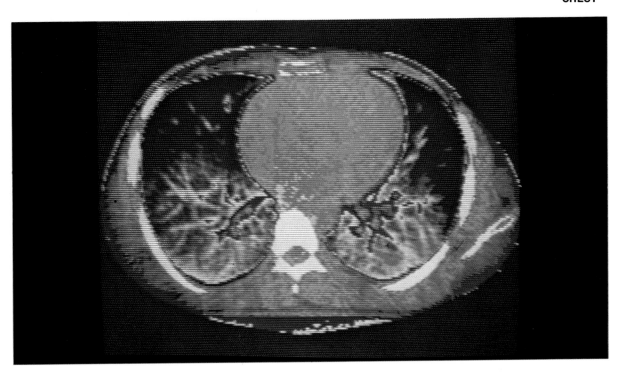

4.63 Color CT scan.

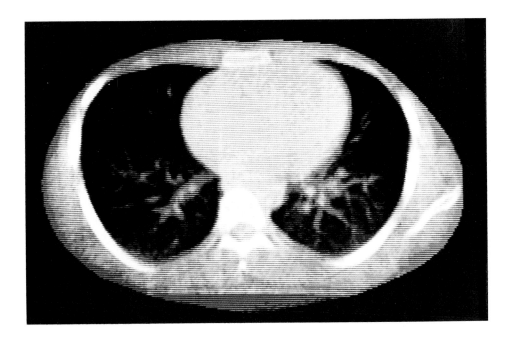

4.64 Black and white CT scan.

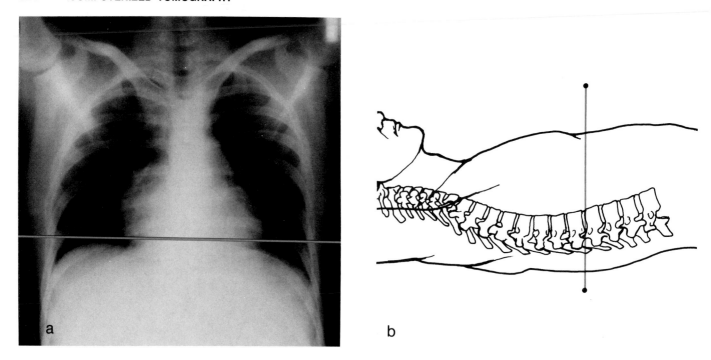

4.65 Scan level. (a) Normal mid-expiration chest roentgenogram; red line shows cross-section level. (b) Schematic drawing of scan level.

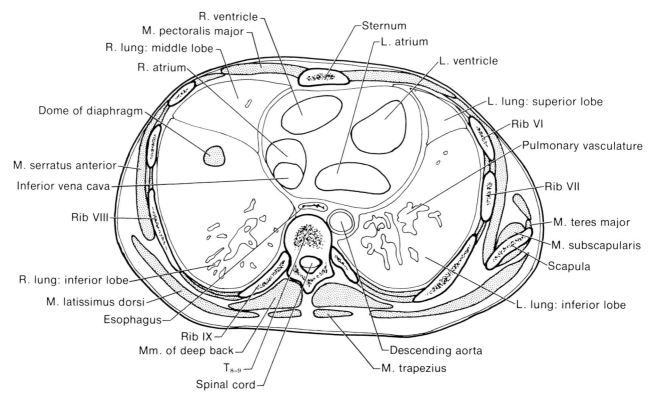

4.66 Anatomical diagram at the level of T_{8-9}.

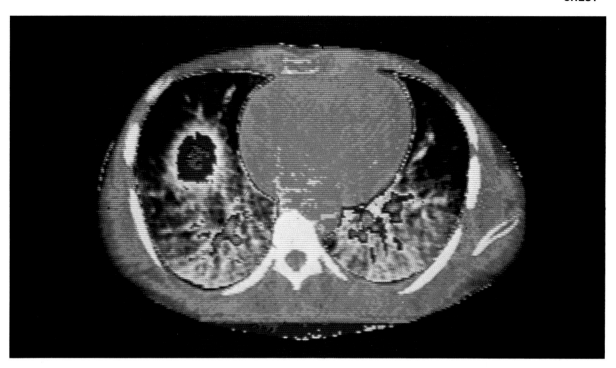

4.67 Color CT scan. Note the appearance of the dome of the right diaphragm.

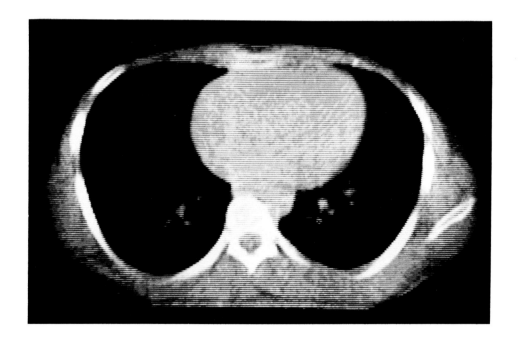

4.68 Black and white CT scan.

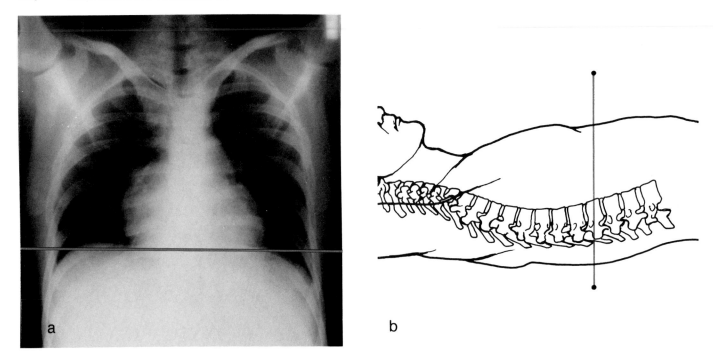

4.69 Scan level. (a) Normal mid-expiration chest roentgenogram; red line shows cross-section level. (b) Schematic drawing of scan level.

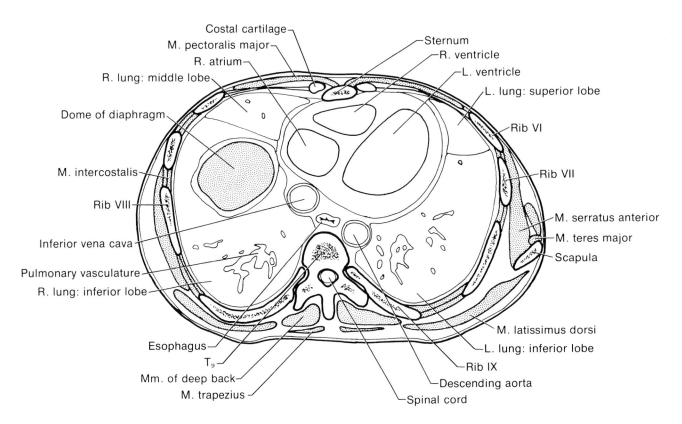

Costal cartilage
M. pectoralis major
R. atrium
R. lung: middle lobe
Dome of diaphragm
M. intercostalis
Rib VIII
Inferior vena cava
Pulmonary vasculature
R. lung: inferior lobe
Esophagus
T₉
Mm. of deep back
M. trapezius

Sternum
R. ventricle
L. ventricle
L. lung: superior lobe
Rib VI
Rib VII
M. serratus anterior
M. teres major
Scapula
M. latissimus dorsi
L. lung: inferior lobe
Rib IX
Descending aorta
Spinal cord

4.70 Anatomical diagram showing the prominence of the left ventricle of the heart at the level T_9.

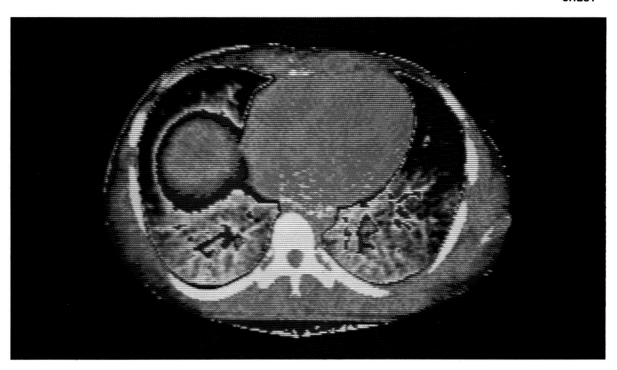

4.71 Color CT scan shows the right dome of the diaphragm depicted in orange within the right lung field.

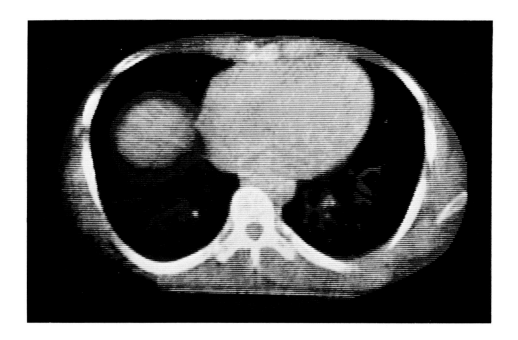

4.72 Black and white CT scan.

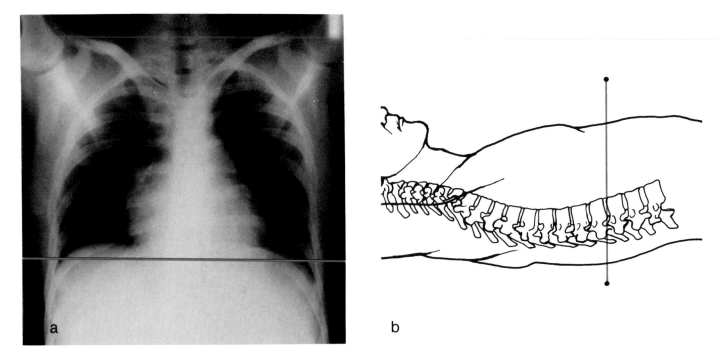

4.73 Scan level. (a) Normal mid-expiration chest roentgenogram; red line shows cross-section level. (b) Schematic drawing of scan level.

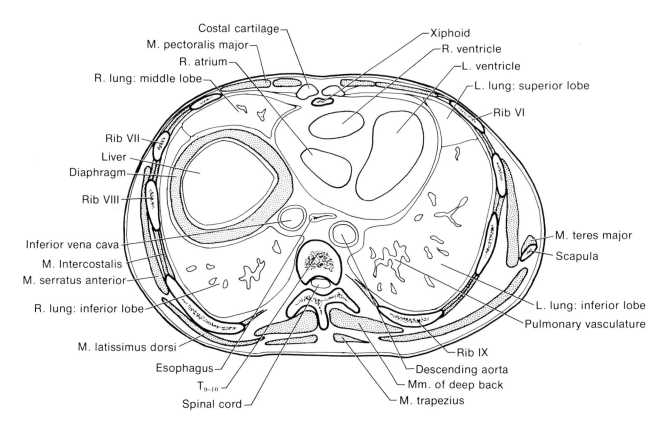

4.74 Anatomical diagram at the level of T$_{9-10}$.

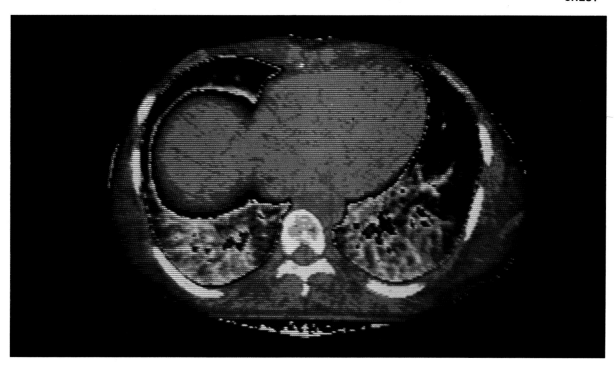

4.75 Color CT scan. Note the right diaphragm dome in the lung field.

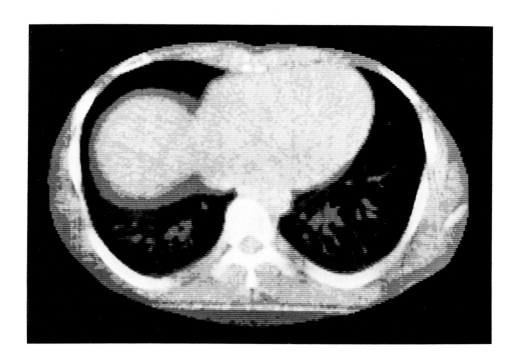

4.76 Black and white CT scan.

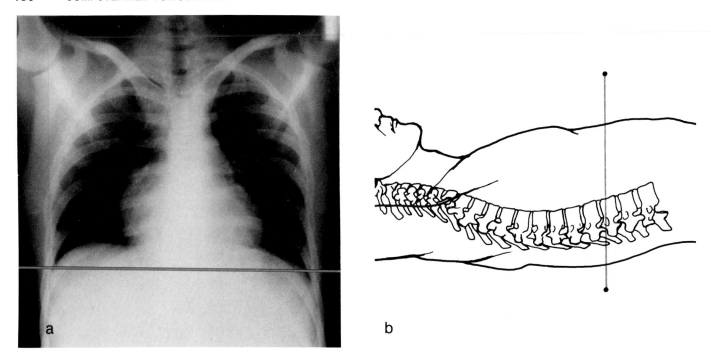

4.77 Scan level. (a) Normal mid-expiration chest roentgenogram; red line shows cross-section level. (b) Schematic drawing of scan level.

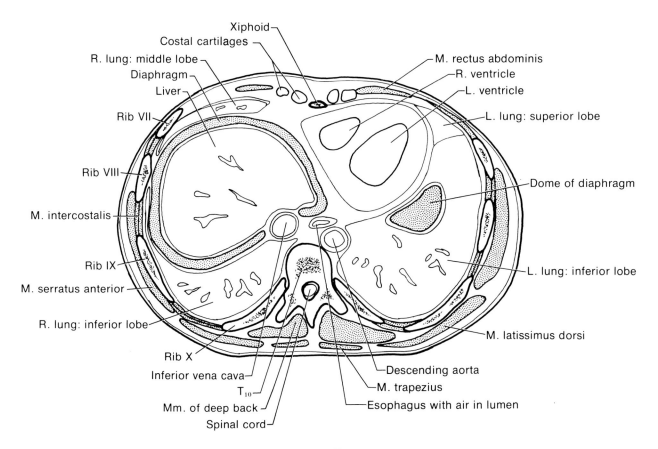

4.78 Anatomical diagram at the level of the xiphoid and T_{10}.

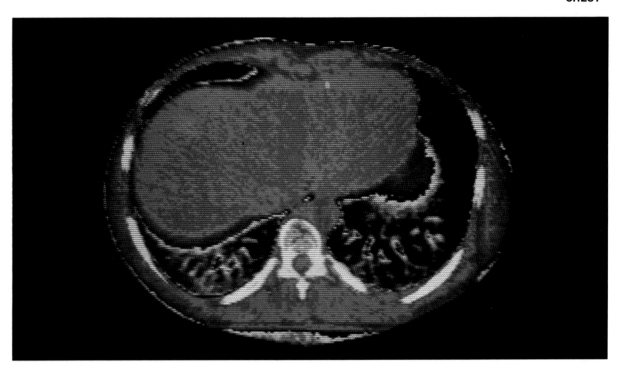

4.79 Color CT scan demonstrating the appearance of the left dome of the diaphragm entering the left lung field.

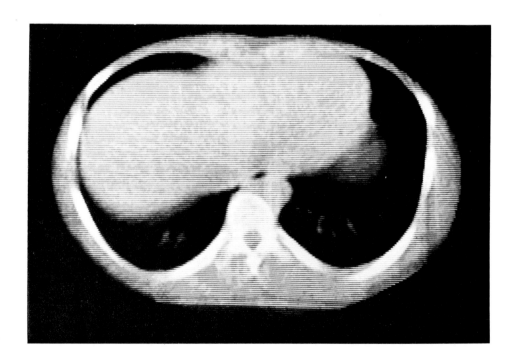

4.80 Black and white CT scan.

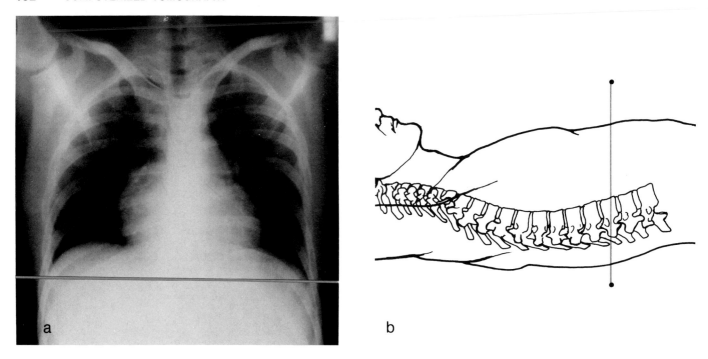

a

b

4.81 Scan level. (a) Normal mid-expiration chest roentgenogram; red line shows cross-section level. (b) Schematic drawing of scan level.

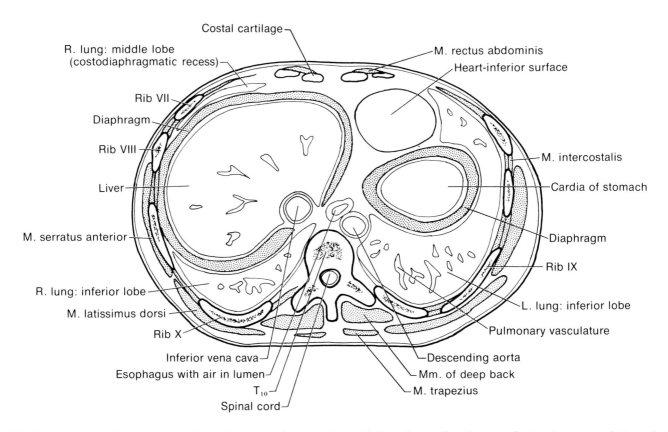

Costal cartilage
R. lung: middle lobe (costodiaphragmatic recess)
M. rectus abdominis
Heart-inferior surface
Rib VII
Diaphragm
Rib VIII
M. intercostalis
Liver
Cardia of stomach
M. serratus anterior
Diaphragm
Rib IX
R. lung: inferior lobe
L. lung: inferior lobe
M. latissimus dorsi
Pulmonary vasculature
Rib X
Inferior vena cava
Descending aorta
Esophagus with air in lumen
Mm. of deep back
T_{10}
M. trapezius
Spinal cord

4.82 Anatomical diagram showing the superior portion of the liver, the base of the heart and the right diaphragmatic dome at the level of T_{10}.

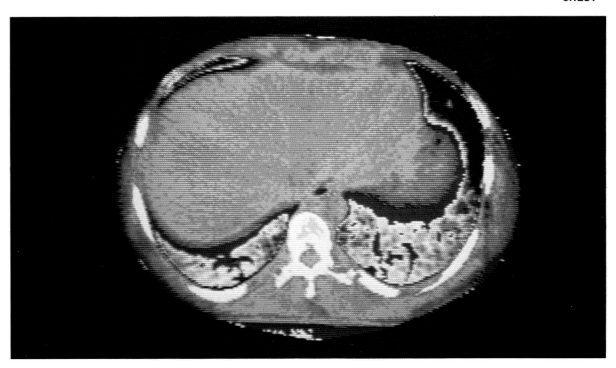

4.83 Color CT scan demonstrating increased density of the lung parenchyma in the dependent, inferior portions of the lower lobes of the lungs and air in the esophagus.

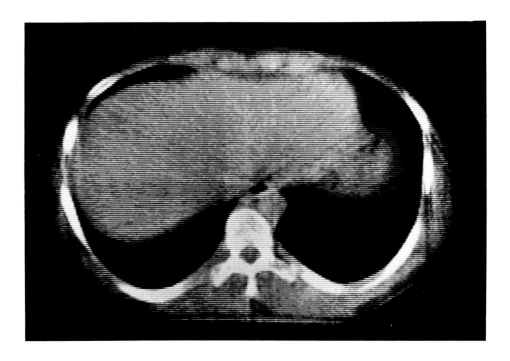

4.84 Black and white CT scan.

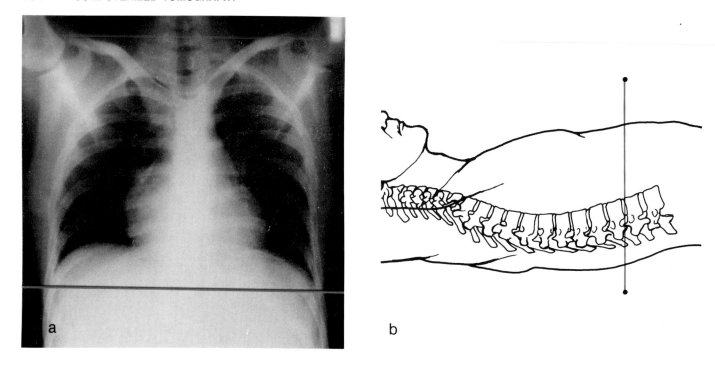

a

b

4.85 Scan level. (a) Normal mid-expiration chest roentgenogram; red line shows cross-section level. (b) Schematic drawing of scan level.

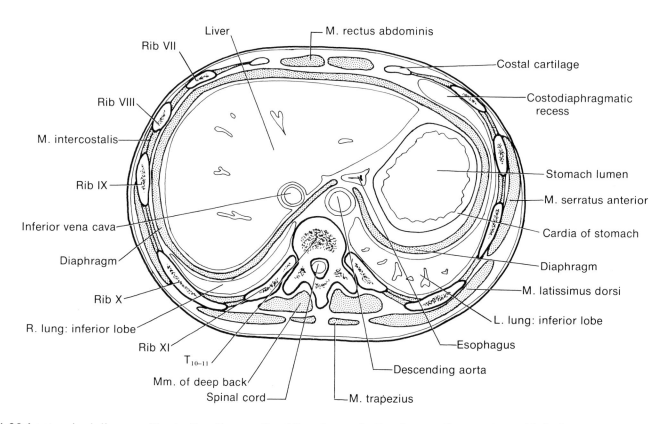

4.86 Anatomical diagram illustrating the cardia of the stomach, the descending aorta and inferior vena cava at the level of T_{10-11}.

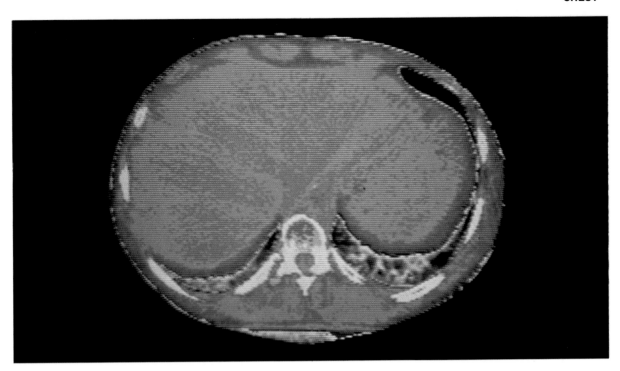

4.87 Color CT scan.

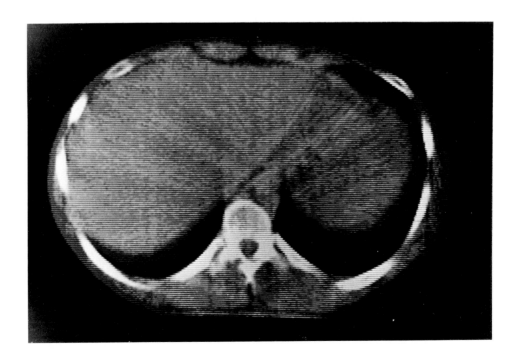

4.88 Black and white CT scan.

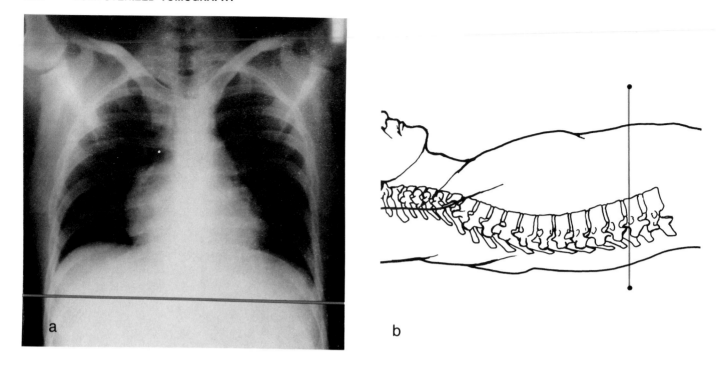

4.89 Scan level. (a) Normal mid-expiration chest roentgenogram; red line shows cross-section level. (b) Schematic drawing of scan level.

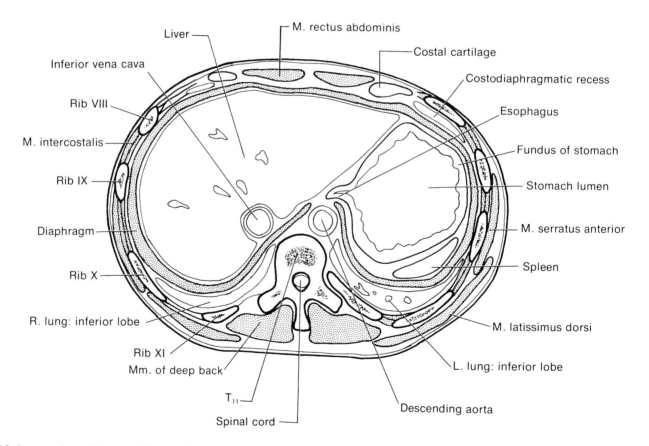

4.90 Anatomical diagram illustrating the gastroesophageal junction, the superior surface of the spleen and the parenchyma of the liver at the level of T_{11}.

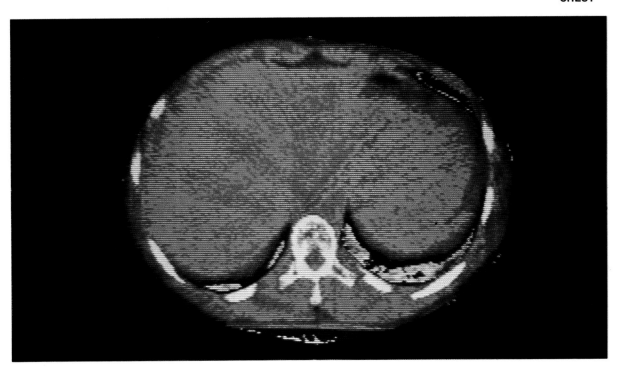

4.91 Color CT scan.

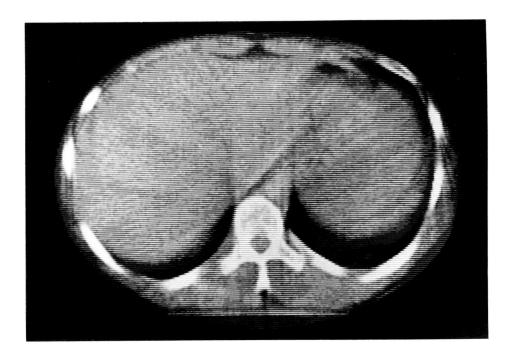

4.92 Black and white CT scan. Note the separation of the spleen from the cardia of the stomach and the appearance of the rectus abdominis muscles in the upper portion of the scan.

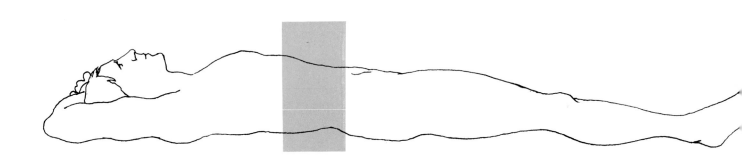

chapter five

Upper Abdomen

This section of the ATLAS ranges from the costodiaphragmatic recesses to the iliac crests, representing the spinal levels from T_{11} to L_4. This region includes most of the abdominal viscera (i.e., liver, spleen, pancreas, kidneys, adrenals, gall bladder, stomach, small bowel, and portions of the colon), the abdominal vasculature (e.g., aorta, inferior vena cava, superior mesenteric artery, renal artery and vein, etc.) and musculature as well as the lower ribs, vertebrae and caudal spinal cord.

CT scanning of the upper abdomen has already proven to be a powerful diagnostic tool. Accurate imaging of the pancreas and retroperitoneal structures can be achieved without the use of special contrast studies or other invasive procedures. The boundaries of most of the upper abdominal organs are quite distinct due to the fact that these structures are invested in thin layers of low density fat. Movement of gas within the bowel can create varying degrees of image degradation, but even in cases where this occurs, the quality of the image remains such that it still provides an abundance of clinical information. Mild anticholinergic drugs minimize these physiological movements and are relatively free of side effects (the use of such drugs is contraindicated in patients having glaucoma and prostatic hypertrophy).

Accurate imaging of the liver and pancreas allows for the establishment of CT criteria for metastic and primary neoplastic involvement of these organs. In particular, cancer of the pancreas, previously one of the most difficult of all abdominal diagnoses, can now be determined using CT methods. The imaging of tumors, cysts, and abscesses of abdominal organs allows for the precise three-dimensional localization of these lesions and has been used to facilitate percutaneous biopsy procedures. The low density of bile within the gall bladder provides a natural source of radiocontrast for the imaging of this structure.

The organs of the upper abdomen are highly mobile structures and as such are prone to a marked degree of anatomical variance. The anatomical diagrams provided with each set of scans represent the anatomy as seen in our subject at a particular time. Thus, when comparing individual patient scans with the figures in this ATLAS, the reader should consider such factors as the patient's size, body build, and parity and the time and content of recent meals. All subjects were scanned in the supine position using a 7.5-mm section thickness at 0° gantry tilt and a scan interval of 1 cm. To minimize gastric air, the subjects were instructed to ingest a fairly large meal prior to the scanning session and consequently have varying degrees of gastric distention as a result. The presence of the examining table can be noted beneath the subjects and results in some compression of the dorsal musculature.

As in other sections, a reference line is provided on a conventional A-P abdominal film and on a body drawing. However, variations between individuals may result in some discrepancies between the structures seen in the scan and the radiograph. In drawing these lines, bony structures were used for alignment purposes.

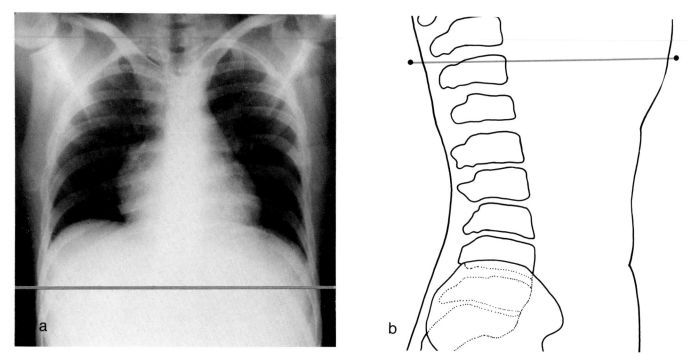

5.1 Scan level. (a) Normal mid-expiration chest roentgenogram; red line shows cross-section level. (b) Schematic diagram of scan level.

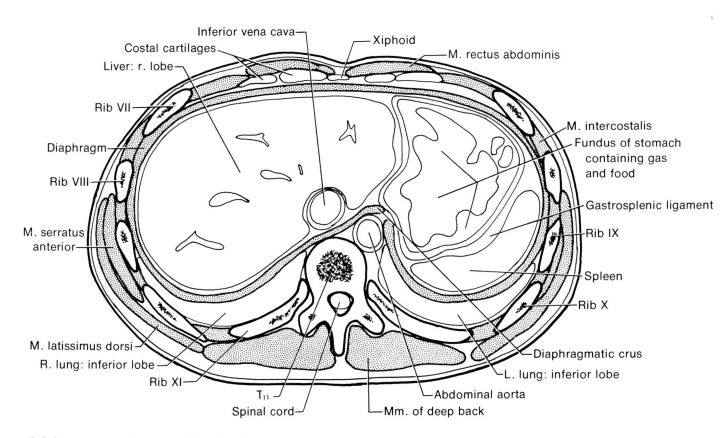

5.2 Anatomical diagram at the level of T$_{11}$.

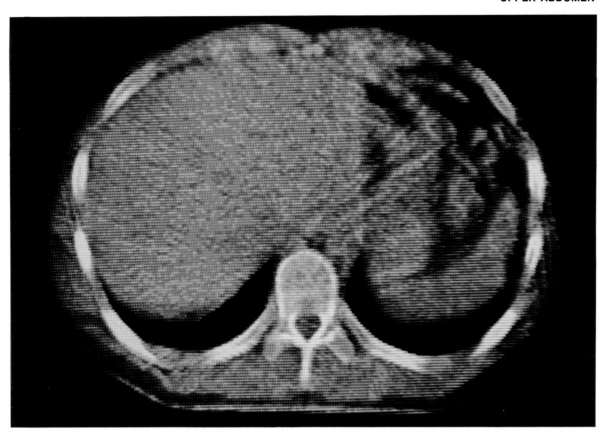

5.3 Color CT scan. Note the appearance of the somewhat distended stomach and its contents.

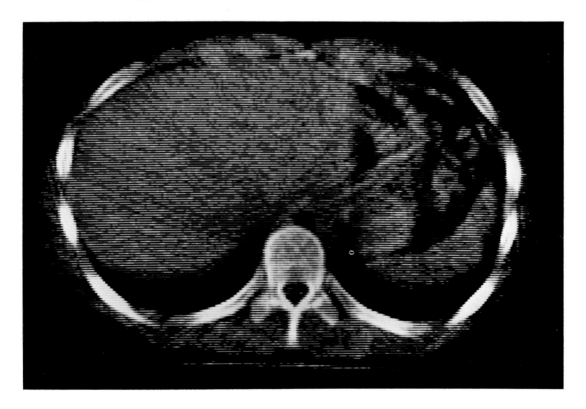

5.4 Black and white CT scan. Note the appearance of the inferior lung field and the spleen.

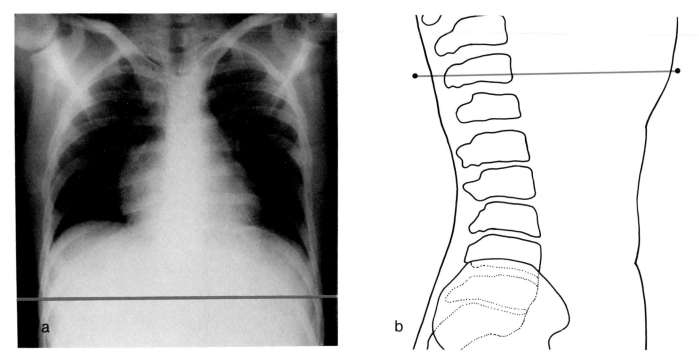

5.5 Scan level. (a) Normal mid-expiration chest roentgenogram; red line shows cross-section level. (b) Schematic diagram of scan level.

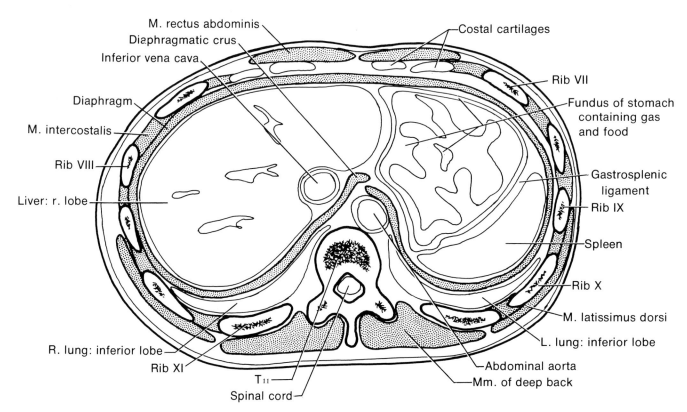

5.6 Anatomical diagram at the level of T_{11}.

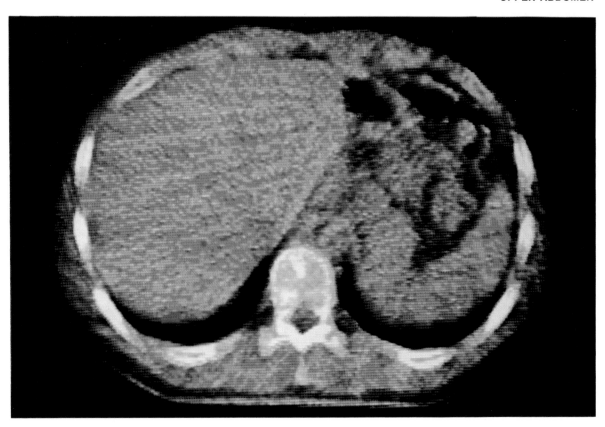

5.7 Color CT scan. Note the presence of food within the stomach as well as the appearance of the spleen and inferior lung fields.

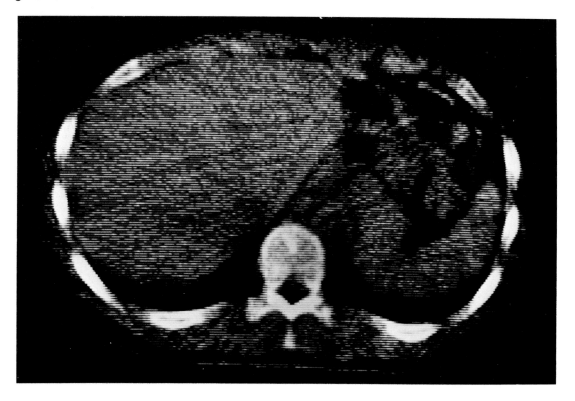

5.8 Black and white CT scan.

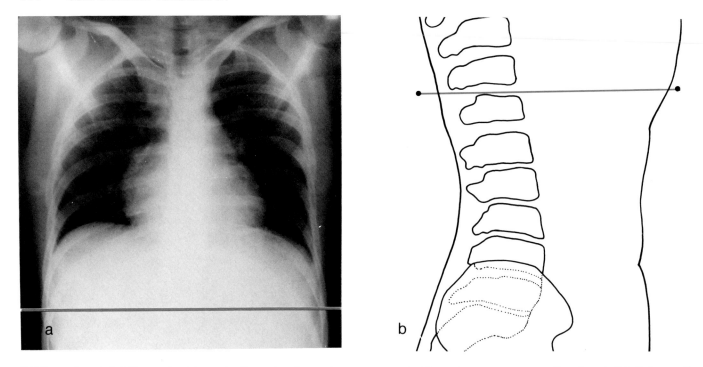

5.9 Scan level. (a) Normal mid-expiration chest roentgenogram; red line shows cross-section level. (b) Schematic diagram of scan level.

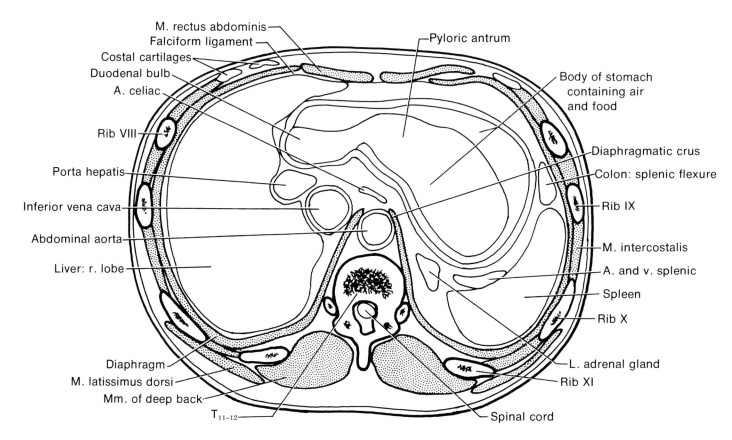

M. rectus abdominis

Falciform ligament

Costal cartilages

Duodenal bulb

A. celiac

Rib VIII

Porta hepatis

Inferior vena cava

Abdominal aorta

Liver: r. lobe

Diaphragm

M. latissimus dorsi

Mm. of deep back

T_{11-12}

Pyloric antrum

Body of stomach containing air and food

Diaphragmatic crus

Colon: splenic flexure

Rib IX

M. intercostalis

A. and v. splenic

Spleen

Rib X

L. adrenal gland

Rib XI

Spinal cord

5.10 Anatomical diagram at the level of T_{11}-T_{12}.

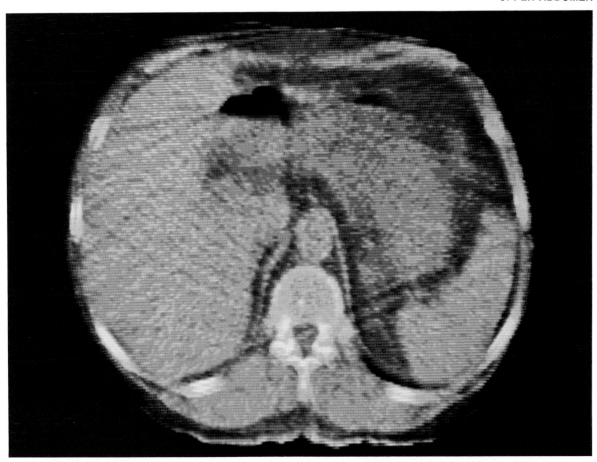

5.11 Color CT scan. Note the superior portion of the celiac artery as it exists from the aorta.

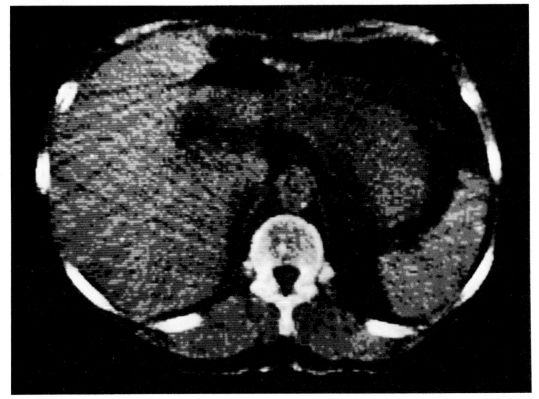

5.12 Black and white CT scan illustrating the liver, spleen and stomach. Note also the presence of the adrenal gland, seen most prominently on the subject's left side.

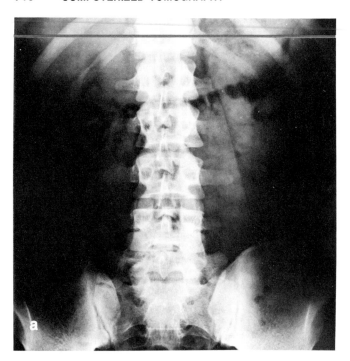

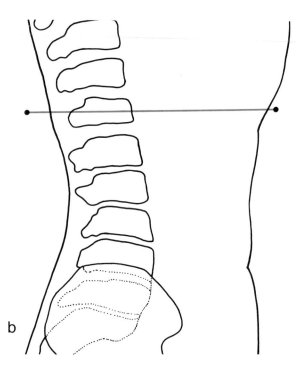

5.13 Scan level. (a) Normal A-P abdominal roentgenogram; red line shows cross-section level. (b) Schematic diagram of scan level.

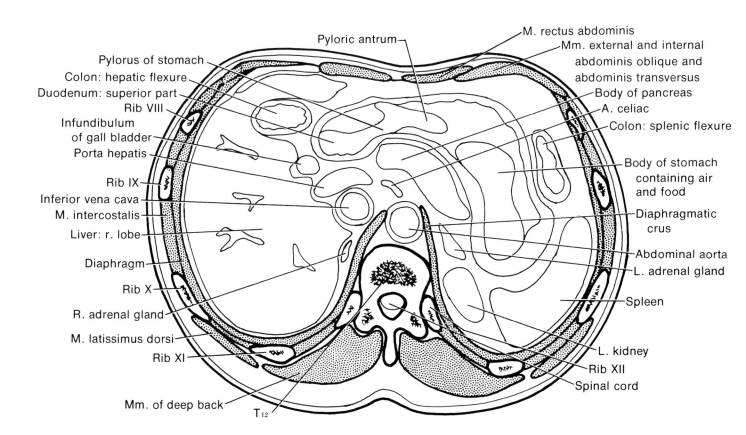

Pyloric antrum

Pylorus of stomach
Colon: hepatic flexure
Duodenum: superior part
Rib VIII
Infundibulum of gall bladder
Porta hepatis
Rib IX
Inferior vena cava
M. intercostalis
Liver: r. lobe
Diaphragm
Rib X
R. adrenal gland
M. latissimus dorsi
Rib XI
Mm. of deep back
T_{12}

M. rectus abdominis
Mm. external and internal abdominis oblique and abdominis transversus
Body of pancreas
A. celiac
Colon: splenic flexure
Body of stomach containing air and food
Diaphragmatic crus
Abdominal aorta
L. adrenal gland
Spleen
L. kidney
Rib XII
Spinal cord

5.14 Anatomical diagram at the level of T_{12}.

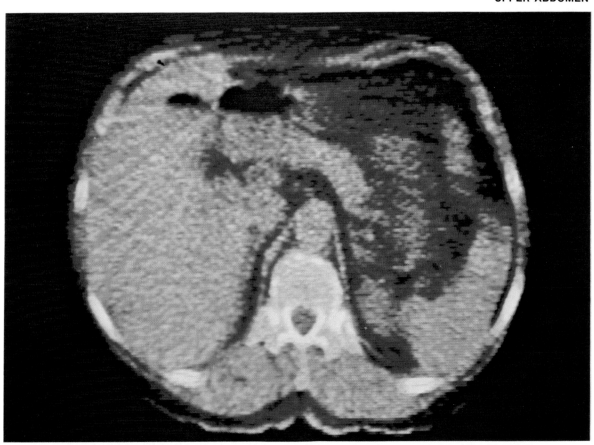

5.15 Color CT scan demonstrating the body of the pancreas, spleen and superior portion of the left kidney.

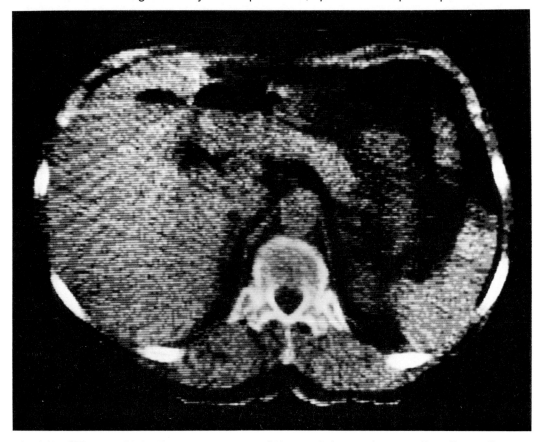

5.16 Black and white CT scan. Note the appearance of the portal vessels as well as the celiac artery.

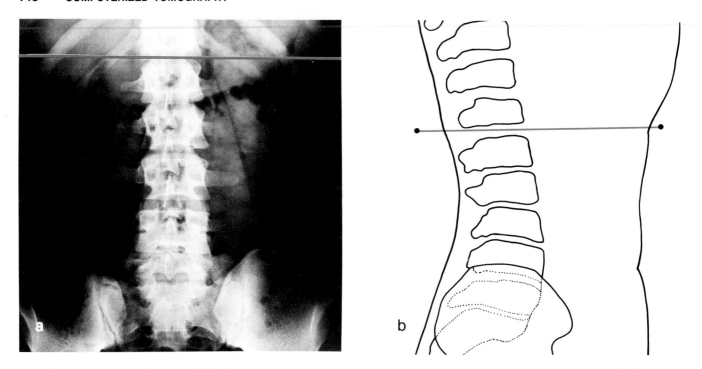

5.17 Scan level. (a) Normal A-P abdominal roentgenogram; red line shows cross-section level. (b) Schematic diagram of scan level.

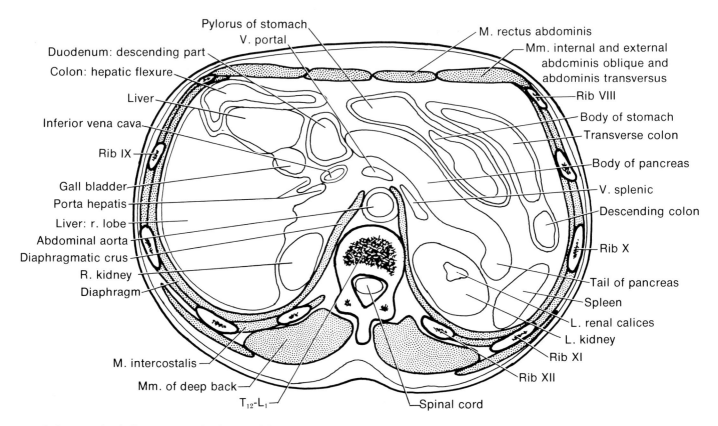

5.18 Anatomical diagram at the level of T_{12}-L_1.

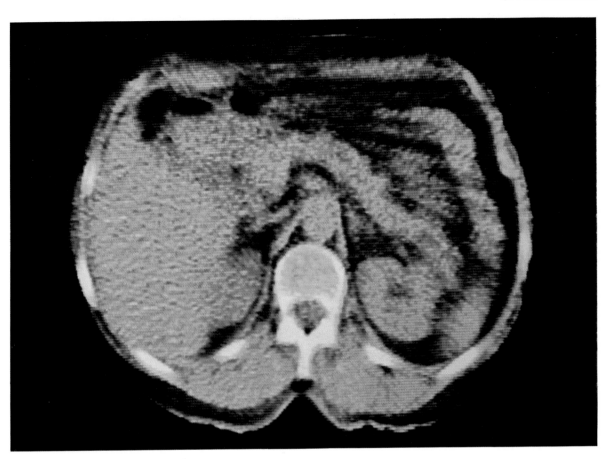

5.19 Color CT scan. Note the appearance of the pancreas in its entirety. This view also demonstrates the hepatic vasculature as well as the inferior pole of the spleen.

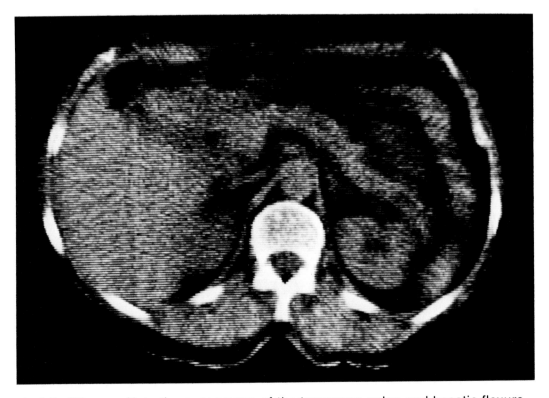

5.20 Black and white CT scan. Note the appearance of the transverse colon and hepatic flexure.

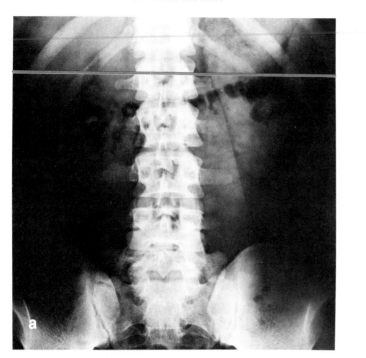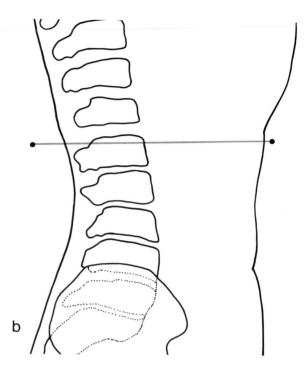

5.21 Scan level. (a) Normal A-P abdominal roentgenogram; red line shows cross-section level. (b) Schematic diagram of scan level.

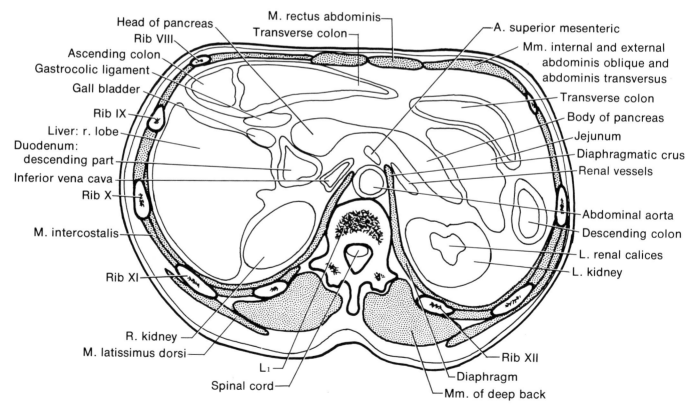

5.22 Anatomical diagram at the level of L₁.

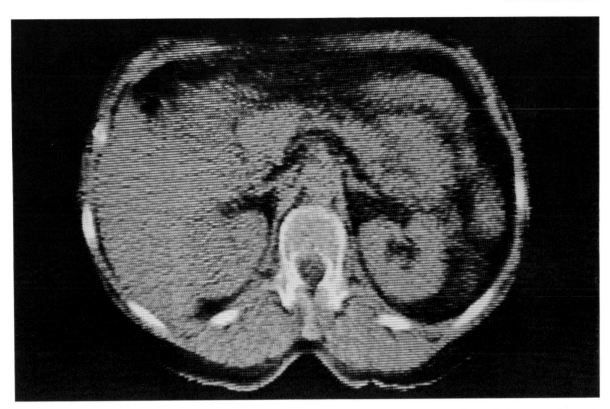

5.23 Color CT scan demonstrating the head of the pancreas and the superior portion of the superior mesenteric artery.

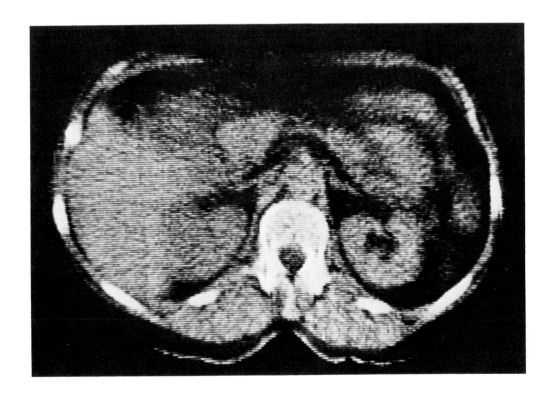

5.24 Black and white CT scan. Note the appearance of the left renal calices.

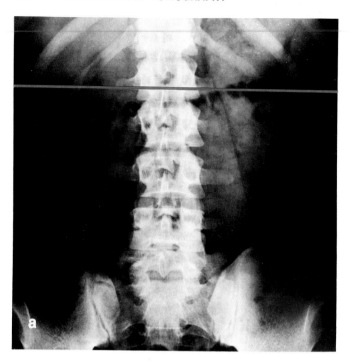

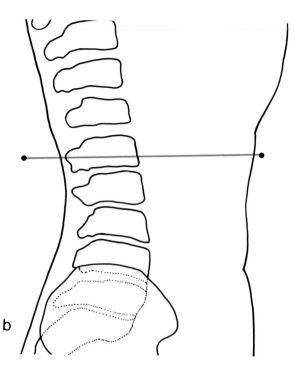

5.25 Scan level. (a) Normal A-P abdominal roentgenogram; red line shows cross-section level. (b) Schematic diagram of scan level.

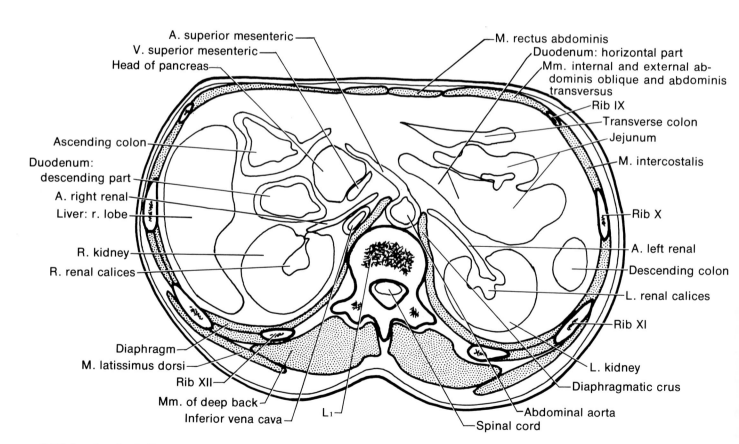

5.26 Anatomical diagram at the level of L₁ illustrating the prominent abdominal vasculature.

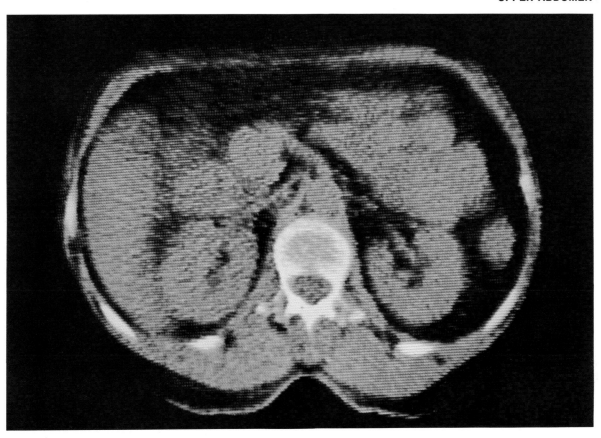

5.27 Color CT scan. Note the appearance of the renal arteries and the superior mesenteric artery which lie in the plane of this cross-section.

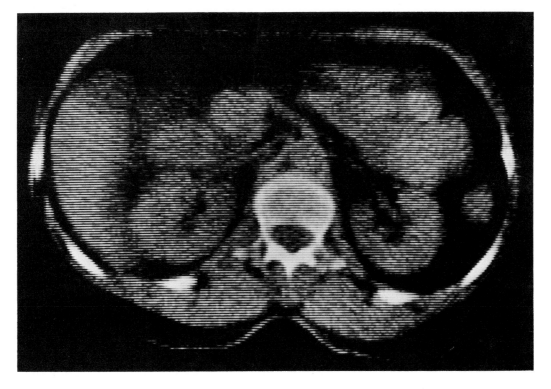

5.28 Black and white CT scan. Note the appearance of the kidneys bilaterally as well as the multiple loops of small bowel occupying the left upper quadrant of the abdomen.

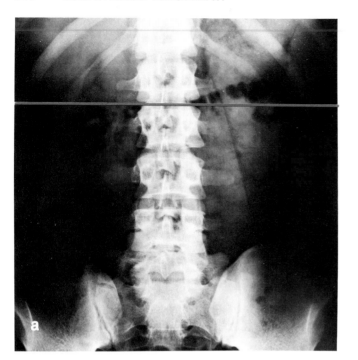
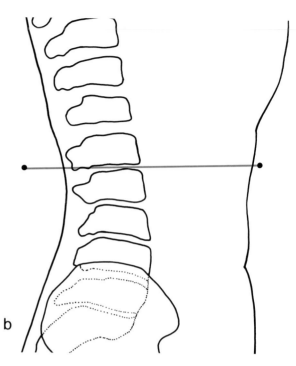

5.29 Scan level. (a) Normal A-P abdominal roentgenogram; red line shows cross-section level. (b) Schematic diagram of scan level.

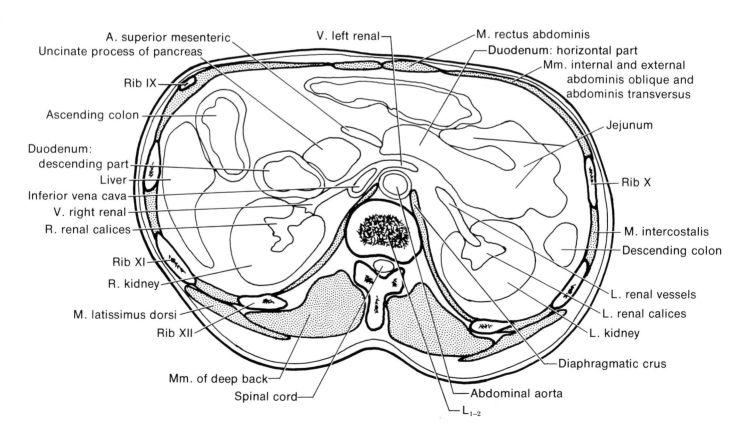

5.30 Anatomical diagram at the level of L_1–L_2. Note the relationship of the duodenum to the head of the pancreas.

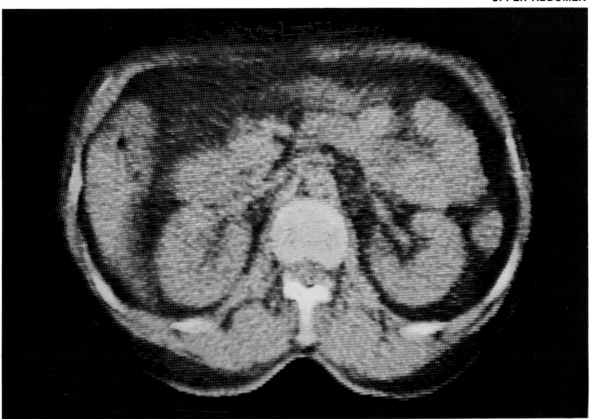

5.31 Color CT scan illustrating the course of the renal veins.

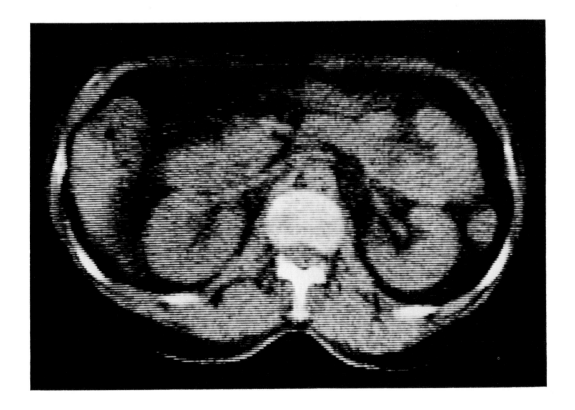

5.32 Black and white CT scan through the mid-portion of the left kidney. Note its close proximity to the descending colon.

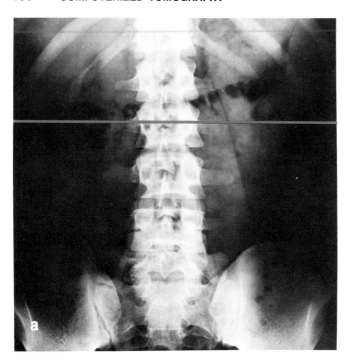
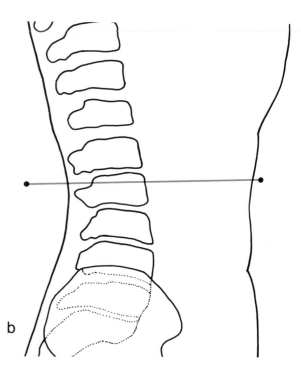

5.33 Scan level. (a) Normal A-P abdominal roentgenogram; red line shows cross-section level. (b) Schematic diagram of scan level.

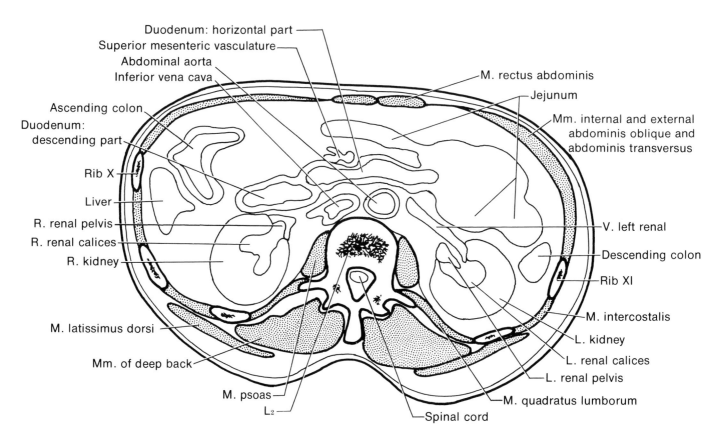

5.34 Anatomical diagram at the level of L$_2$.

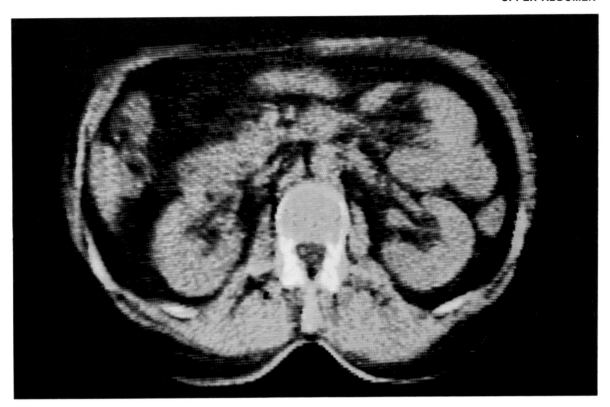

5.35 Color CT scan demonstrating the course of the renal veins.

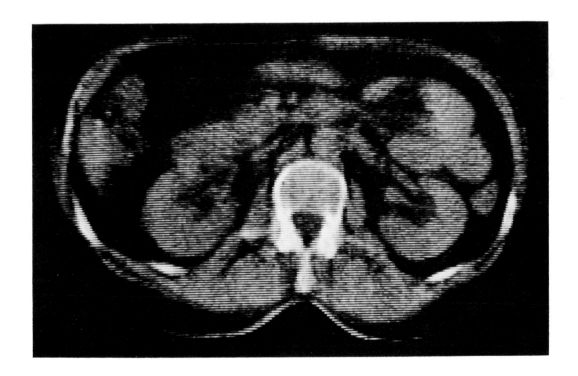

5.36 Black and white CT scan. Note the presence of the inferior pole of the liver.

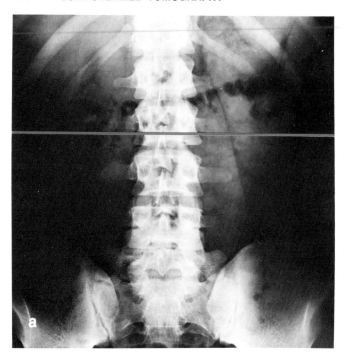

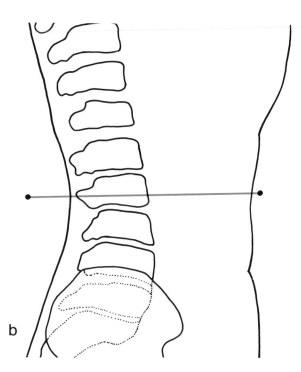

5.37 Scan level. (a) Normal A-P abdominal roentgenogram; red line shows cross-section level. (b) Schematic diagram of scan level.

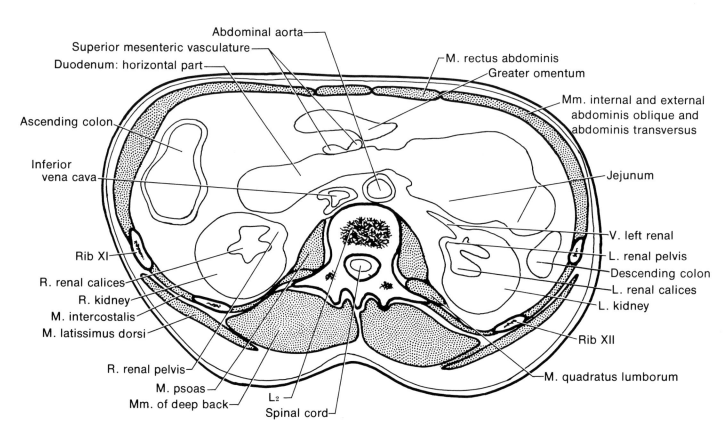

5.38 Anatomical diagram at the level of L$_2$.

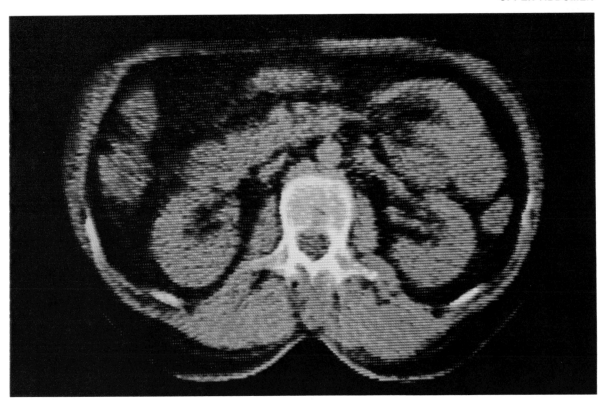

5.39 Color CT scan demonstrating the horizontal part of the duodenum and the mid-portion of the kidneys.

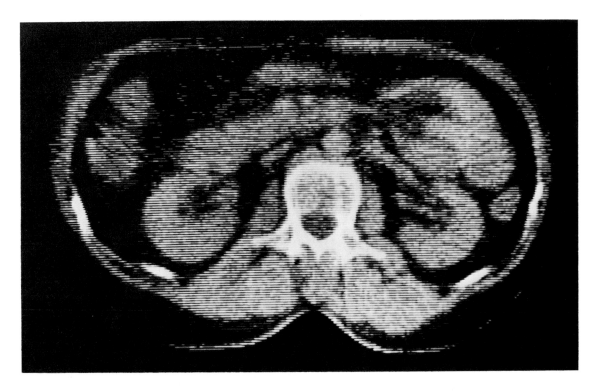

5.40 Black and white CT scan. Note the branches of the superior mesenteric vessels just anterior to the horizontal part of the duodenum.

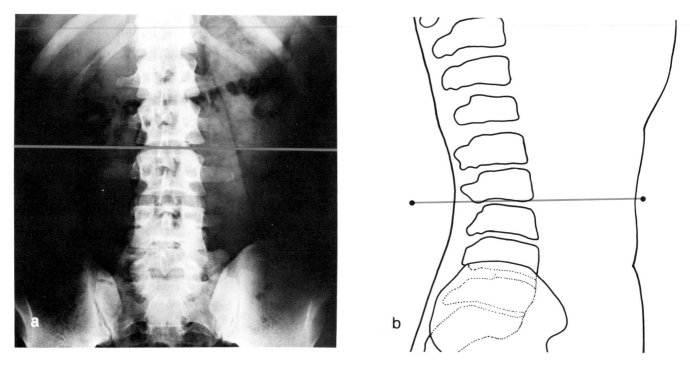

5.41 Scan level. (a) Normal A-P abdominal roentgenogram; red line shows cross-section level. (b) Schematic diagram of scan level.

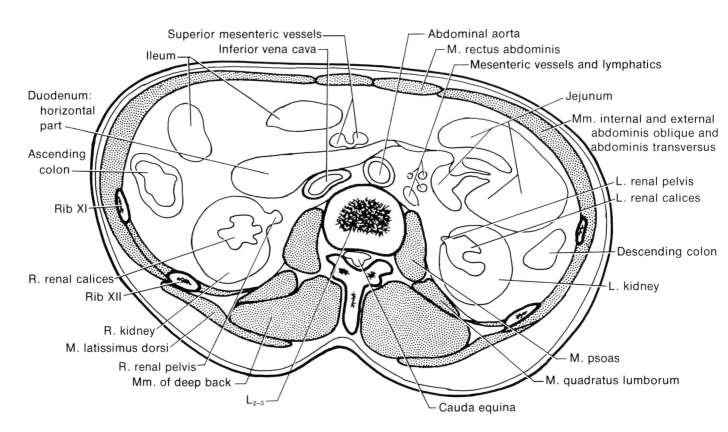

5.42 Anatomical diagram at the level of L₂–L₃.

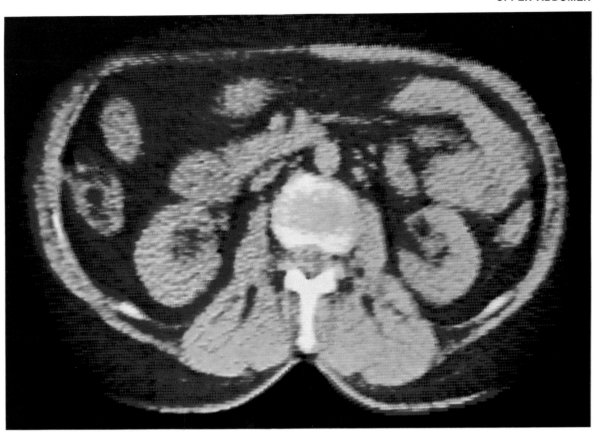

5.43 Color CT scan. Note the appearance of the branches of the superior mesenteric vessels and the presence of the ascending and descending colon.

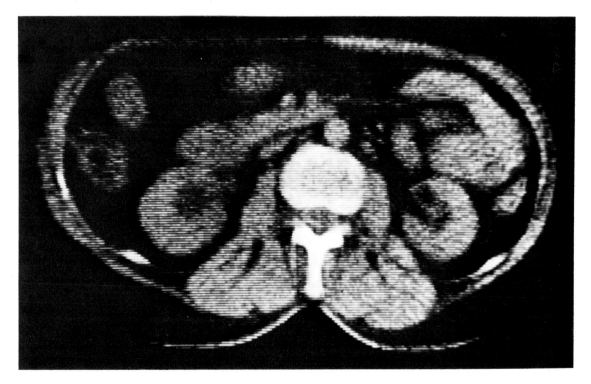

5.44 Black and white CT scan.

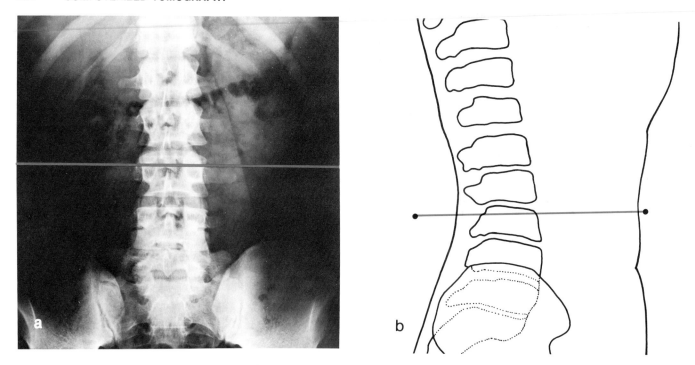

5.45 Scan level. (a) Normal A-P abdominal roentgenogram; red line shows cross-section level. (b) Schematic diagram of scan level.

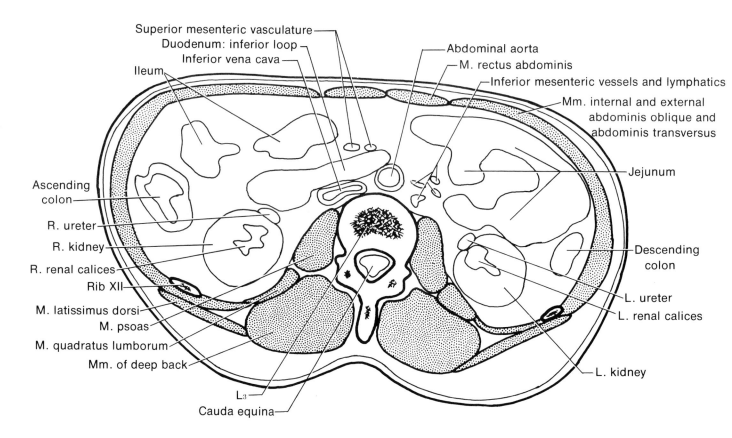

Superior mesenteric vasculature
Duodenum: inferior loop
Inferior vena cava
Ileum

Abdominal aorta
M. rectus abdominis
Inferior mesenteric vessels and lymphatics
Mm. internal and external abdominis oblique and abdominis transversus

Ascending colon
R. ureter
R. kidney
R. renal calices
Rib XII
M. latissimus dorsi
M. psoas
M. quadratus lumborum
Mm. of deep back

Jejunum

Descending colon

L. ureter
L. renal calices

L. kidney

L_3
Cauda equina

5.46 Anatomical diagram at the level of L_3.

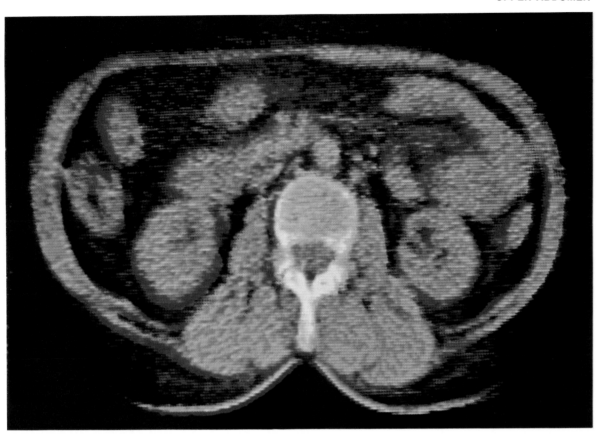

5.47 Color CT scans demonstrating the appearance of the psoas muscles just lateral to the vertebral body.

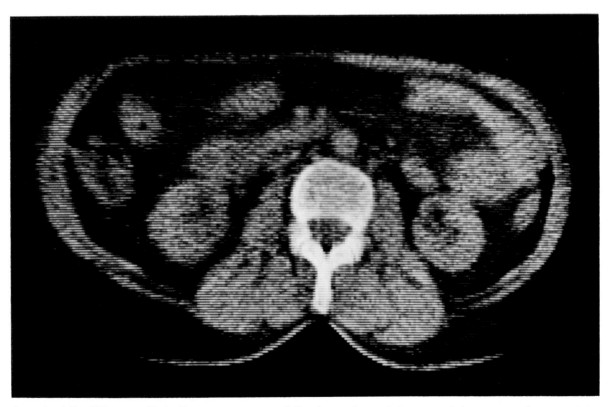

5.48 Black and white CT scan. Note the appearance of the branches of the superior mesenteric vasculature just anterior to the horizontal part of the duodenum.

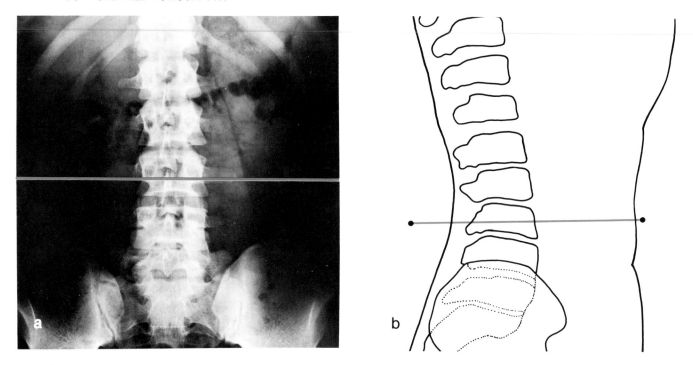

5.49 Scan level. (a) Normal A-P abdominal roentgenogram; red line shows cross-section level. (b) Schematic diagram of scan level.

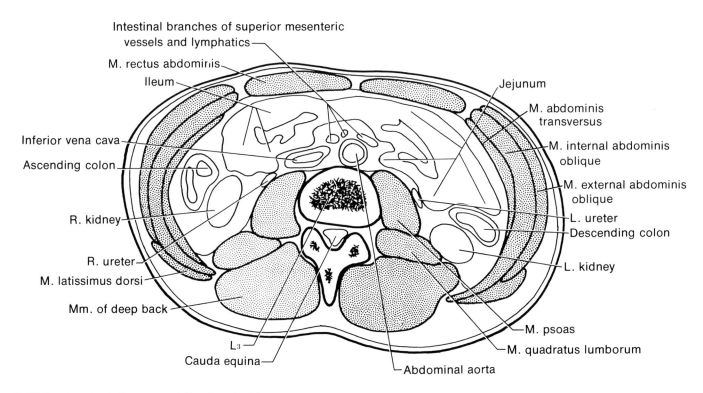

5.50 Anatomical diagram at the level of L₃.

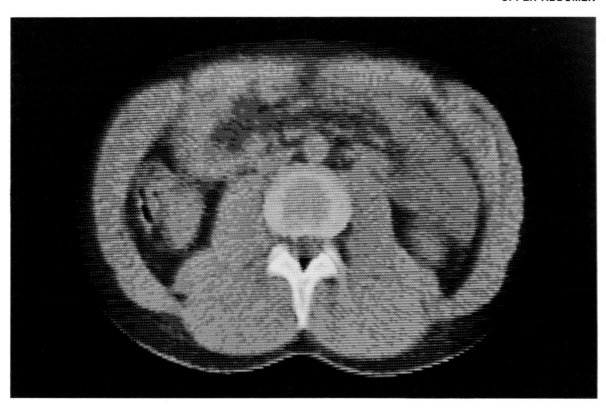

5.51 Color CT scan. Note the appearance of the somewhat flattened inferior vena cava relative to the circular abdominal aorta in this supine subject. This scan also demonstrates the intervertebral joints.

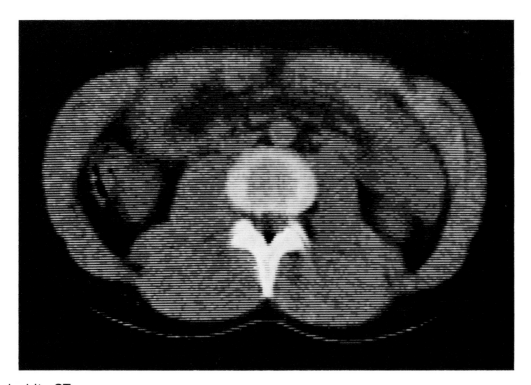

5.52 Black and white CT scan.

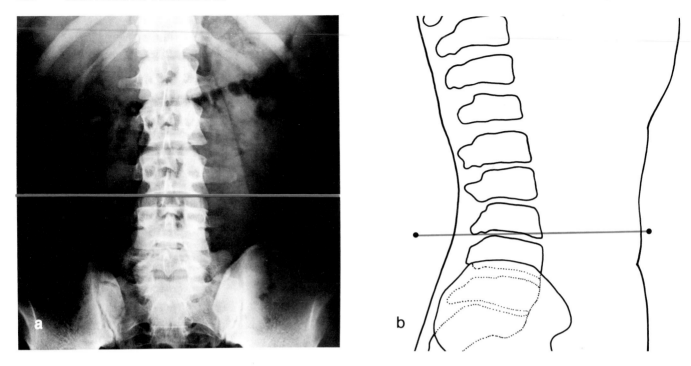

5.53 Scan level. (a) Normal A-P abdominal roentgenogram; red line shows cross-section level. (b) Schematic diagram of scan level.

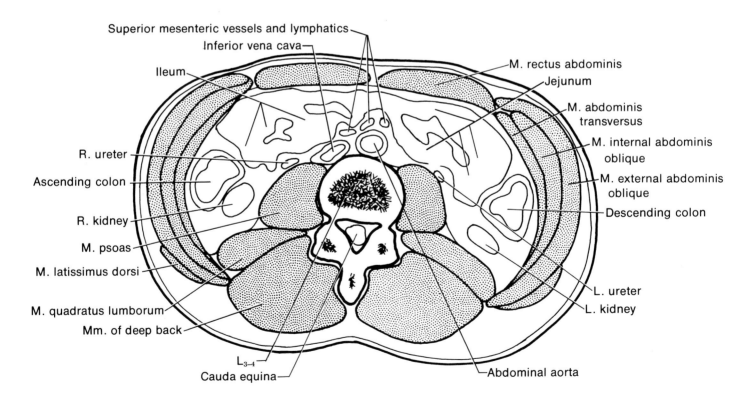

5.54 Anatomical diagram at the level of L_3–L_4.

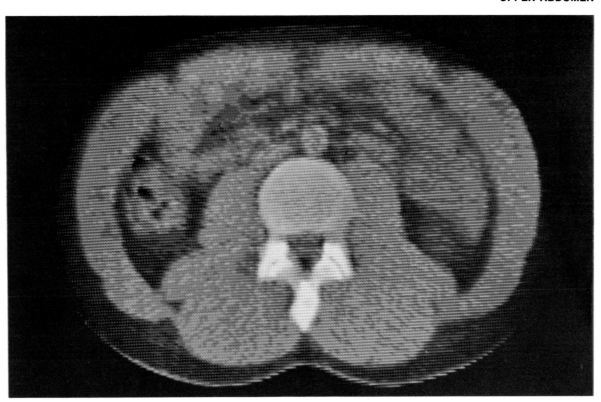

5.55 Color CT scan. Note the inferior pole of the kidney and the ascending and descending colon as well as the intervertebral joints.

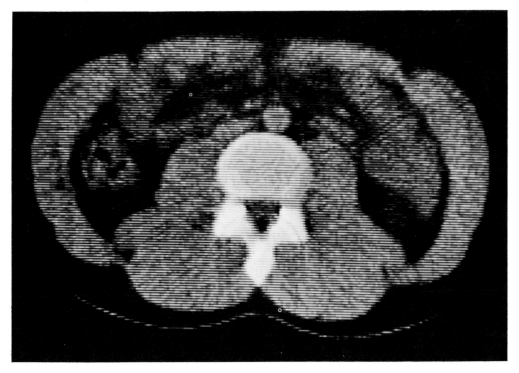

5.56 Black and white CT scan. Note the multiple loops of small bowel in the central portion of the peritoneal cavity.

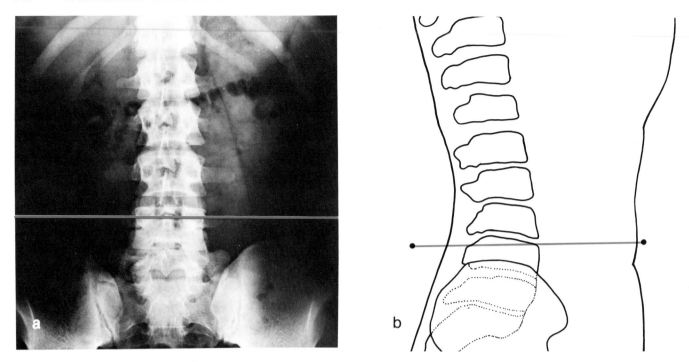

5.57 Scan level. (a) Normal A-P abdominal roentgenogram; red line shows cross-section level. (b) Schematic diagram of scan level.

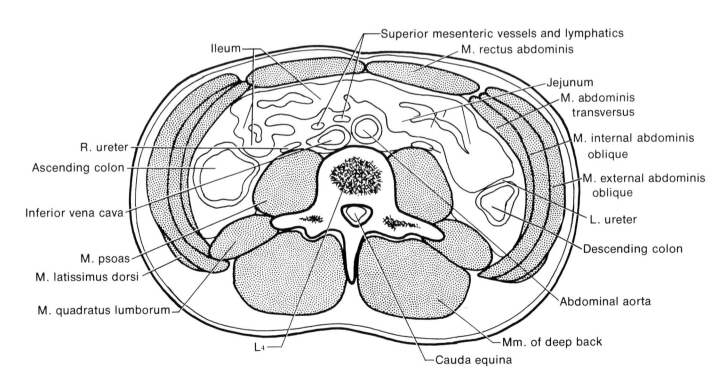

5.58 Anatomical diagram at the level of L₄.

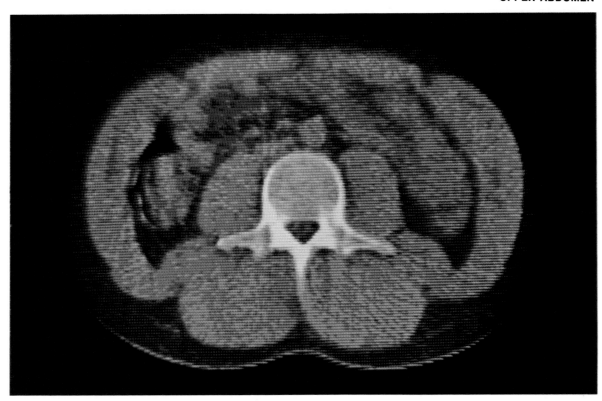

5.59 Color CT scan. Note the appearance of the psoas muscles as well as the musculature of the anterior and lateral abdominal walls.

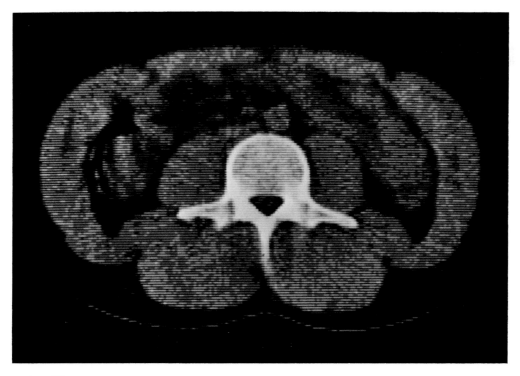

5.60 Black and white CT scan.

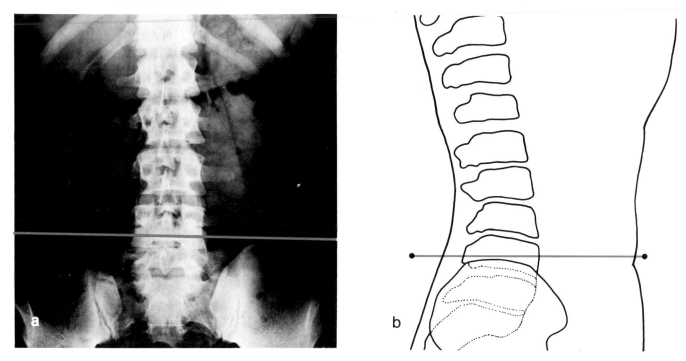

5.61 Scan level. (a) Normal A-P abdominal roentgenogram; red line shows cross-section level. (b) Schematic diagram of scan level.

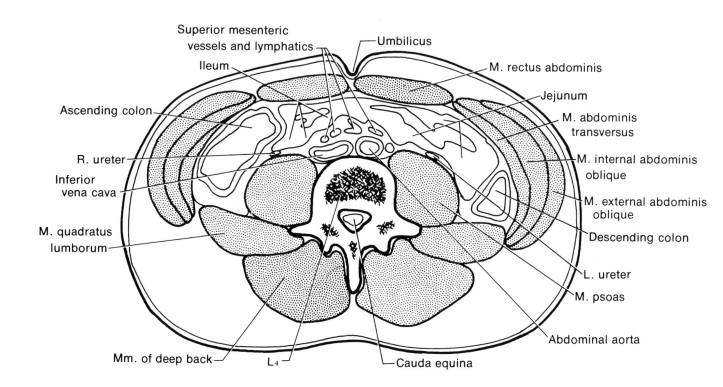

5.62 Anatomical diagram at the level of L₄.

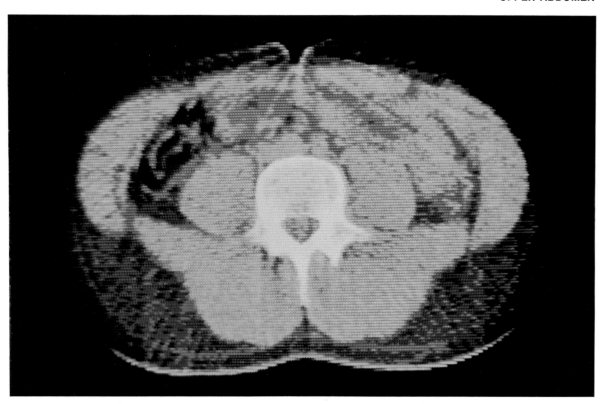

5.63 Color CT scan through the umbilicus. Note the presence of the descending colon and the ascending colon which contain some fecal material in this subject.

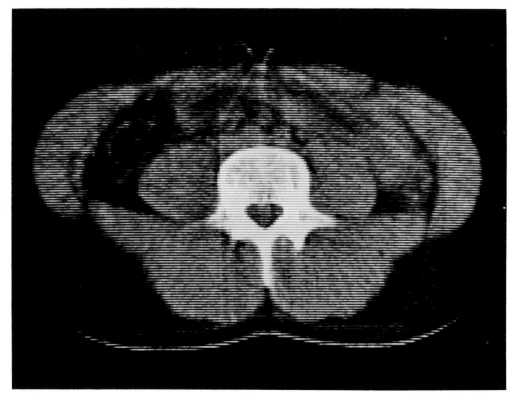

5.64 Black and white CT scan demonstrating the very prominent psoas musculature as well as the musculature of the lower back.

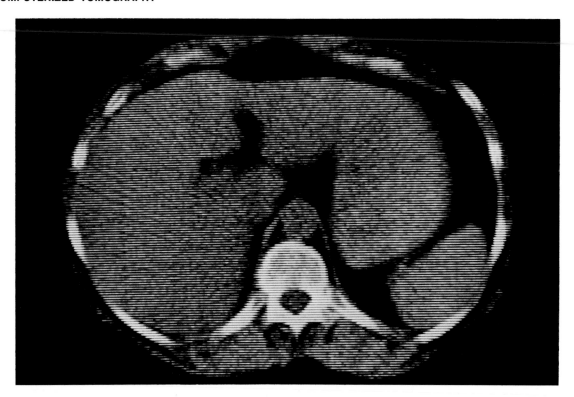

5.65 ABNORMAL black and white CT scan of a patient 5 years postoperative from a cholecystectomy and demonstrating the architecture of the liver lobes as well as the spleen, abdominal vasculature and the somewhat distended stomach.

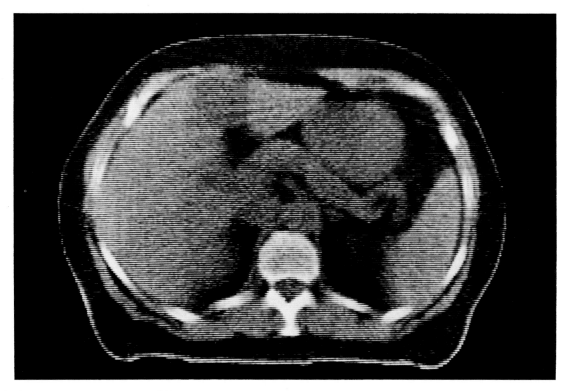

5.66 ABNORMAL black and white CT scan in a patient with a benign cyst of the liver. The cyst occupies the junction between the left and right liver lobes. Also note in this scan the fundus of the stomach, the body of the pancreas, the spleen, the left adrenal gland and the superior poles of both kidneys.

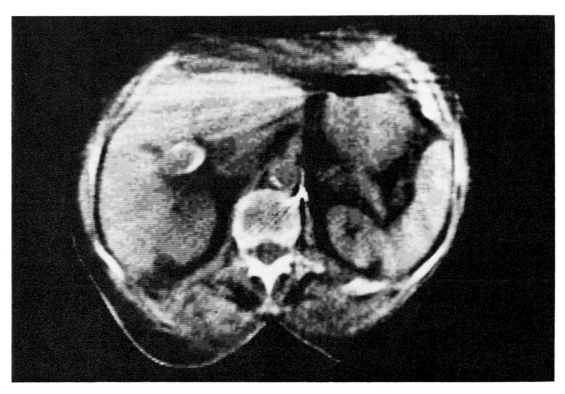

5.67 ABNORMAL black and white CT scan of a patient demonstrating the condition known as porcelain gall bladder. This patient also has aortic calcifications.

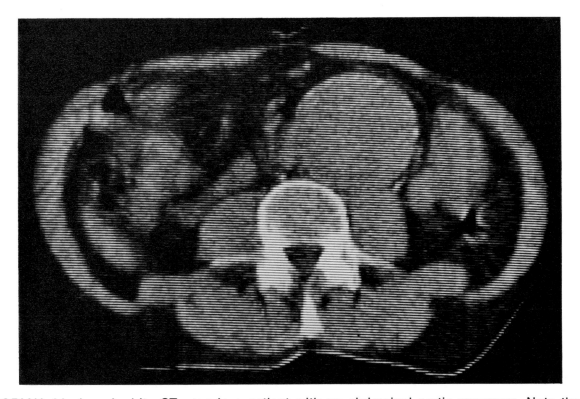

5.68 ABNORMAL black and white CT scan in a patient with an abdominal aortic aneurysm. Note the cross-sectional area of this aneurysm, the thin rim of calcification within its wall and the displacement of the normal abdominal structures due to its presence.

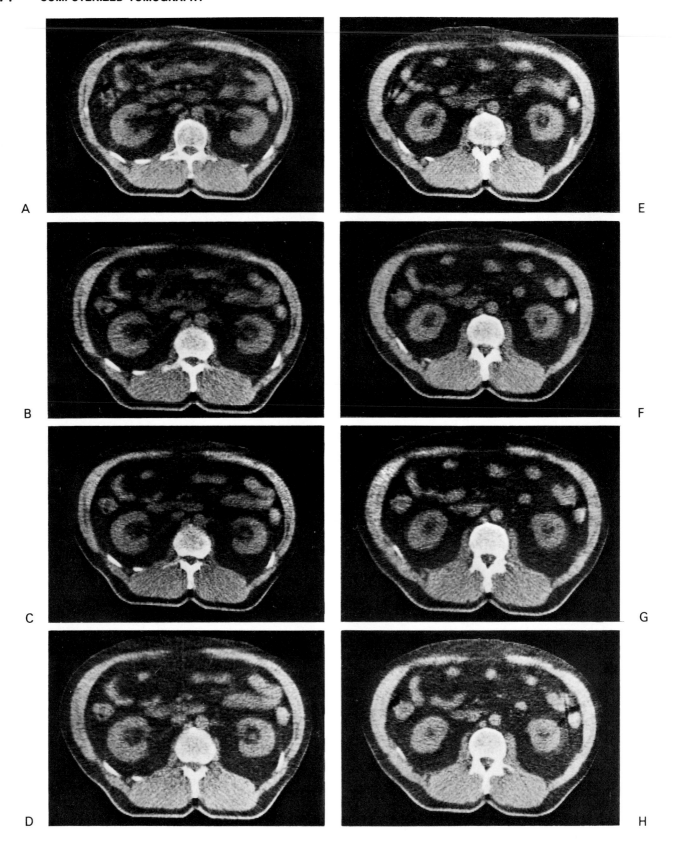

5.69 A serial set of 16 black and white CT scans made with a 3-mm scan thickness and including the vertebral levels: L_2 (A–B), the L_{2-3} disc space (C-F) and L_3 (G-O) and corresponding to Figures 5.37 through 5.48 in this chapter. The series demonstrates the inferior halves of both kidneys, the ascending and descending colon as well as the small bowel and the abdominal vasculature.

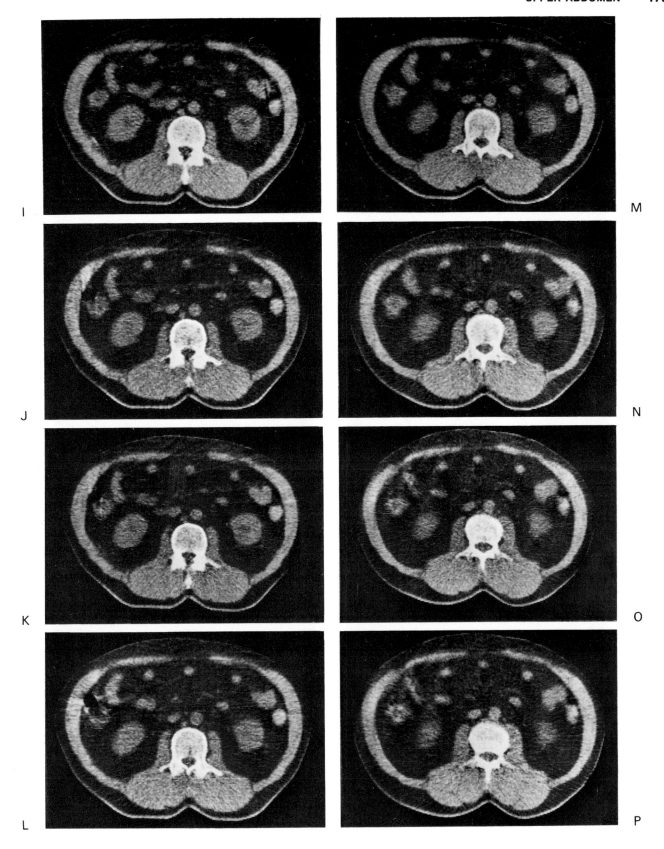

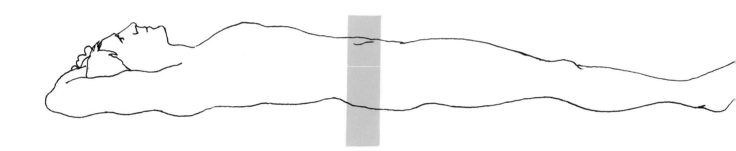

chapter six

Lower Abdomen

This section of the ATLAS represents the region of the body between the iliac crests and the pelvic brim, and encompasses the spinal levels from L_4 to the mid-sacrum, including the bifurcations of both the aorta and inferior vena cava, the ascending, descending, and sigmoid segments of the colon, the distal portions of the small intestine, the caecum, and the gluteal and anterior abdominal musculature and their associated neurovascular supplies. Tumors of this region, such as lymphomas involving the periaortic lymphatic system, can be examined by the CT scan. In addition, pelvic tumors with extension into the lower abdomen may be detected.

All subjects were scanned in the supine position, using a section thickness of 7.5 mm at $0°$ gantry tilt and a scan interval of 1 cm. As in other sections of the ATLAS, a reference line has been drawn on each conventional X-ray image to correspond with the level shown on the CT scan and diagram. The presence of the examining table may be seen under the subjects and some compression of the posterior structures results.

Adjacent loops of small bowel are grouped under a common label and have been divided into jejunum and ileum by region. This division is somewhat arbitrary due to the mobility of these structures and represents an estimate of where the organs lie in the supine adult.

Bony landmarks are again provided for patient positioning and these correspond with the following figure numbers:

Iliac crest . . . . Figure 6.2–6.6
Anterior superior iliac spine Figure 6.10–6.14
Anterior inferior iliac spine Figure 6.30–6.40

In the subjects used for this ATLAS, the distance between the iliac crest and the anterior superior iliac spine is 2 cm, the distance from the superior to inferior anterior iliac spine is 5–6 cm.

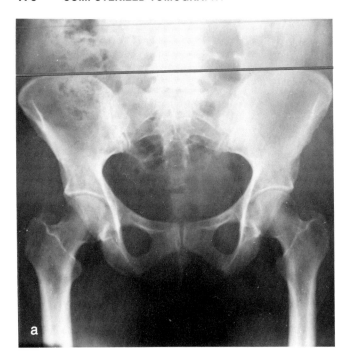
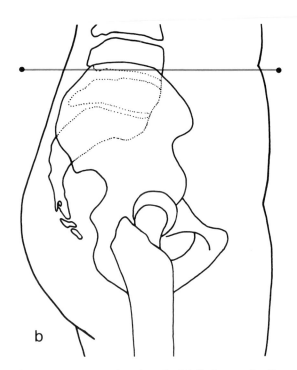

6.1 Scan level. (a) Normal A-P pelvic roentgenogram; red line shows cross-section level. (b) Schematic diagram of scan level.

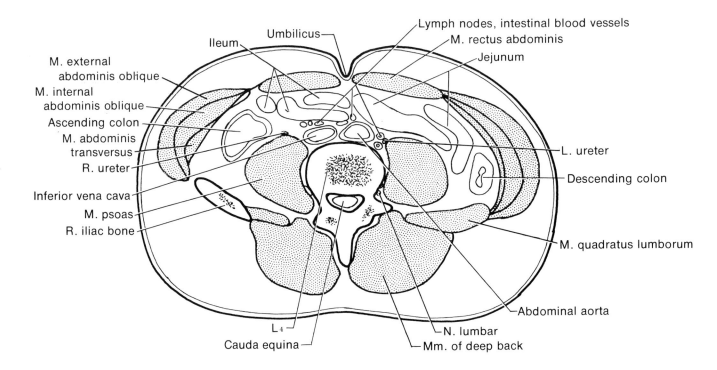

6.2 Anatomical diagram at the level of the iliac crest.

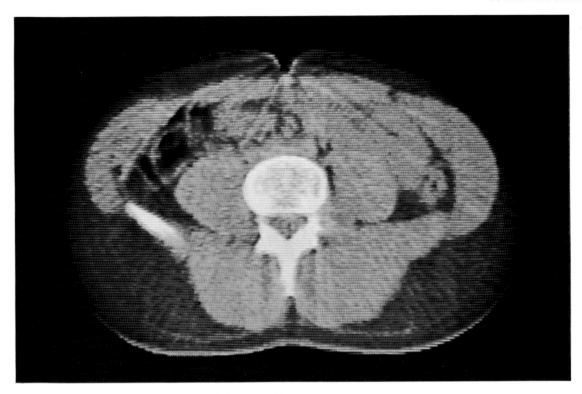

6.3 Color CT scan. Note the appearance of the umbilicus.

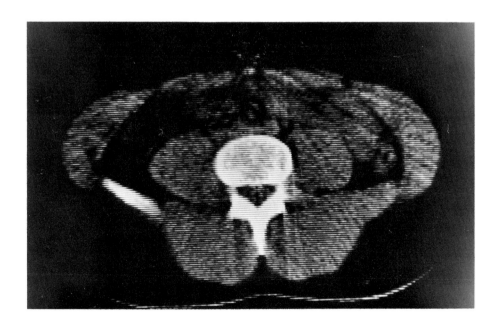

6.4 Black and white CT scan.

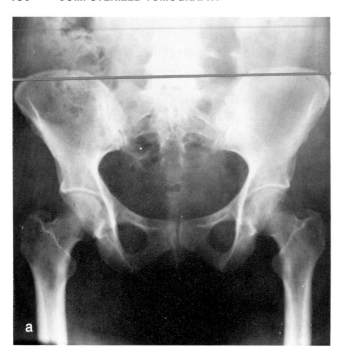

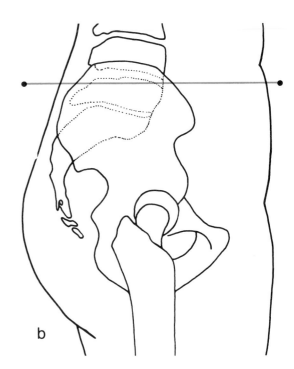

6.5 Scan level. (a) Normal A-P pelvic roentgenogram; red line shows cross-section level. (b) Schematic diagram of scan level.

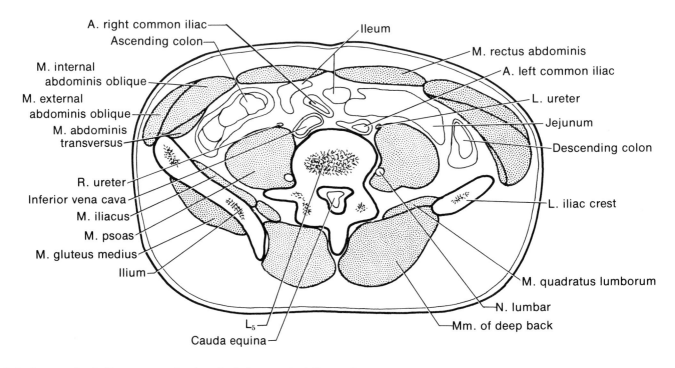

6.6 Anatomical diagram at the level of the aortic bifurcation.

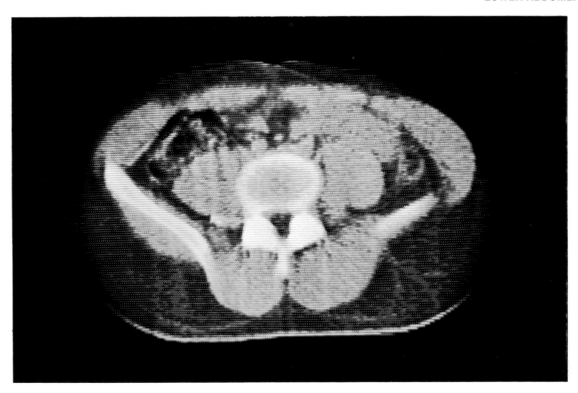

6.7 Color CT scan. Note the ascending and descending colon outlined in green.

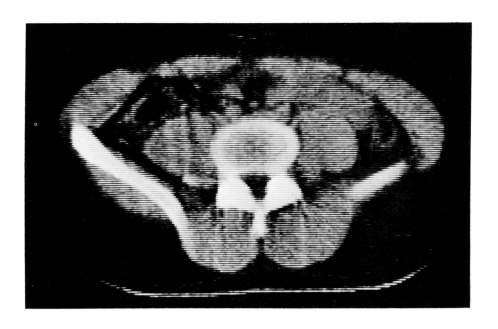

6.8 Black and white CT scan.

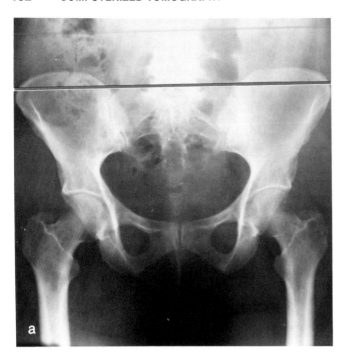
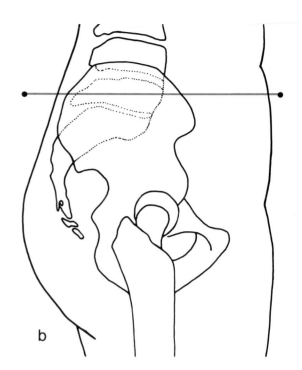

6.9 Scan level. (a) Normal A-P pelvic roentgenogram; red line shows cross-section level. (b) Schematic diagram of scan level.

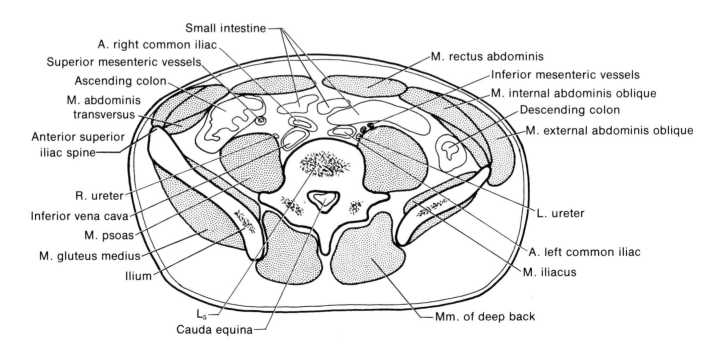

6.10 Anatomical diagram.

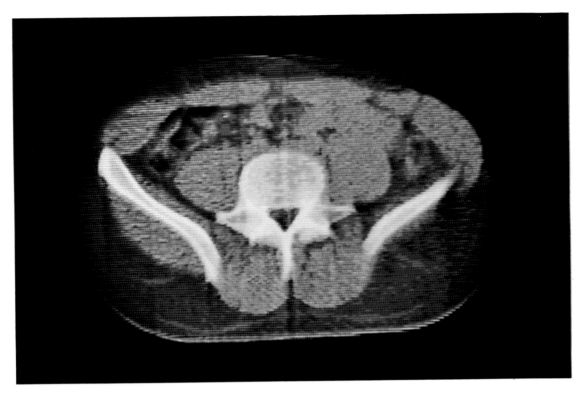

6.11 Color CT scan illustrating the psoas muscles in green.

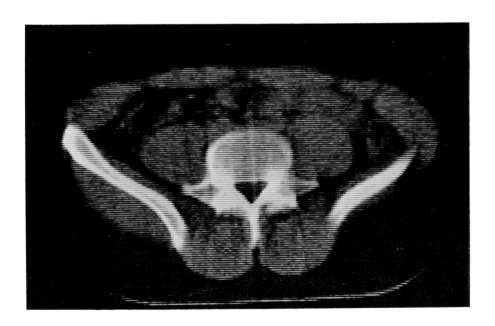

6.12 Black and white CT scan.

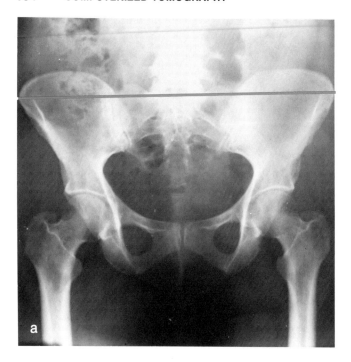
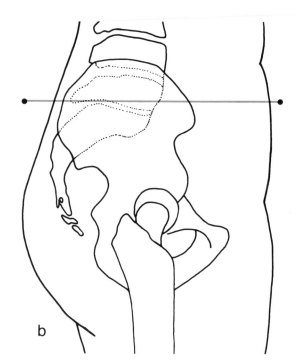

6.13 Scan level. (a) Normal A-P pelvic roentgenogram; red line shows cross-section level. (b) Schematic diagram of scan level.

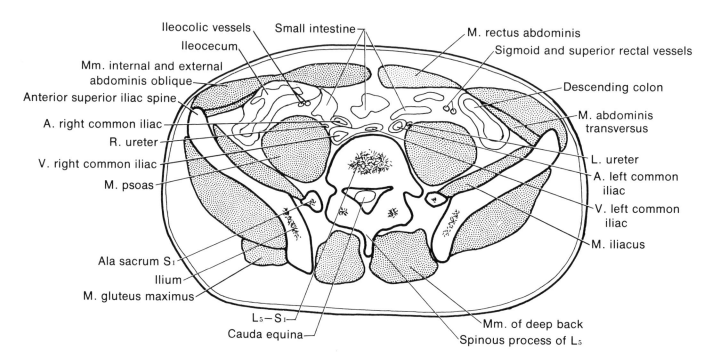

6.14 Anatomical diagram of the L_5–S_1 vertebral level.

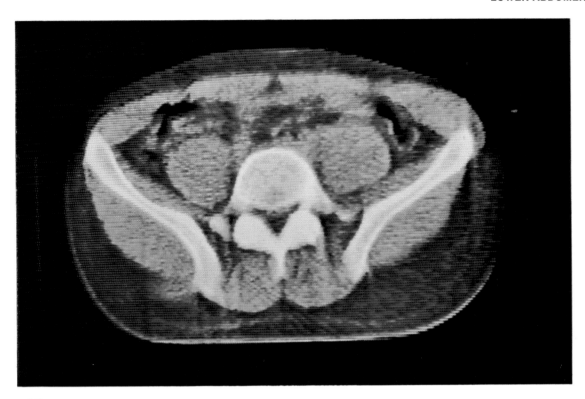

6.15 Color CT scan.

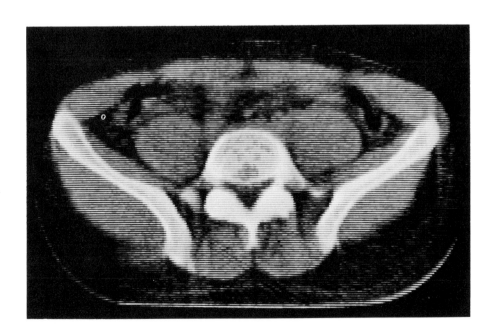

6.16 Black and white CT scan.

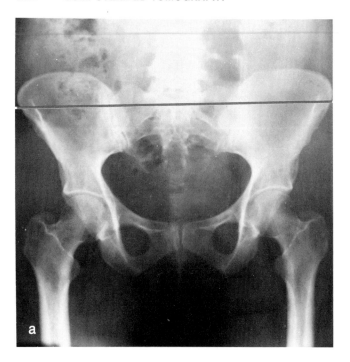

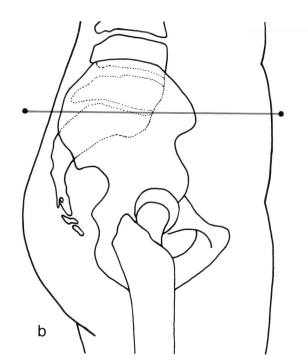

6.17 Scan level. (a) Normal A-P pelvic roentgenogram; red line shows cross-section level. (b) Schematic diagram of scan level.

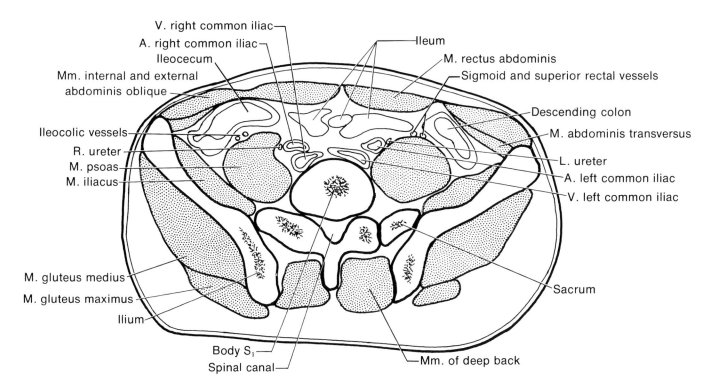

6.18 Anatomical diagram at the level of S_1.

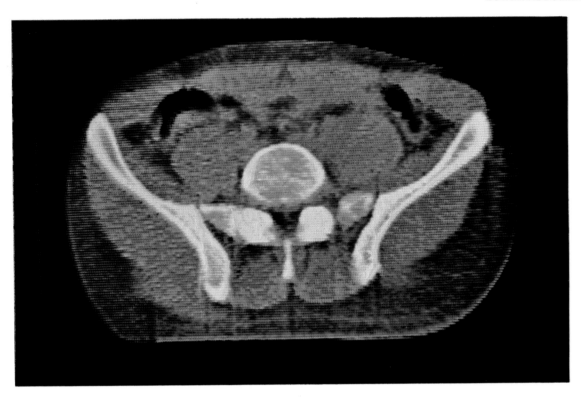

6.19 Color CT scan showing the superior border of the sacroiliac joint.

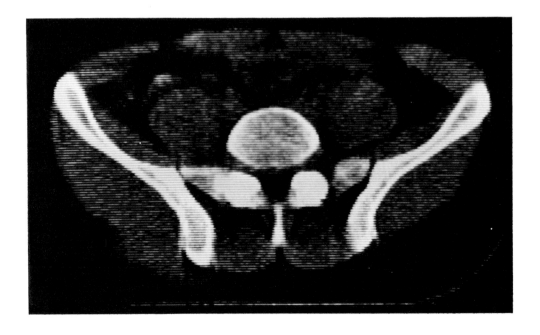

6.20 Black and white CT scan.

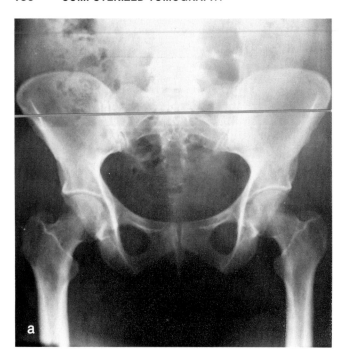

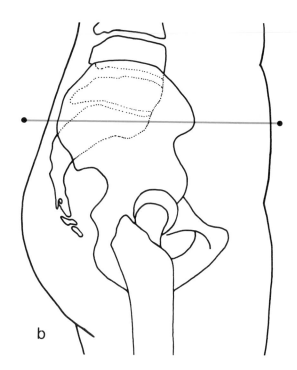

6.21 Scan level. (a) Normal A-P pelvic roentgenogram; red line shows cross-section level. (b) Schematic diagram of scan level.

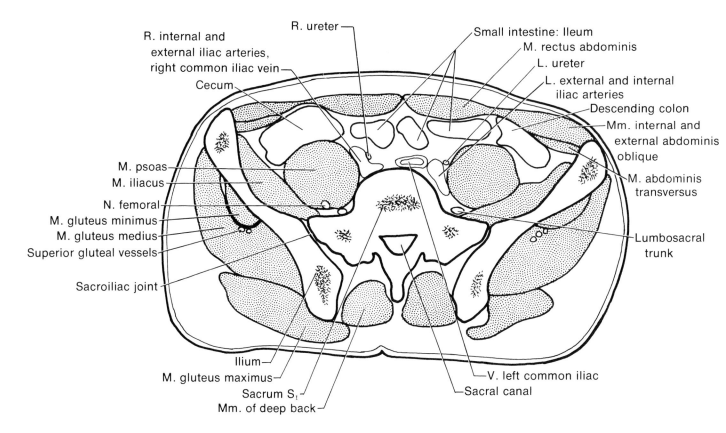

6.22 Anatomical diagram at the level of S_1.

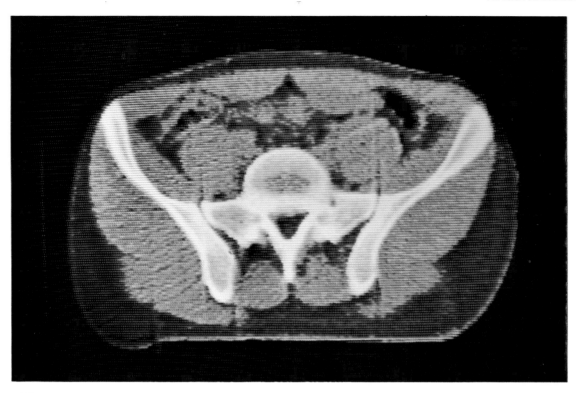

6.23 Color CT scan demonstrating the iliopsoas muscles in green.

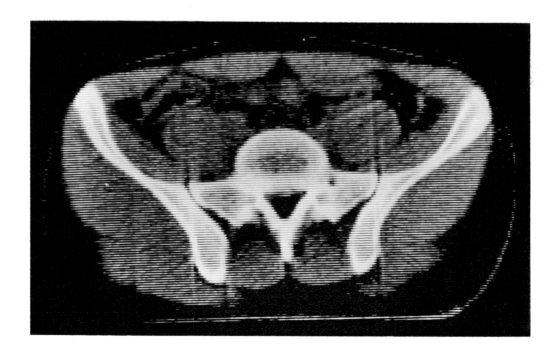

6.24 Black and white CT scan demonstrating the sacroiliac joint.

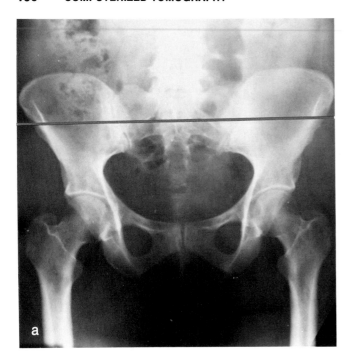

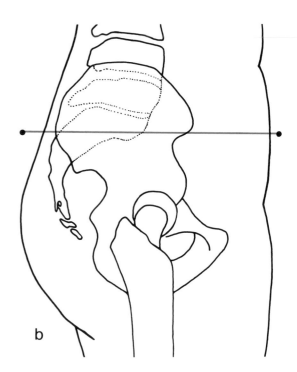

6.25 Scan level. (a) Normal A-P pelvic roentgenogram; red line shows cross-section level. (b) Schematic diagram of scan level.

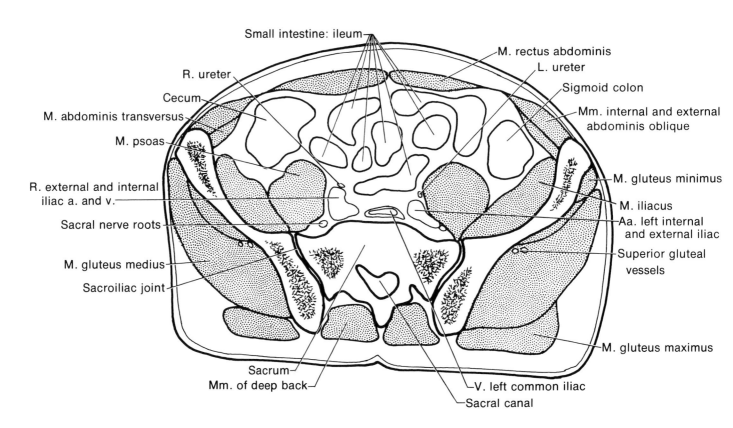

6.26 Anatomical diagram through the sacroiliac joint.

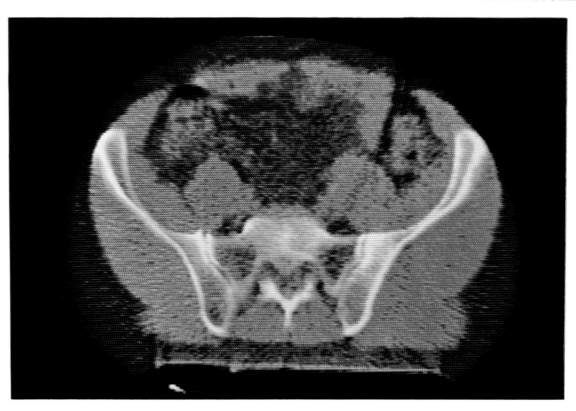

6.27 Color CT scan demonstrating the descending colon and the cecum.

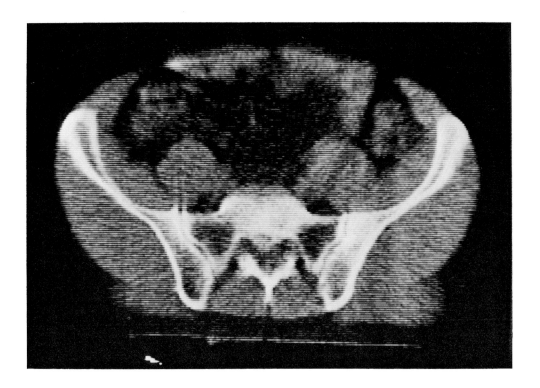

6.28 Black and white CT scan. Note the appearance of the sacroiliac joint.

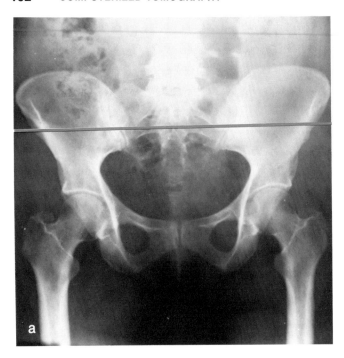
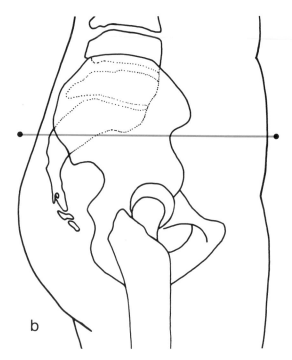

6.29 Scan level. (a) Normal A-P pelvic roentgenogram; red line shows cross-section level. (b) Schematic diagram of scan level.

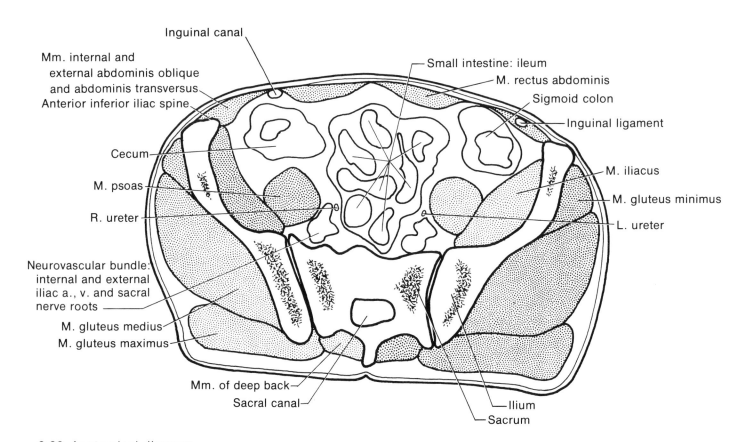

6.30 Anatomical diagram.

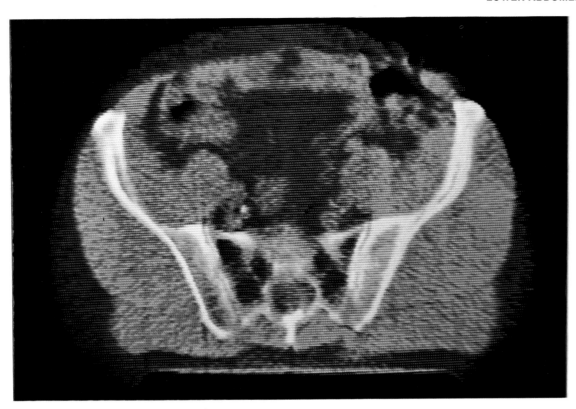

6.31 Color CT scan. Note the flattening of the gluteal musculature due to the examining table beneath subject.

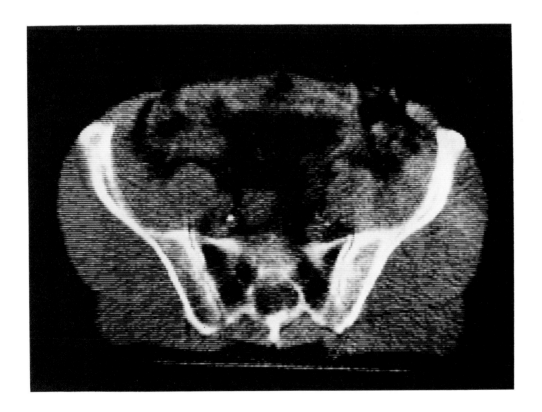

6.32 Black and white CT scan.

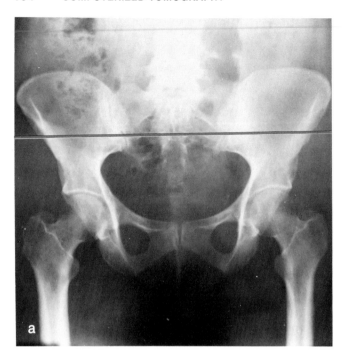
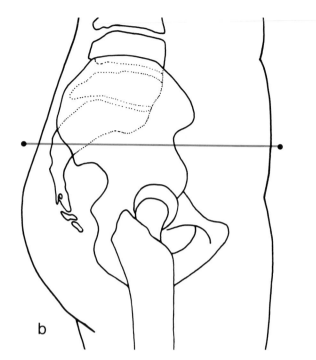

6.33 Scan level. (a) Normal A-P pelvic roentgenogram; red line shows cross-section level. (b) Schematic diagram of scan level.

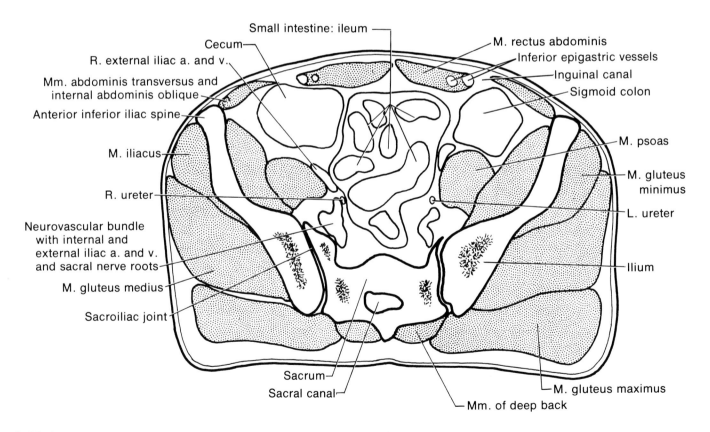

6.34 Anatomical diagram. Note the anterior migration of the external iliac vessels.

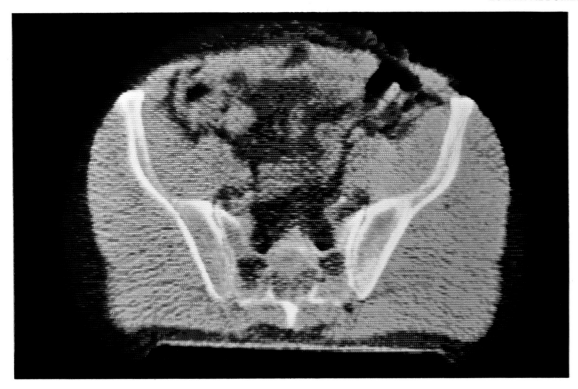

6.35 Color CT scan. Note the appearance of the multiple loops of small bowel.

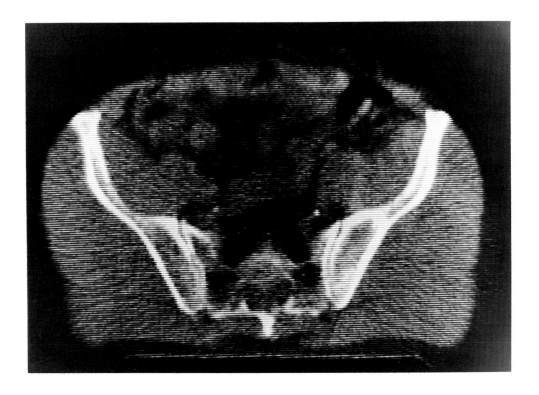

6.36 Black and white CT scan.

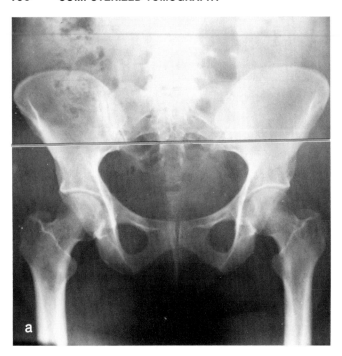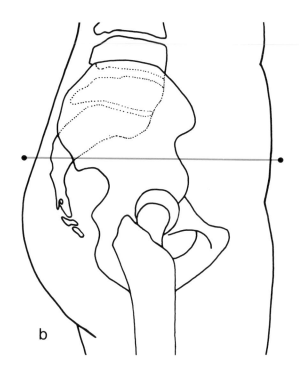

6.37 Scan level. (a) Normal A-P pelvic roentgenogram; red line shows cross-section level. (b) Schematic diagram of scan level.

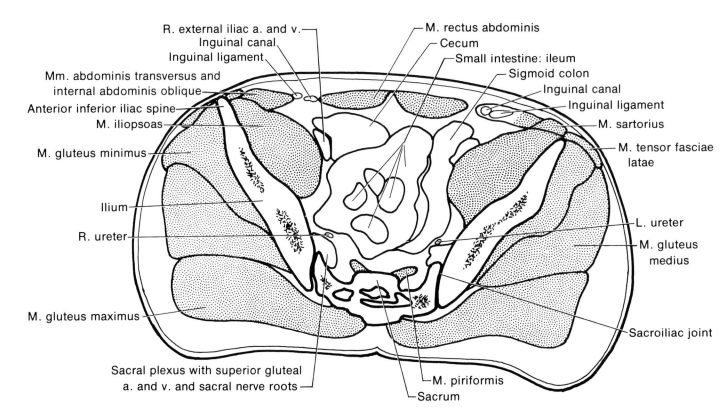

6.38 Anatomical diagram through the mid-sacrum.

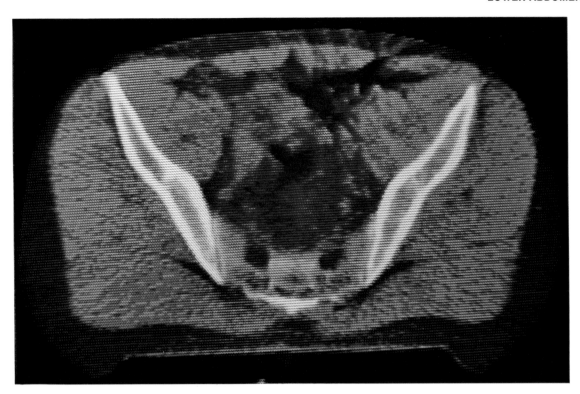

6.39 Color CT scan showing the inferior portion of the sacroiliac joint.

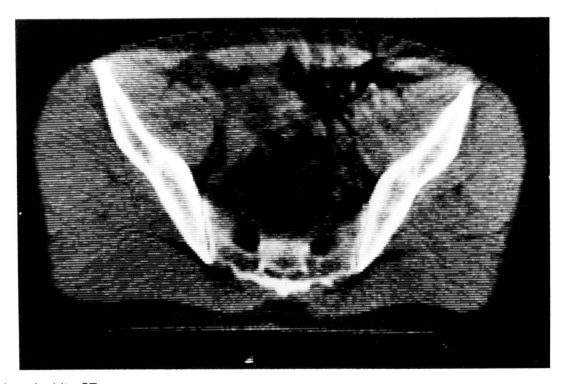

6.40 Black and white CT scan.

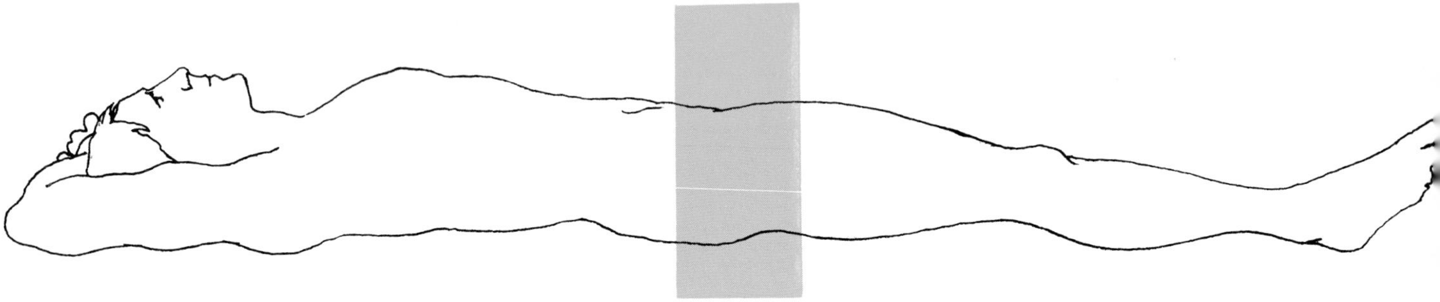

chapter seven

Male Pelvis

This section of the ATLAS includes scans through the entire male pelvis, including such structures as the rectum, anus, bladder, prostate, the hip joint with its associated musculature, and the male reproductive tract. The scans in this region range from the pelvic brim to the lesser trochanter of the femur.

CT studies can provide accurate imaging of the pelvic organs and are particularly useful for the evaluation of prostatic and bladder tumors. However, in order to be visualized using conventional radiographic techniques, practically all of the soft tissue within the pelvis requires contrast studies. When these contrast studies techniques are adapted and combined with the capabilities of the CT scanner, even more precise details of the distal ureters, bladder, and prostatic urethra will be seen. As in the lower abdomen, pelvic primary tumors and metastatic spread of local and systemic (lymphoma) tumors can be visualized using CT methods.

CT scanning of the hip joint results in excellent images of the bony components, the articular capsule, and the extensive musculature which inserts on the greater and lesser trochanters of the femur. With the increase in prosthetic replacement of this joint, CT scanning can become an additional source of information in determining the need for surgical intervention in diseases of the hip. In addition to allowing for the visualization of the bony pelvis and hip, CT scan can be analyzed numerically to determine quantitative changes in bone calcium density, thereby providing objective data in the study of osteoporosis and pathological bone alteration. This can be especially helpful in cases of lytic and blastic bony metastases, which are so prevalent in the pelvic region.

Subjects scanned in this region were lying in the supine position; a 7.5-mm section thickness was used with a 0° gantry tilt and a 1-cm scan interval. Subjects for this section were at least 50 years of age. All muscles have been named individually with the exception of the anterior abdominal musculature (M. transversus and internal oblique). The loops of bowel comprising the distal segment of the ileum are also collectively grouped under one label. As in other sections, the presence of the examining table can be seen under the subjects scanned and results in some compression of the posterior musculature.

Two palpable bony landmarks, the coccyx and the greater trochanter of the femur, are encountered in this region. Both landmarks lie at a level which corresponds to Figures 7.22–7.32. The upper limit of this section (Figure 7.1) was found to be 6 cm above these landmarks in our subject population.

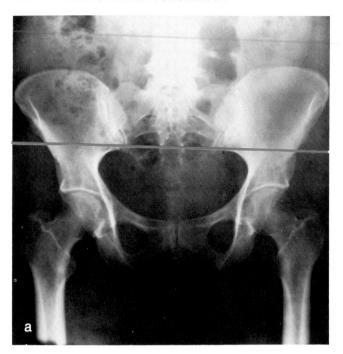

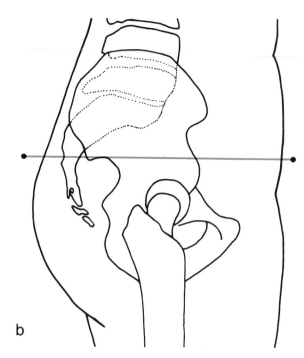

7.1 Scan level. (a) Normal A-P pelvic roentgenogram; red line shows cross-section level. (b) Schematic diagram of scan level.

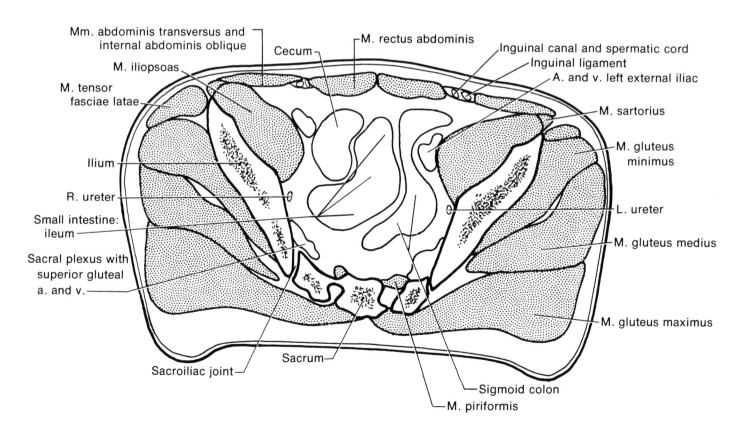

7.2 Anatomical diagram at the level of the inferior sacroiliac joint.

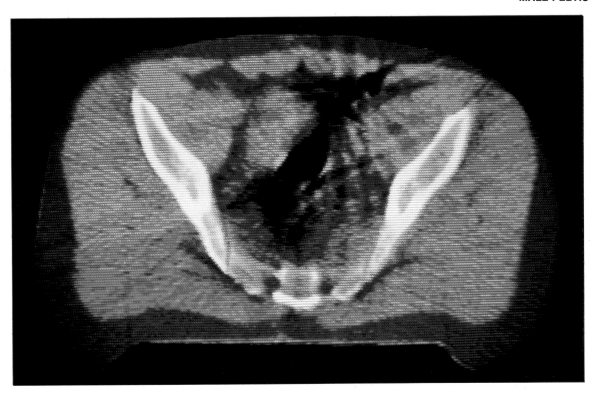

7.3 Color CT scan. Note the appearance of the sacroiliac joint.

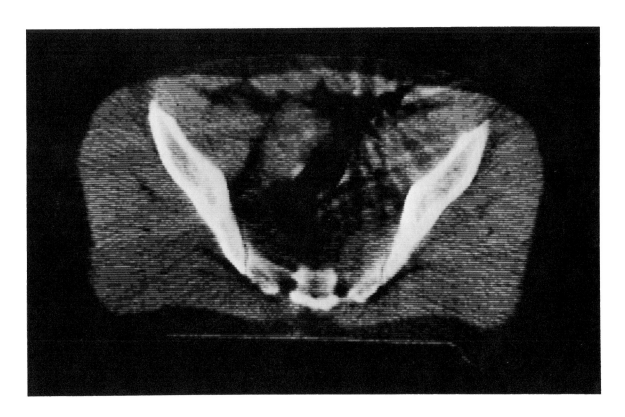

7.4 Black and white CT scan.

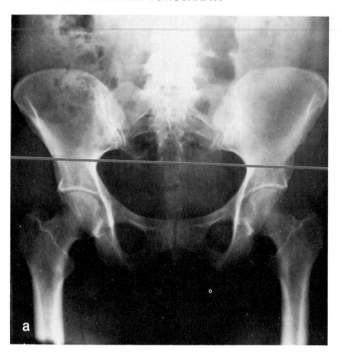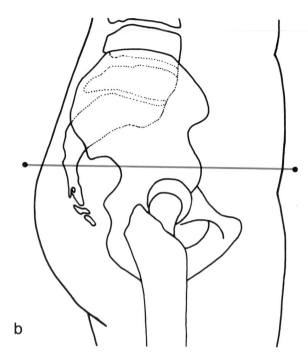

7.5 Scan level. (a) Normal A-P pelvic roentgenogram; red line shows cross-section level. (b) Schematic diagram of scan level.

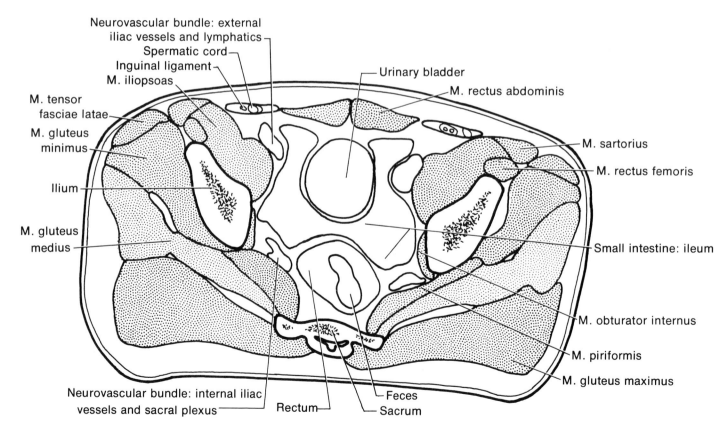

7.6 Anatomical diagram.

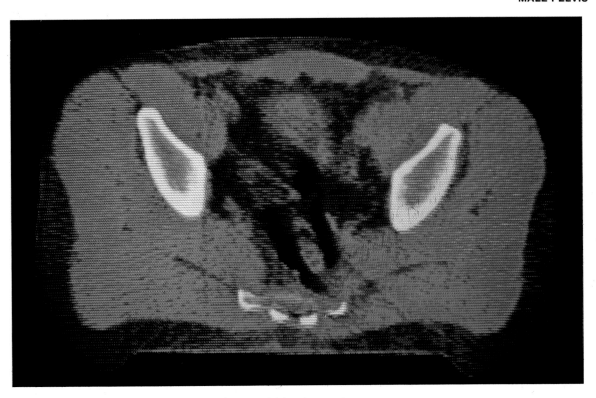

7.7 Color CT scan. Note the appearance of gas within the rectum.

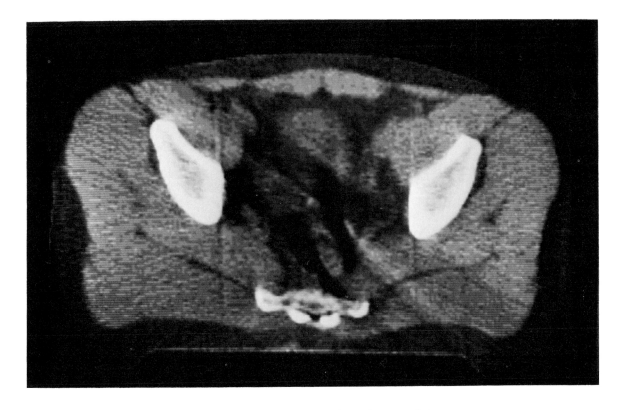

7.8 Black and white CT scan. Note the separation of the gluteal musculature.

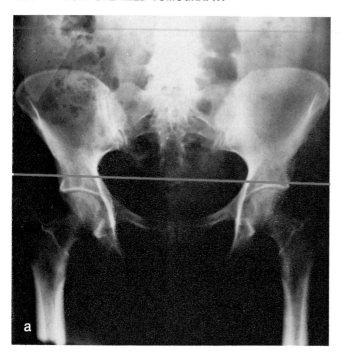

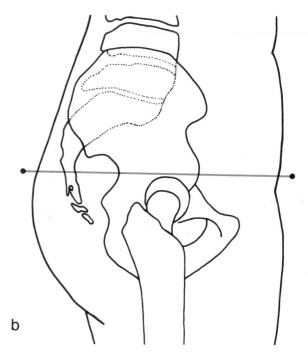

7.9 Scan level. (a) Normal A-P pelvic roentgenogram; red line shows cross-section level. (b) Schematic diagram of scan level.

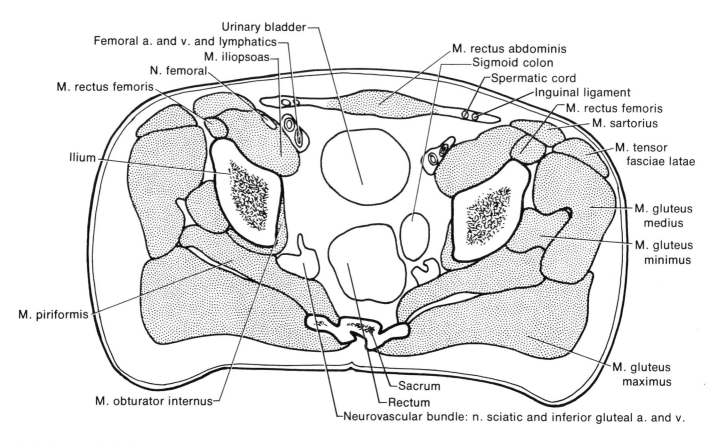

Urinary bladder

Femoral a. and v. and lymphatics

M. iliopsoas

N. femoral

M. rectus femoris

M. rectus abdominis

Sigmoid colon

Spermatic cord

Inguinal ligament

M. rectus femoris

M. sartorius

M. tensor fasciae latae

Ilium

M. gluteus medius

M. gluteus minimus

M. piriformis

M. gluteus maximus

M. obturator internus

Sacrum

Rectum

Neurovascular bundle: n. sciatic and inferior gluteal a. and v.

7.10 Anatomical diagram. Note the relationships of the muscles of the hip joint and upper leg.

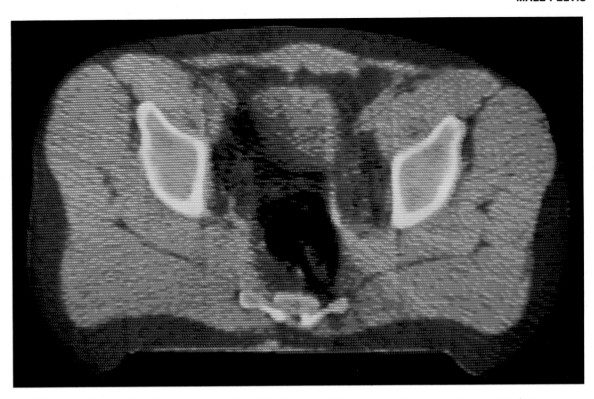

7.11 Color CT scan illustrating the dome of the bladder and the musculature of the upper leg.

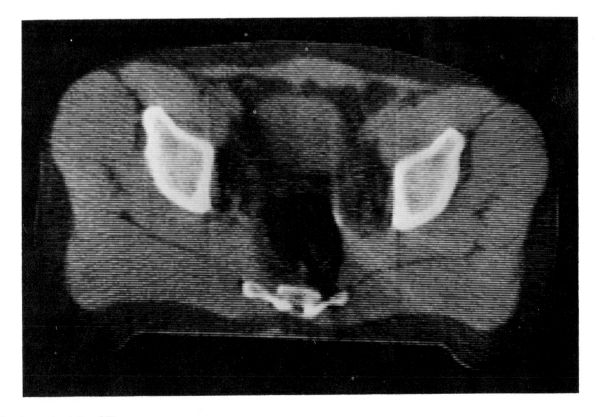

7.12 Black and white CT scan.

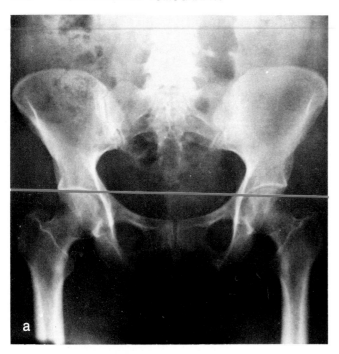 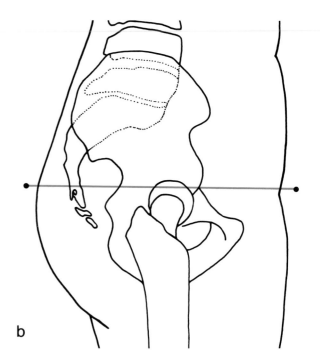

7.13 Scan level. (a) Normal A-P pelvic roentgenogram; red line shows cross-section level. (b) Schematic diagram of scan level.

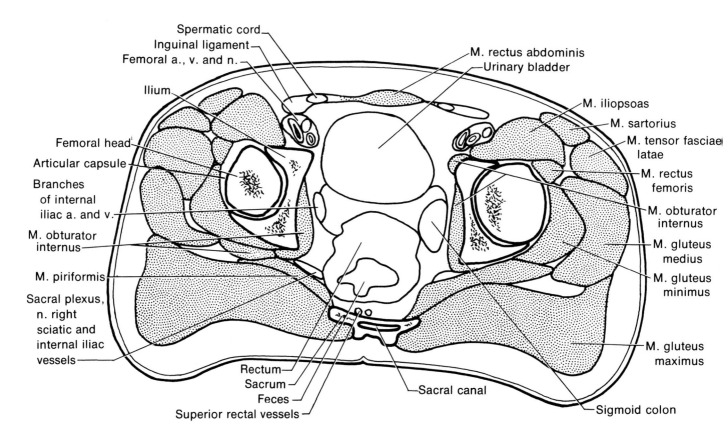

Spermatic cord
Inguinal ligament
Femoral a., v. and n.
Ilium
Femoral head
Articular capsule
Branches of internal iliac a. and v.
M. obturator internus
M. piriformis
Sacral plexus, n. right sciatic and internal iliac vessels
Rectum
Sacrum
Feces
Superior rectal vessels

M. rectus abdominis
Urinary bladder
M. iliopsoas
M. sartorius
M. tensor fasciae latae
M. rectus femoris
M. obturator internus
M. gluteus medius
M. gluteus minimus
M. gluteus maximus
Sigmoid colon
Sacral canal

7.14 Anatomical diagram at the superior border of the hip joint.

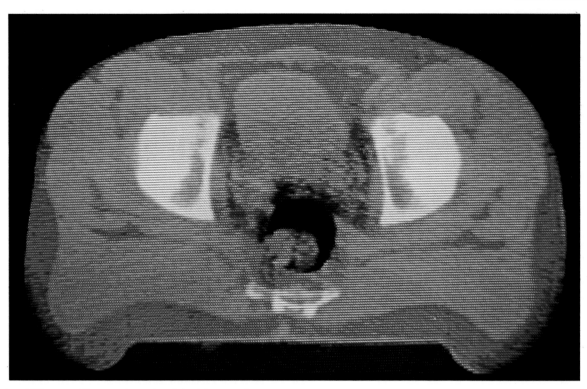

7.15 Color CT scan illustrating the bladder and rectum.

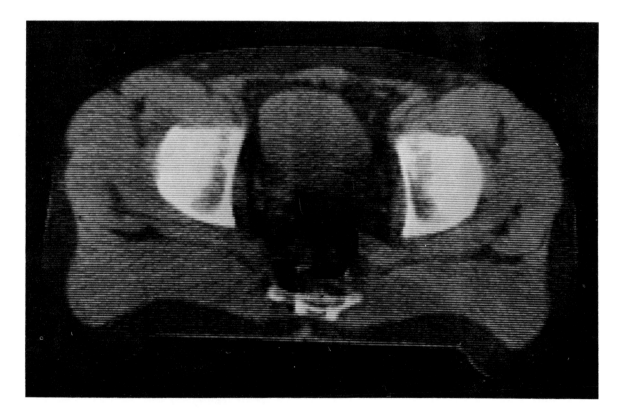

7.16 Black and white CT scan. Note the compression of the gluteal musculature due to the presence of the examining table beneath the subject.

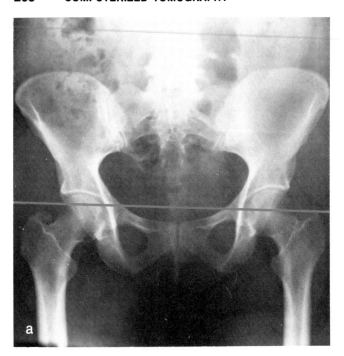
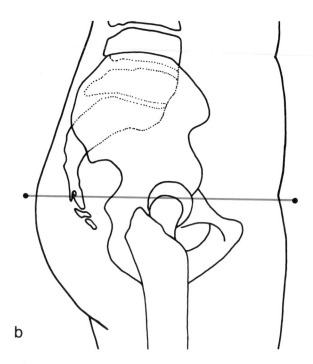

7.17 Scan level. (a) Normal A-P pelvic roentgenogram; red line shows cross-section level. (b) Schematic diagram of scan level.

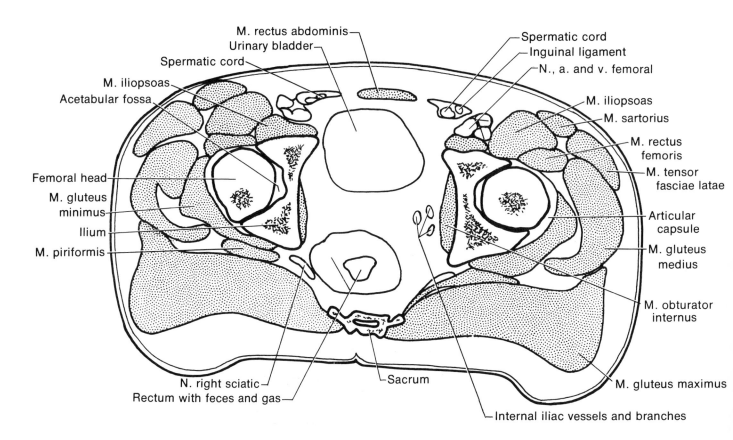

7.18 Anatomical diagram at the level of the hip joint.

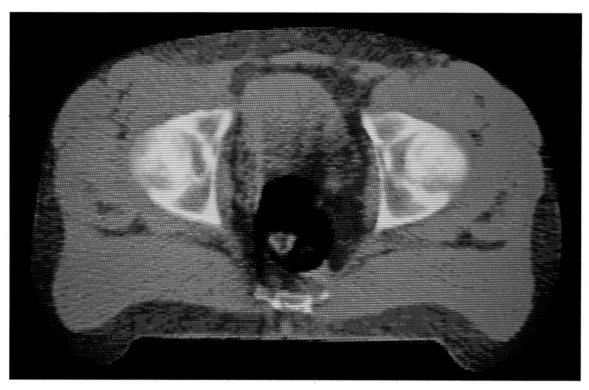

7.19 Color CT scan illustrating the features of the hip joint and the musculature of the upper thigh.

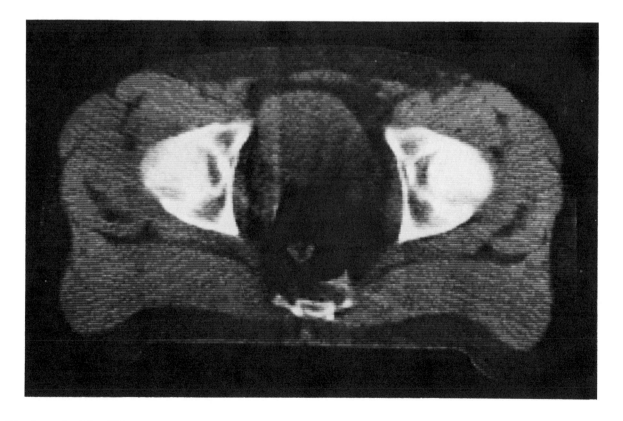

7.20 Black and white CT scan.

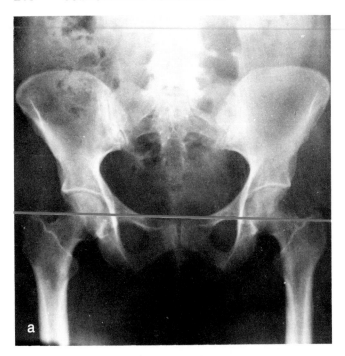

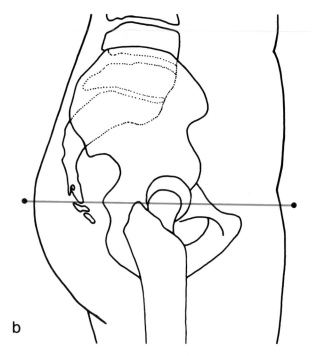

7.21 Scan level. (a) Normal A-P pelvic roentgenogram; red line shows cross-section level. (b) Schematic diagram of scan level.

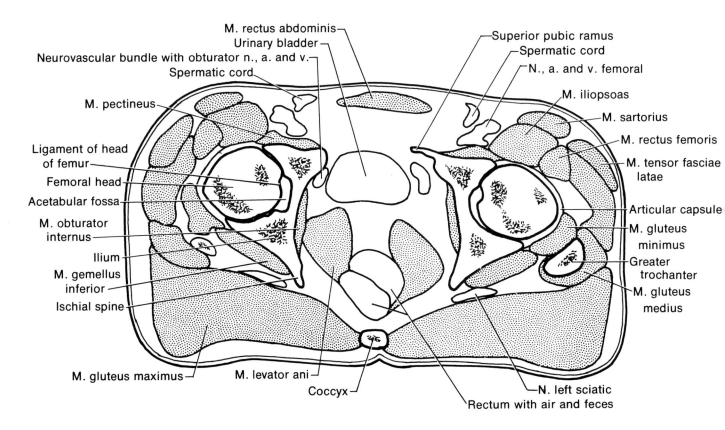

7.22 Anatomical diagram at the level of the hip joint.

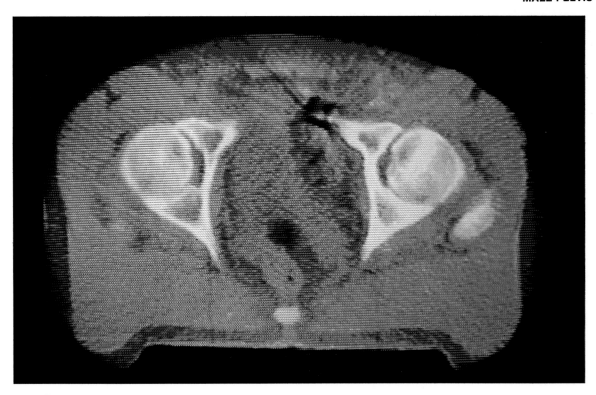

7.23 Color CT scan. Note the presence of the greater trochanter of the femur and the details of the hip joint.

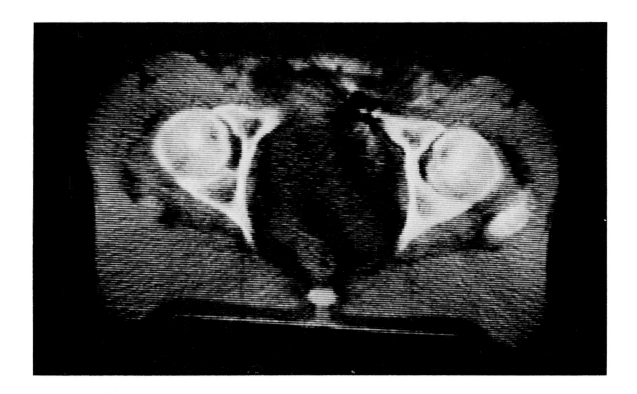

7.24 Black and white CT scan. Note that there is some rotation of the subject, the left side being slightly elevated relative to the right side.

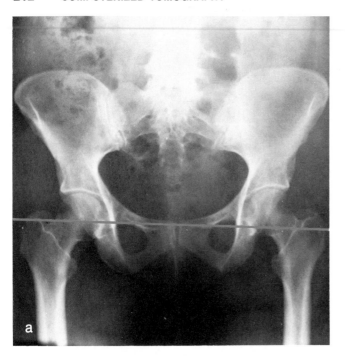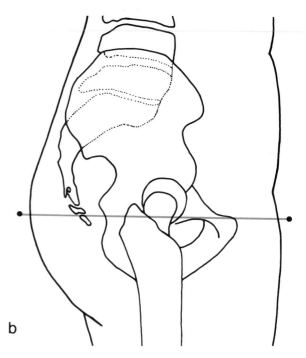

7.25 Scan level. (a) Normal A-P pelvic roentgenogram; red line shows cross-section level. (b) Schematic diagram of scan level.

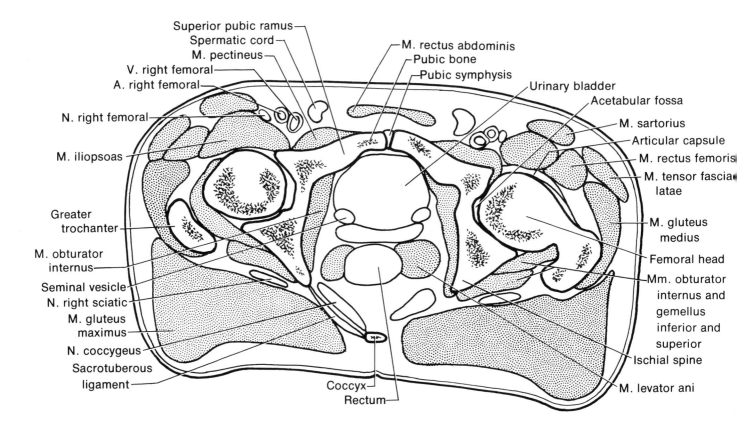

Superior pubic ramus
Spermatic cord
M. pectineus
V. right femoral
A. right femoral
N. right femoral
M. iliopsoas
Greater trochanter
M. obturator internus
Seminal vesicle
N. right sciatic
M. gluteus maximus
N. coccygeus
Sacrotuberous ligament
M. rectus abdominis
Pubic bone
Pubic symphysis
Urinary bladder
Acetabular fossa
M. sartorius
Articular capsule
M. rectus femoris
M. tensor fasciae latae
M. gluteus medius
Femoral head
Mm. obturator internus and gemellus inferior and superior
Ischial spine
M. levator ani
Coccyx
Rectum

7.26 Anatomical diagram through the hip joint illustrating the seminal vesicles, bladder and rectum.

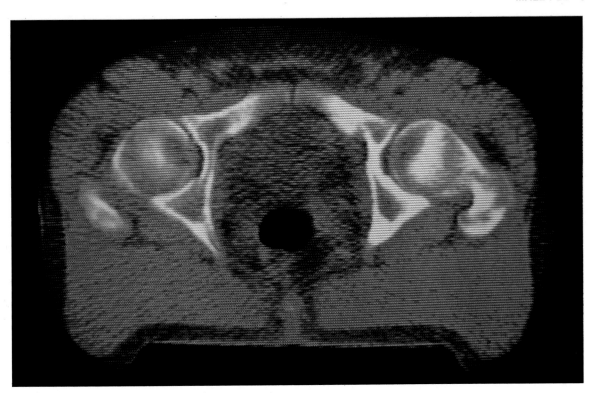

7.27 Color CT scan at the level of the symphysis pubis and the superior pubic ramus.

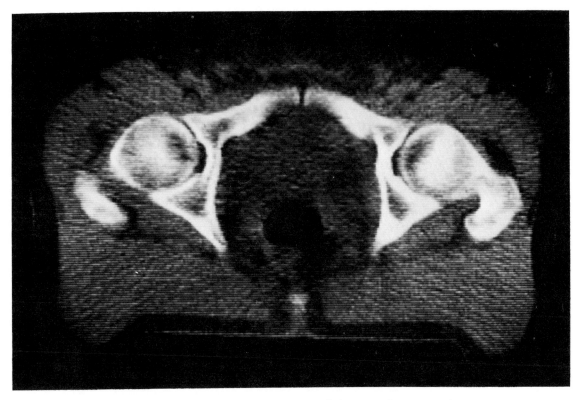

7.28 Black and white CT scan illustrating the musculature of the anterior upper leg.

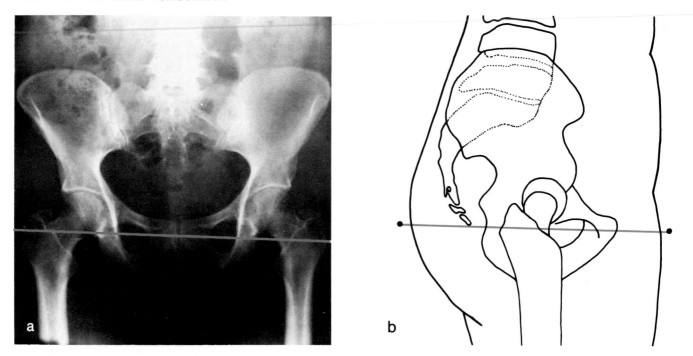

7.29 Scan level. (a) Normal A-P pelvic roentgenogram; red line shows cross-section level. (b) Schematic diagram of scan level.

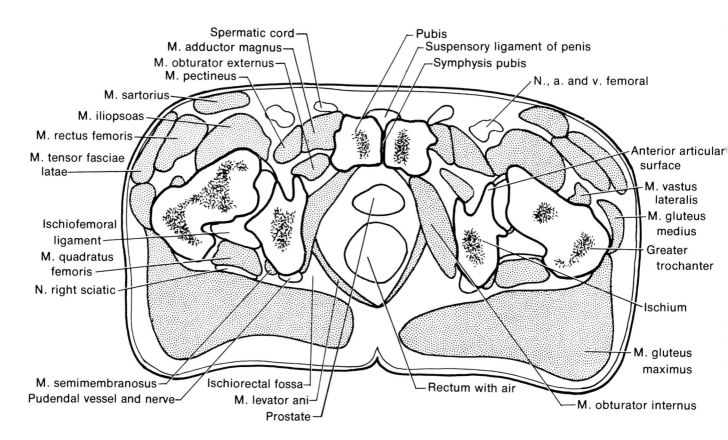

Spermatic cord
M. adductor magnus
M. obturator externus
M. pectineus
M. sartorius
M. iliopsoas
M. rectus femoris
M. tensor fasciae latae
Ischiofemoral ligament
M. quadratus femoris
N. right sciatic
M. semimembranosus
Pudendal vessel and nerve
Ischiorectal fossa
M. levator ani
Prostate
Rectum with air
Pubis
Suspensory ligament of penis
Symphysis pubis
N., a. and v. femoral
Anterior articular surface
M. vastus lateralis
M. gluteus medius
Greater trochanter
Ischium
M. gluteus maximus
M. obturator internus

7.30 Anatomical diagram through the inferior portion of the hip joint.

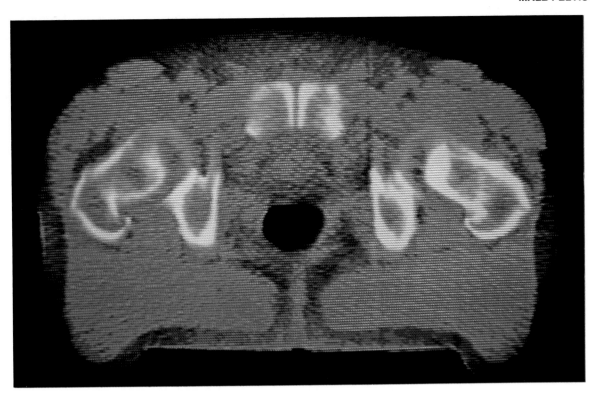

7.31 Color CT scan illustrating in light green the complex musculature of the hip joint. Also note the appearance of the prostate gland just posterior to the symphysis pubis.

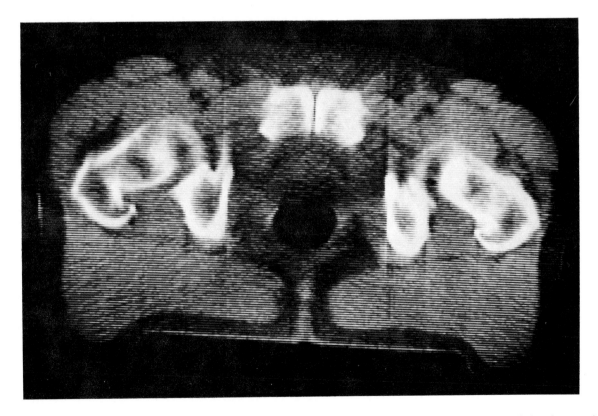

7.32 Black and white CT scan. Note the anterior thigh musculature and the appearance of the femoral vessels and nerves.

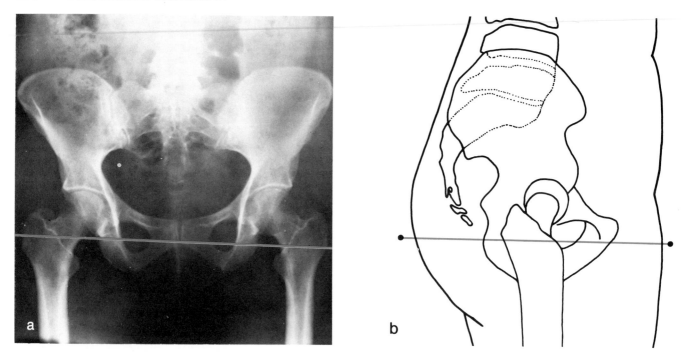

7.33 Scan level. (a) Normal A-P pelvic roentgenogram; red line shows cross-section level. (b) Schematic diagram of scan level.

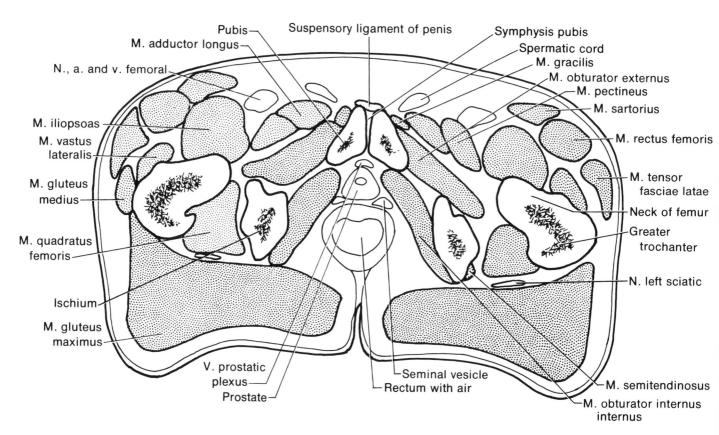

7.34 Anatomical diagram through the inferior portion of the symphysis pubis.

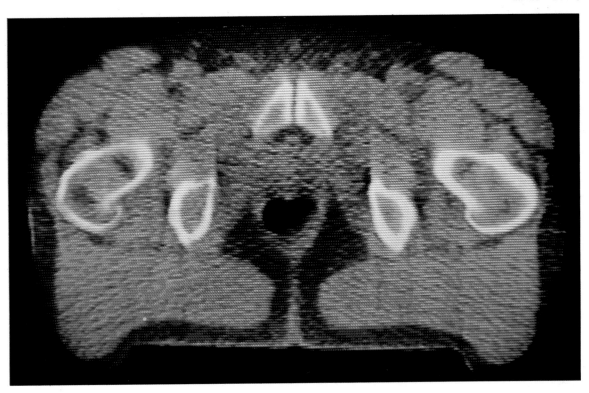

7.35 Color CT scan. Note the appearance of the prostate gland, lying just posterior to the retropubic space.

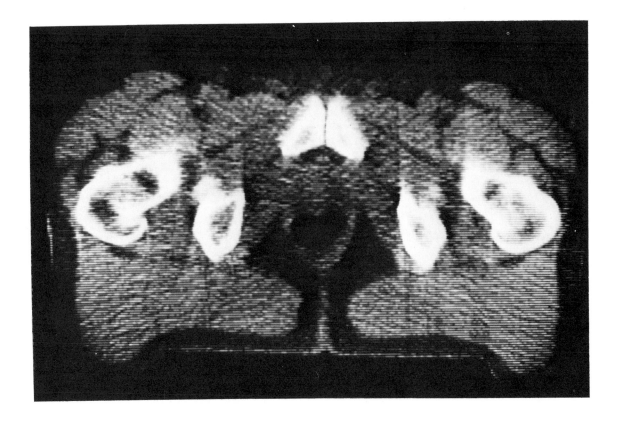

7.36 Black and white CT scan demonstrating the musculature of the hip joint and upper leg.

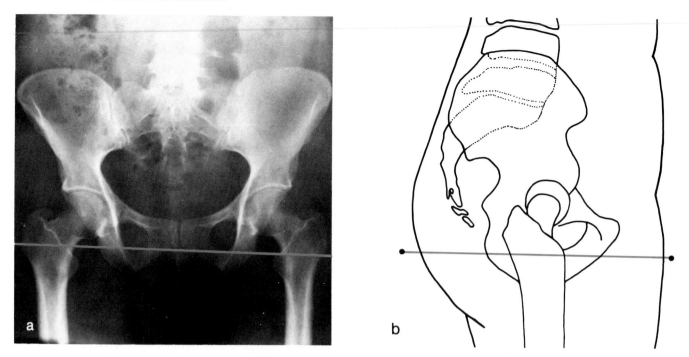

7.37 Scan level. (a) Normal A-P pelvic roentgenogram; red line shows cross-section level. (b) Schematic diagram of scan level.

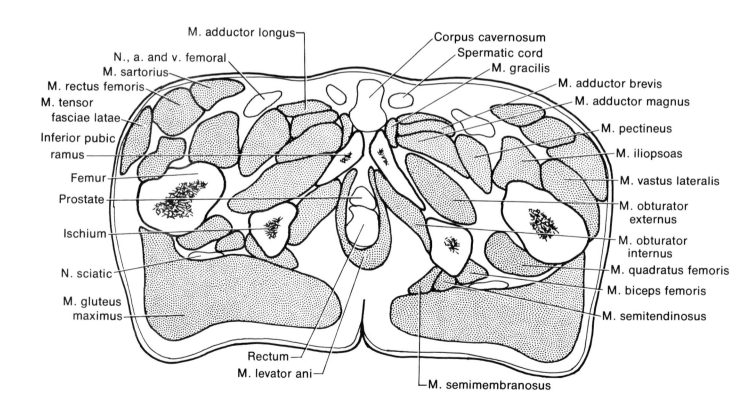

7.38 Anatomical diagram at the level of the inferior pubic ramus.

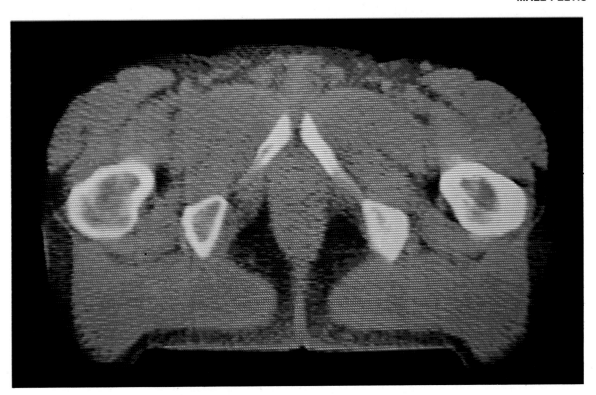

7.39 Color CT scan. Note the appearance of the spermatic cords just lateral to the corpus cavernosum penis.

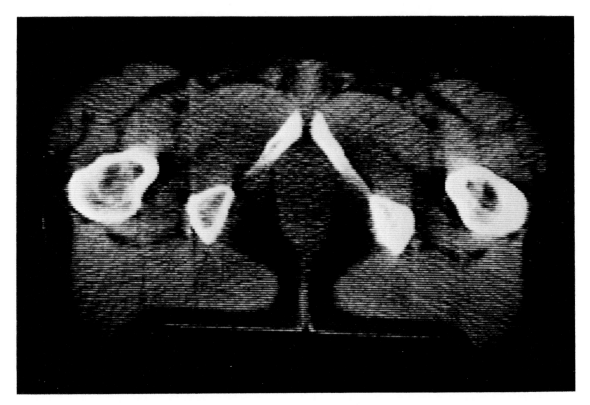

7.40 Black and white CT scan. Note the flattening of the gluteal musculature due to the presence of the examining table dorsal to the subject.

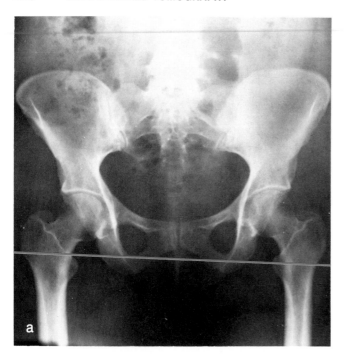

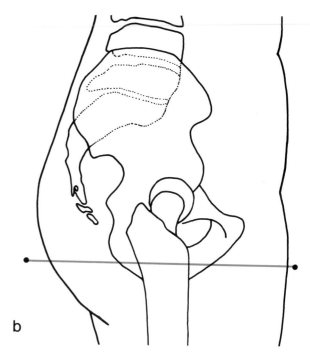

7.41 Scan level. (a) Normal A-P pelvic roentgenogram; red line shows cross-section level. (b) Schematic diagram of scan level.

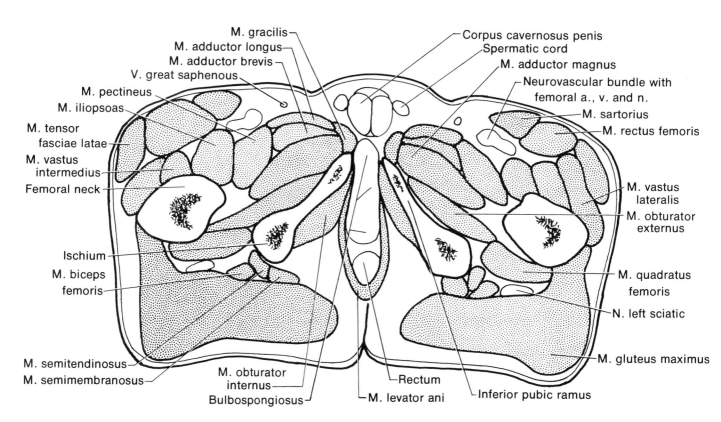

7.42 Anatomical diagram at the level of the inferior pubic ramus.

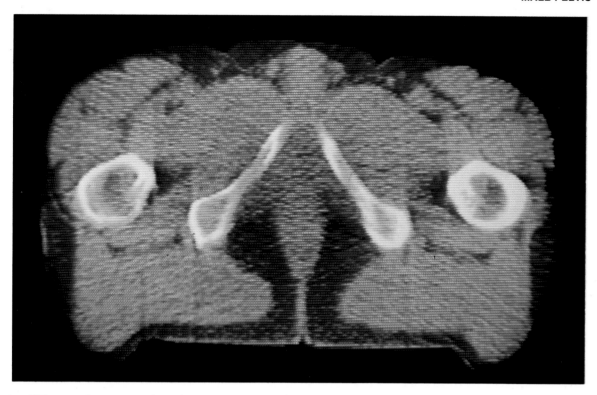

7.43 Color CT scan demonstrating the corpus cavernosum urethrae, which appears in longitudinal sections in this scan and is located posterior to the inferior pubic rami.

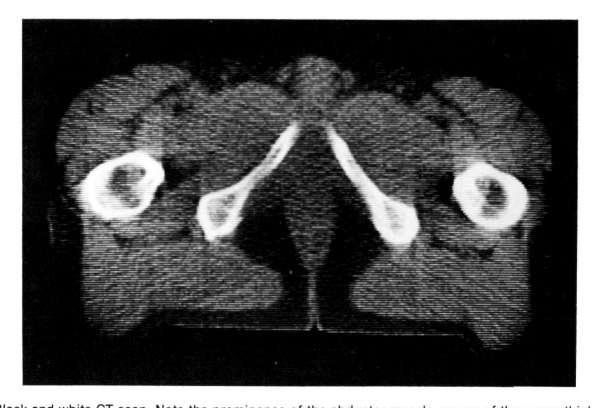

7.44 Black and white CT scan. Note the prominence of the abductor muscle groups of the upper thigh.

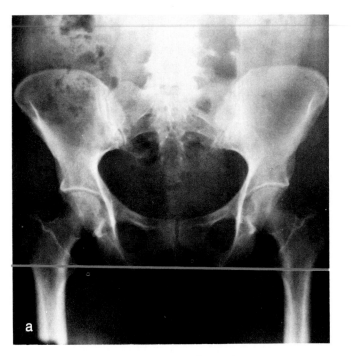
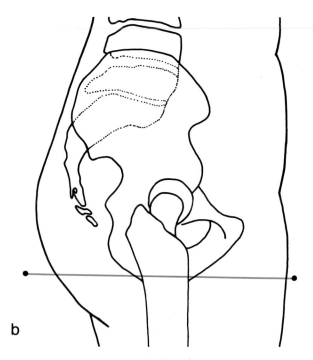

7.45 Scan level. (a) Normal A-P pelvic roentgenogram; red line shows cross-section level. (b) Schematic diagram of scan level.

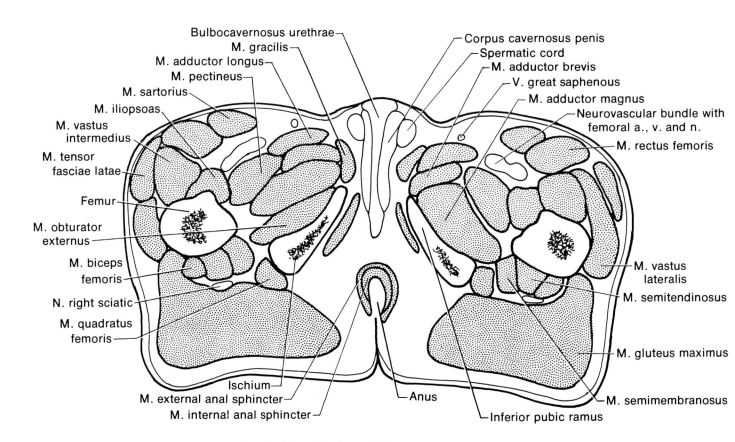

7.46 Anatomical diagram at the level of the inferior pubic ramus.

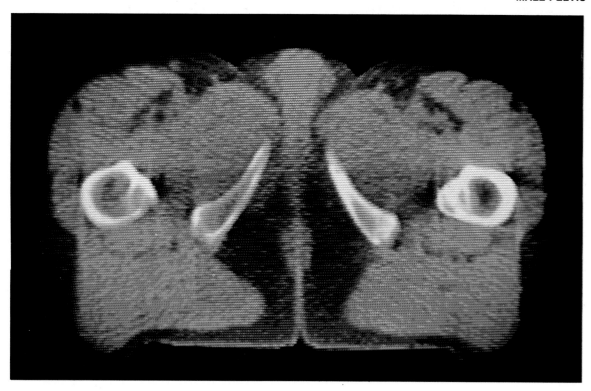

7.47 Color CT scan demonstrating in green the musculature of the upper leg, the spermatic cords and the corpus cavernosum penis.

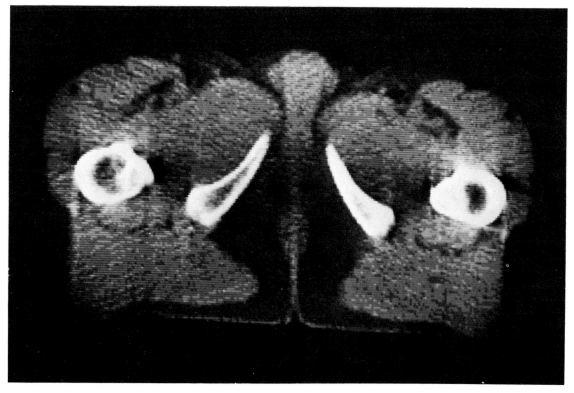

7.48 Black and white CT scan.

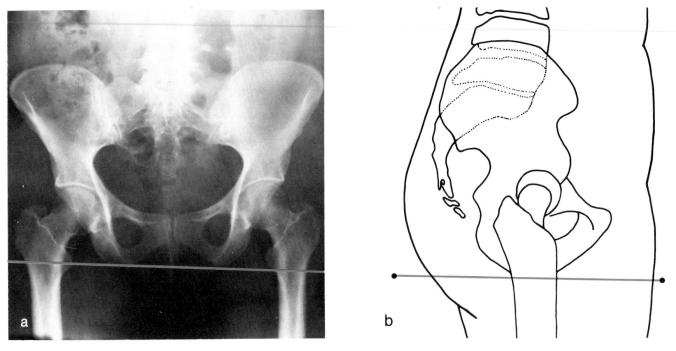

7.49 Scan level. (a) normal A-P pelvic roentgenogram; red line shows corss-section level. (b) Schematic diagram of scan level.

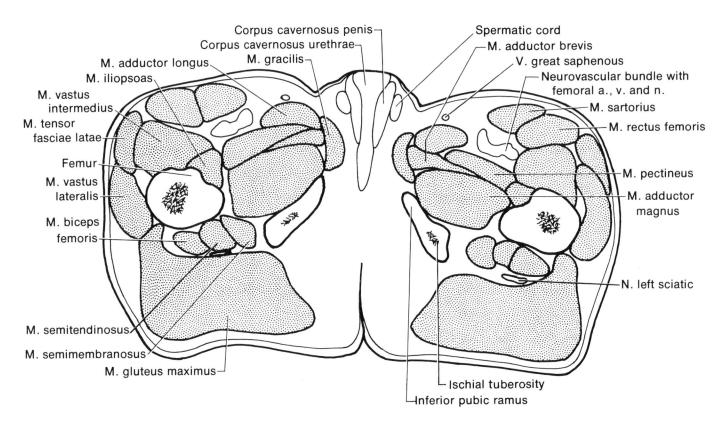

7.50 Anatomical diagram through the inferior pubic ramus.

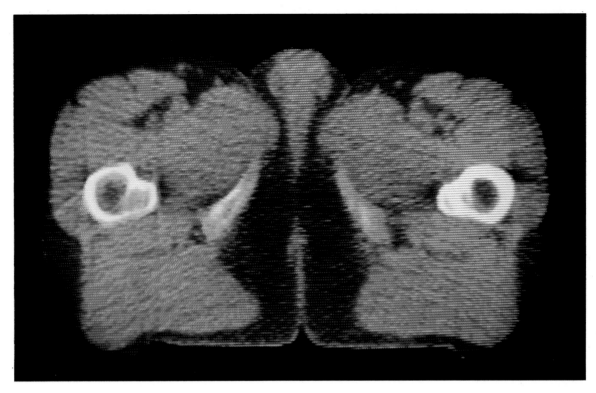

7.51 Color CT scan. Note the appearance of the femoral vessels and nerves and the musculature of the upper leg.

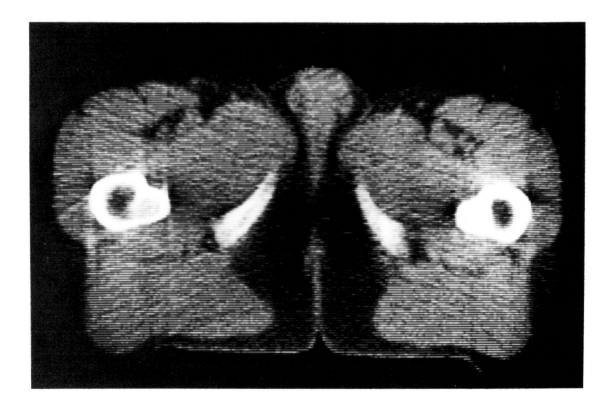

7.52 Black and white CT scan.

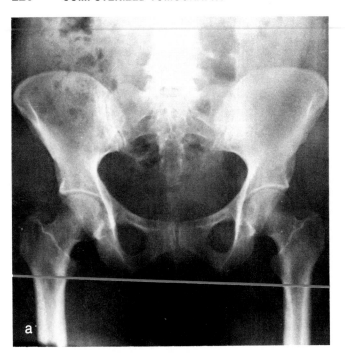
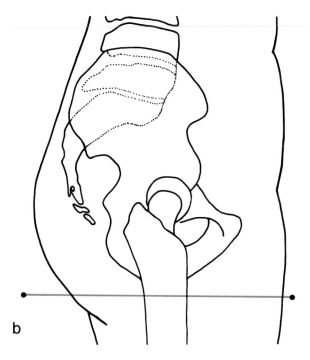

7.53 Scan level. (a) Normal A-P pelvic roentgenogram; red line shows cross-section level. (b) Schematic diagram of scan level.

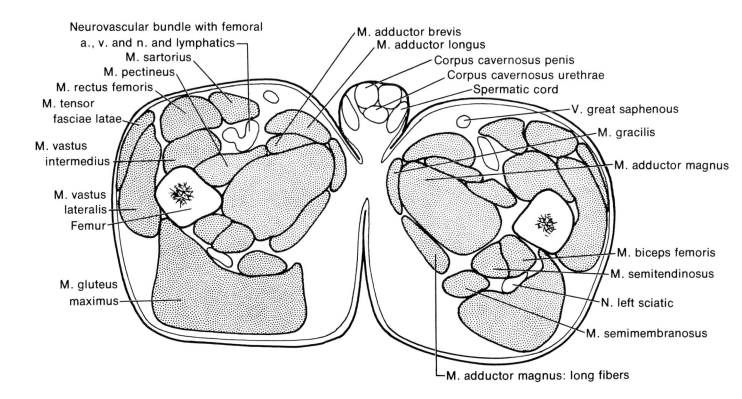

Neurovascular bundle with femoral
a., v. and n. and lymphatics
M. sartorius
M. pectineus
M. rectus femoris
M. tensor
fasciae latae
M. vastus
intermedius
M. vastus
lateralis
Femur
M. gluteus
maximus

M. adductor brevis
M. adductor longus
Corpus cavernosus penis
Corpus cavernosus urethrae
Spermatic cord
V. great saphenous
M. gracilis
M. adductor magnus
M. biceps femoris
M. semitendinosus
N. left sciatic
M. semimembranosus
M. adductor magnus: long fibers

7.54 Anatomical diagram at a level just inferior to the ischial tuberosities.

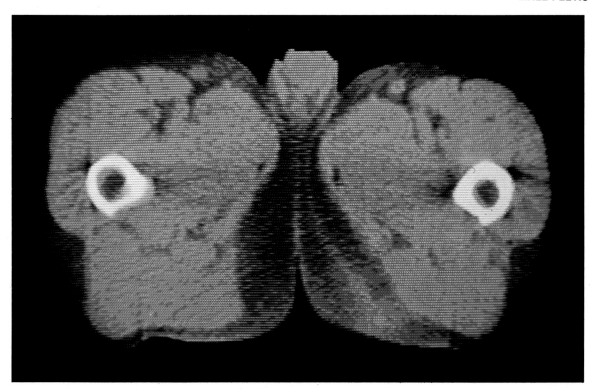

7.55 Color CT scan. Note the appearance of the spermatic cords as they enter into the superior portion of the scrotum.

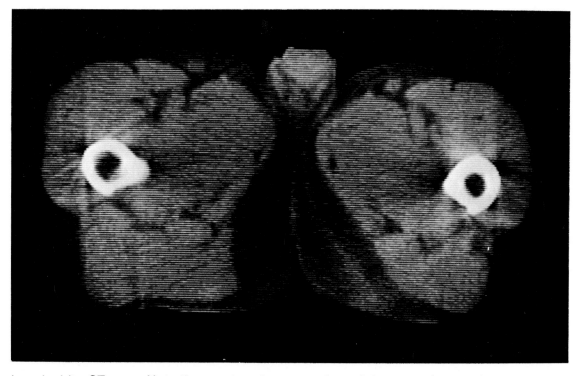

7.56 Black and white CT scan. Note the great saphenous vein and the musculature of the upper leg.

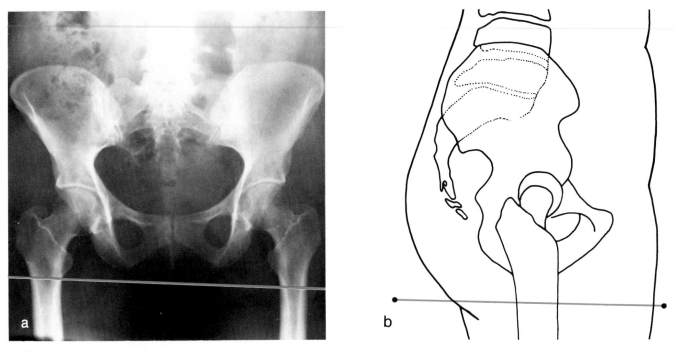

7.57 Scan level. (a) Normal A-P pelvic roentgenogram; red line shows cross-section level. (b) Schematic diagram of scan level.

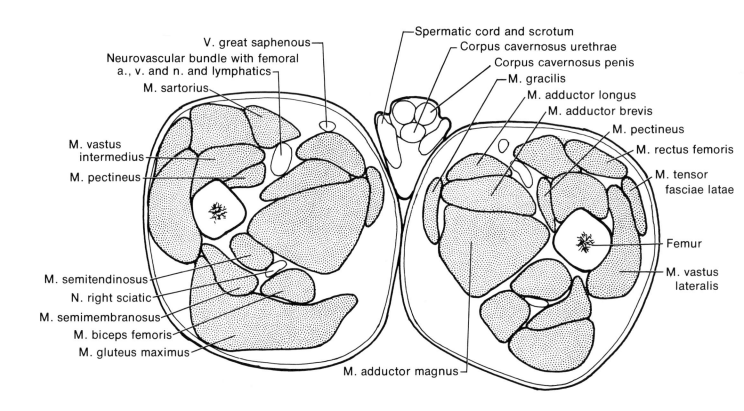

V. great saphenous
Neurovascular bundle with femoral
a., v. and n. and lymphatics
M. sartorius

Spermatic cord and scrotum
Corpus cavernosus urethrae
Corpus cavernosus penis
M. gracilis
M. adductor longus
M. adductor brevis
M. pectineus
M. rectus femoris

M. vastus
intermedius
M. pectineus

M. tensor
fasciae latae

Femur

M. semitendinosus
N. right sciatic
M. semimembranosus
M. biceps femoris
M. gluteus maximus

M. vastus
lateralis

M. adductor magnus

7.58 Anatomical diagram through the superior portion of the femur.

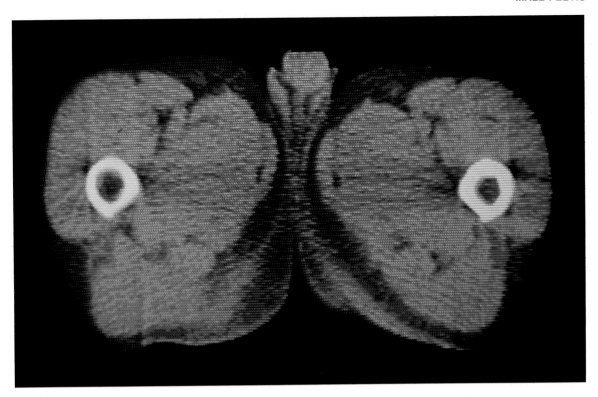

7.59 Color CT scan demonstrating the musculature of the thigh. Note the large adductor muscle groups in the medial portion of the thigh.

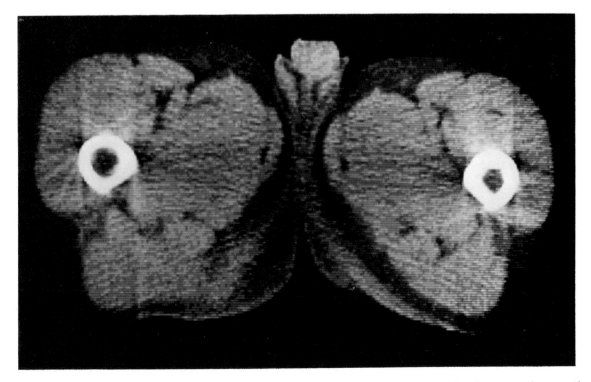

7.60 Black and white CT scan. Note the presence of the spermatic cords within the superior portion of the scrotum.

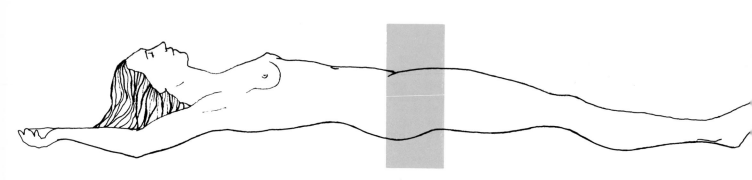

chapter eight

Female Pelvis

This section of the ATLAS extends from the pelvic brim to the upper thigh and includes the sigmoid colon, rectum, uterus, vagina, urinary bladder, the pelvic musculature and vasculature, and the hip joints.

CT methods delineate pelvic structures directly and with a high degree of detail. Tumors of the pelvic organs can be visualized, including those of the uterus and lymphatic masses in the inguinal regions. For known cancer of the uterus or cervix, where radiotherapy is being considered, CT scanning, in conjunction with intravenous contrast procedures, can provide accurate anatomical cross-sections for radiotherapy planning. In addition to visualizing the tumors themselves, the radiosensitive pelvic organs (e.g., rectum, bladder and ureters) can also be imaged.

As in the male pelvis, CT scanning provides exceptional detail of the hip joints, their capsules, and their extensive musculature. Osteoporosis of postmenopausal females can be evaluated using the qualitative and quantitative CT methods described in the previous section of this ATLAS. As in the male, CT scanning can provide a useful preoperative study in the planning of prosthetic hip replacement surgery. Similarly, bony pathological changes (e.g., blastic and lytic metastases) can be studied by CT scans.

The female pelvis represents another region of great anatomic variation which is proportional to the patient's size, prior surgery, degree of bowel preparation, distention of the bladder, and the patient's parity. Relative amounts of uterine and vesicular prolapse alter the interpretation of the scan at the levels encompassing these structures. All subjects were scanned in the supine position using a 7.5-mm section thickness, 0° gantry tilt and a scan interval of 1 cm. Subjects for this region were at least 50 years of age. The presence of the examining table is apparent in the scans of this section and results in some compression of the gluteal musculature.

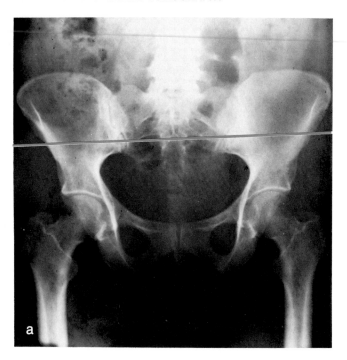
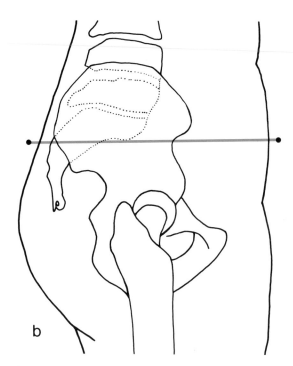

8.1 Scan level. (a) Normal A-P pelvic roentgenogram; red line shows cross-section level. (b) Schematic diagram of scan level.

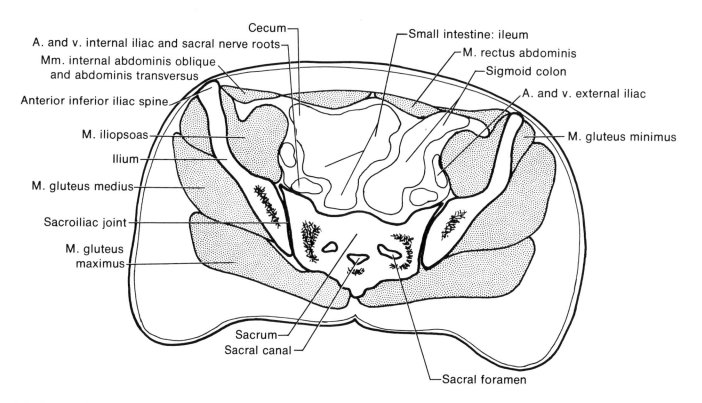

8.2 Anatomical diagram through the inferior portion of the sacroiliac joint.

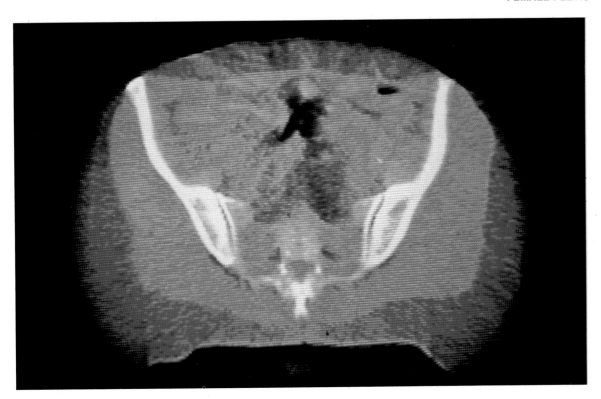

8.3 Color CT scan illustrating multiple loops of small bowel.

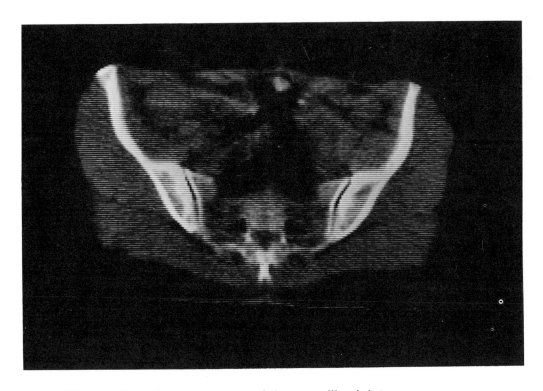

8.4 Black and white CT scan. Note the appearance of the sacroiliac joint.

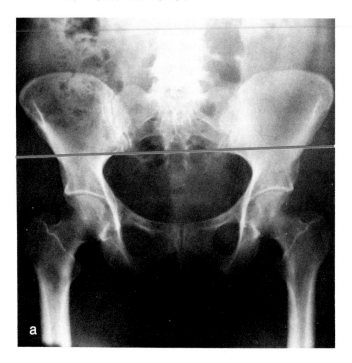
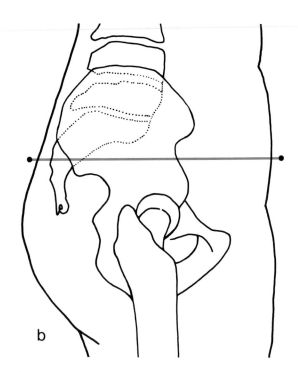

8.5 Scan level. (a) Normal A-P pelvic roentgenogram; red line shows cross-section level. (b) Schematic diagram of scan level.

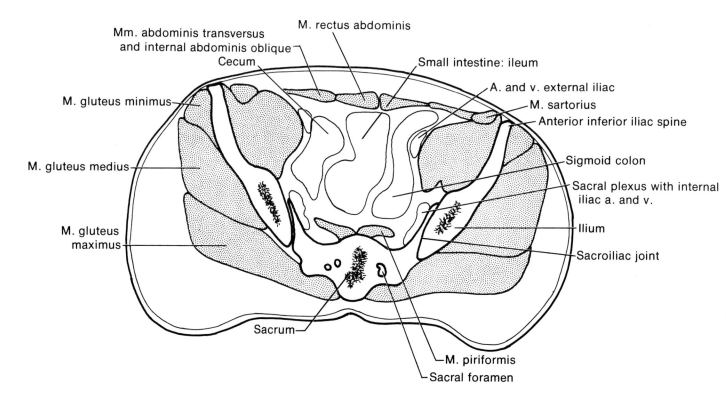

8.6 Anatomical diagram through the inferior portion of the sacroiliac joint.

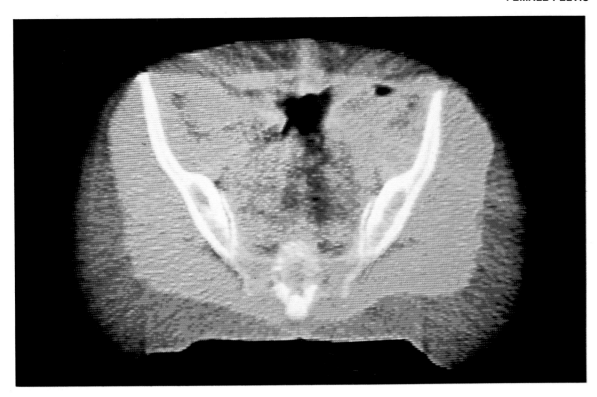

8.7 Color CT scan.

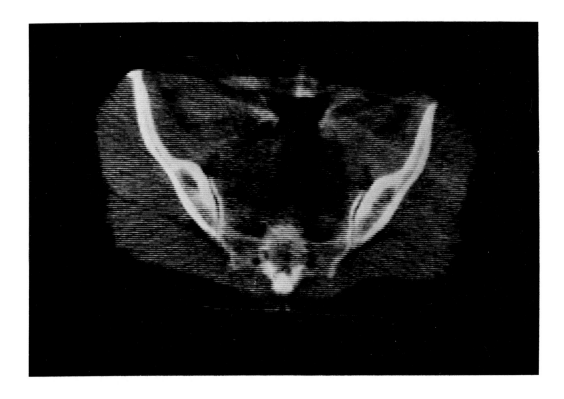

8.8 Black and white CT scan. Note the appearance of the sacroiliac joint.

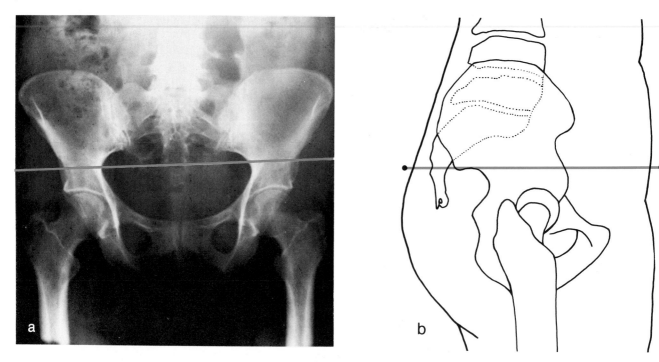

8.9 Scan level. (a) Normal A-P pelvic roentgenogram; red line shows cross-section level. (b) Schematic diagram of scan level.

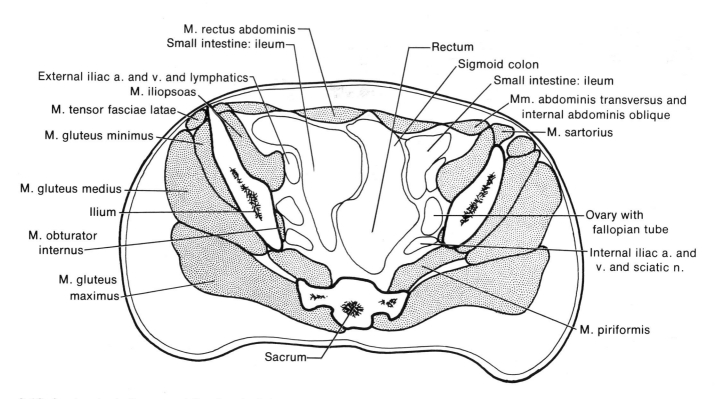

8.10 Anatomical diagram at the level of the ovary.

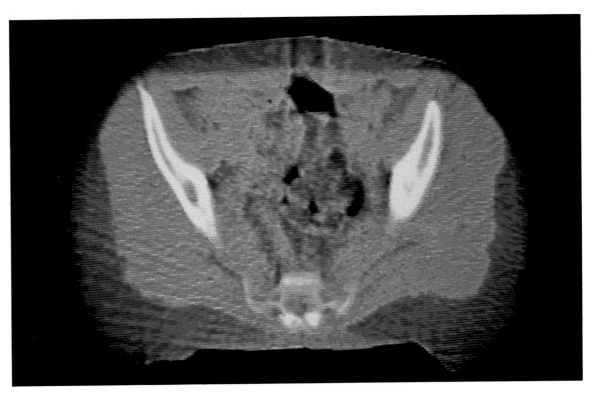

8.11 Color CT scan. Note the appearance of the ovary with attached fallopian tubes just medial to the posterior portion of the iliac bones.

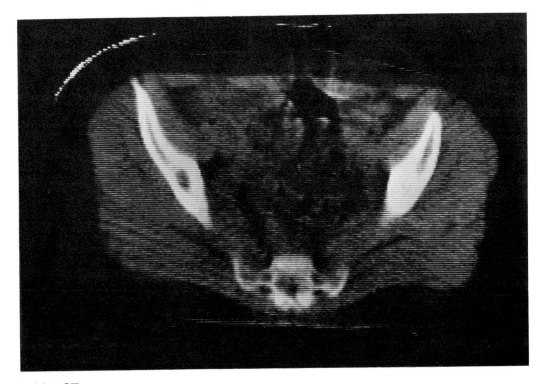

8.12 Black and white CT scan.

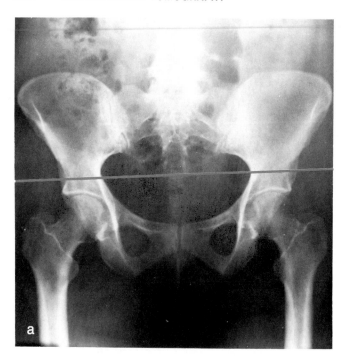
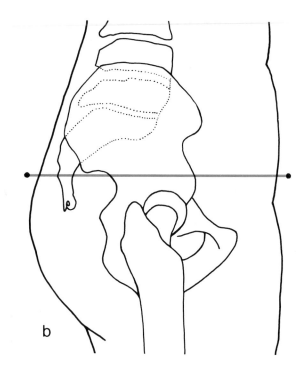

8.13 Scan level. (a) Normal A-P pelvic roentgenogram; red line shows cross-section level. (b) Schematic diagram of scan level.

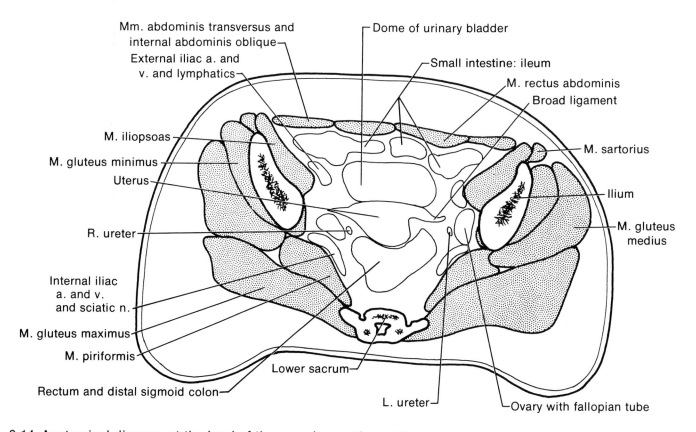

8.14 Anatomical diagram at the level of the superior portion of the uterus.

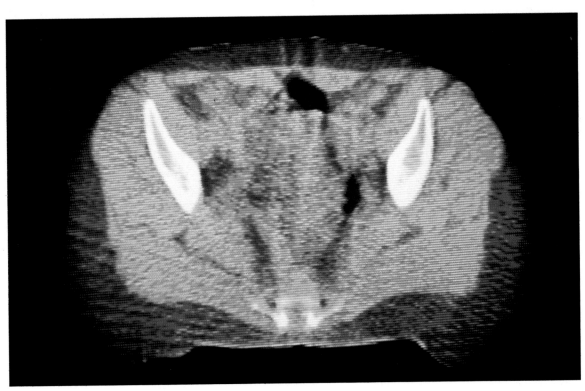

8.15 Color CT scan. Note the presence of the ovary and attached fallopian tubes medial to the posterior portion of the iliac bones.

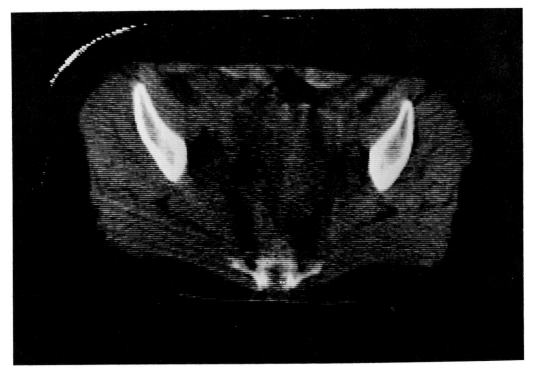

8.16 Black and white CT scan. Note that there is some dorsal flattening due to the presence of the examining table beneath the subject.

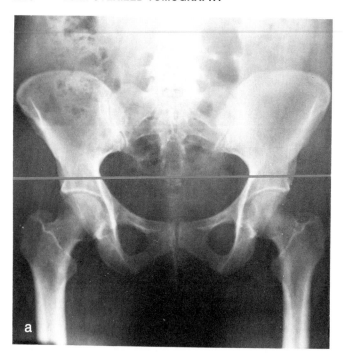

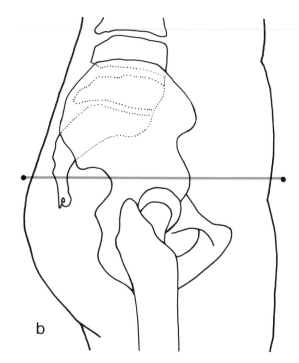

8.17 Scan level. (a) Normal A-P pelvic roentgenogram; red line shows cross-section level. (b) Schematic diagram of scan level.

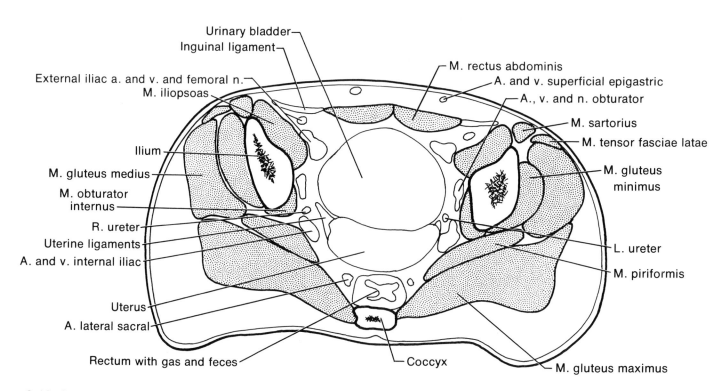

8.18 Anatomical diagram at the level of the superior portion of the uterus.

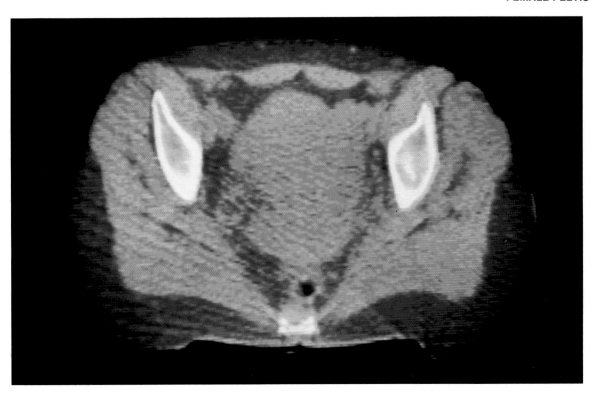

8.19 Color CT scan demonstrating the uterus, rectum and bladder (bladder is somewhat extended in this subject).

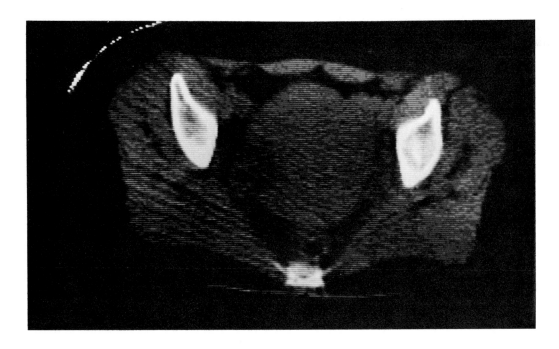

8.20 Black and white CT scan.

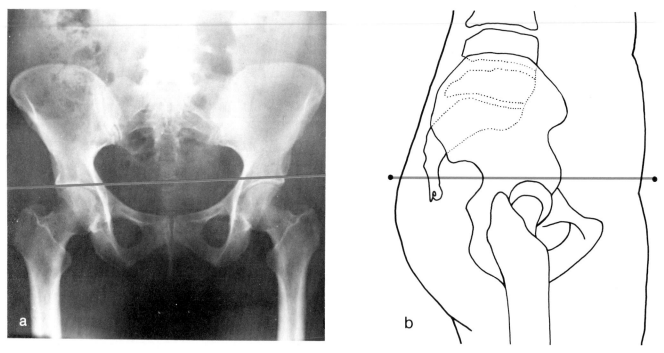

8.21 Scan level. (a) Normal A-P pelvic roentgenogram; red line shows cross-section level. (b) Schematic diagram of scan level.

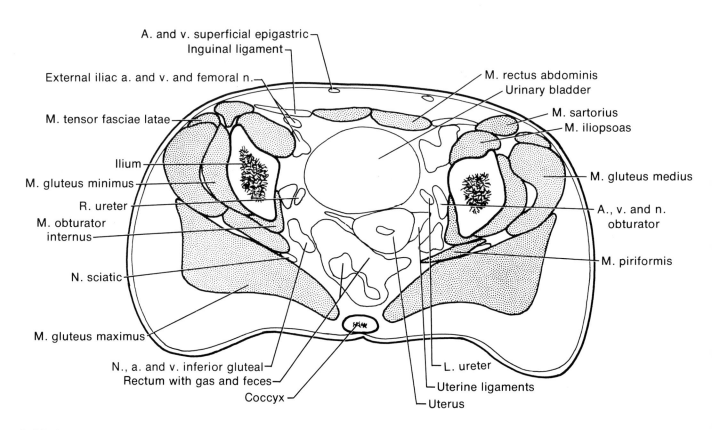

8.22 Anatomical diagram at a level just superior to the hip joint.

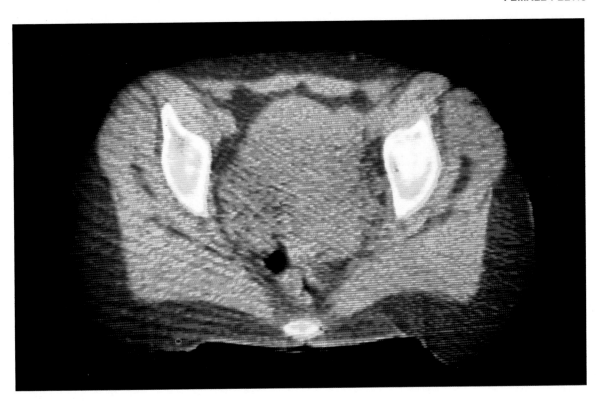

8.23 Color CT scan demonstrating the bladder, uterus and rectum. The rectum is somewhat redundant in this patient and the bladder somewhat distended.

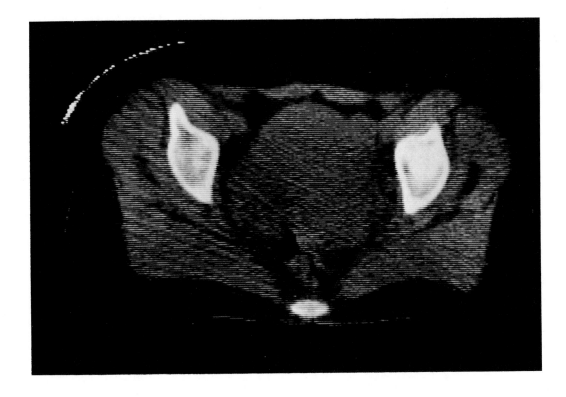

8.24 Black and white CT scan. Note the musculature of the hip joint and upper thigh.

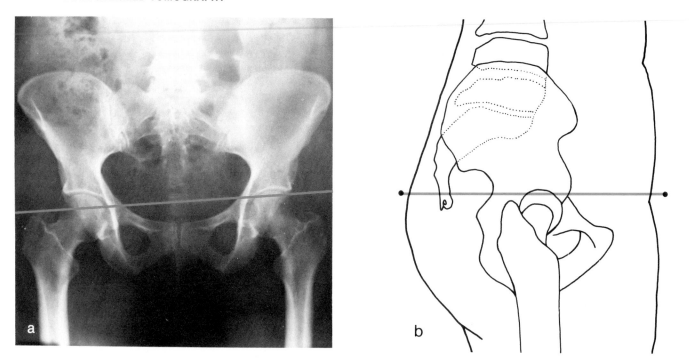

8.25 Scan level. (a) Normal A-P pelvic roentgenogram; red line shows cross-section level. (b) Schematic diagram of scan level.

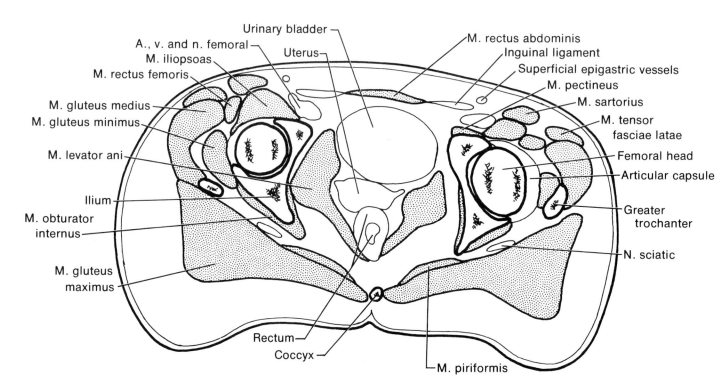

8.26 Anatomical diagram at the level of the superior portion of the hip joint.

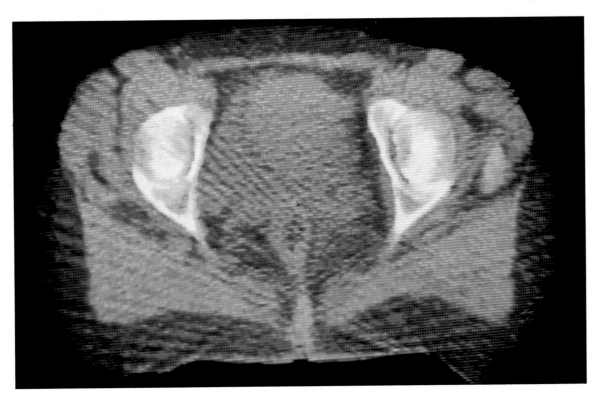

8.27 Color CT scan. Note the details of the hip joint and its articular capsule as well as the appearance of the greater trochanter.

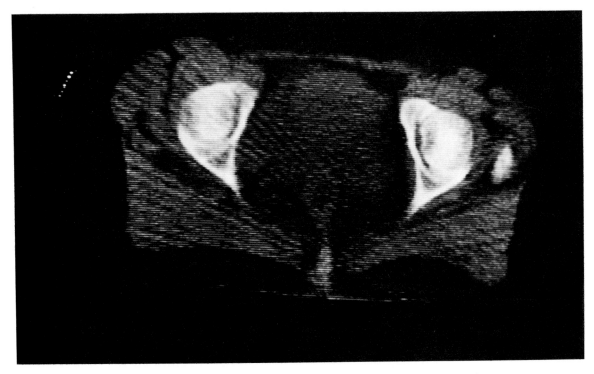

8.28 Black and white CT scan illustrating the bladder, uterus and rectum.

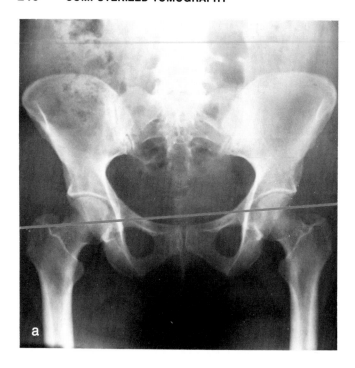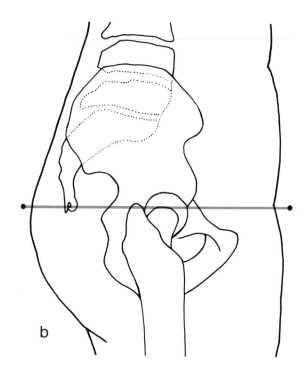

8.29 Scan level. (a) Normal A-P pelvic roentgenogram; red line shows cross-section level. (b) Schematic diagram of scan level.

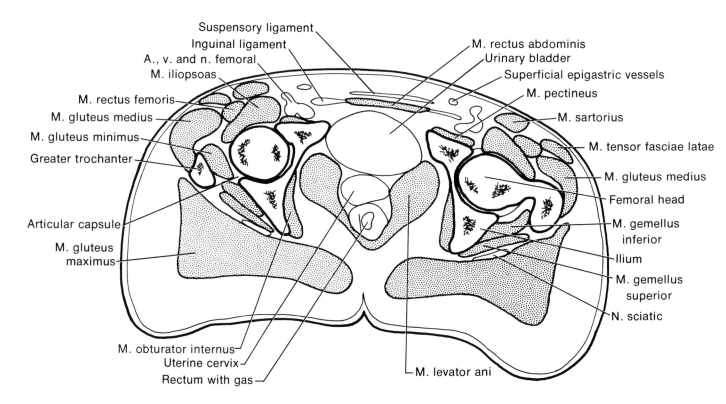

8.30 Anatomical diagram through the mid-portion of the hip joint.

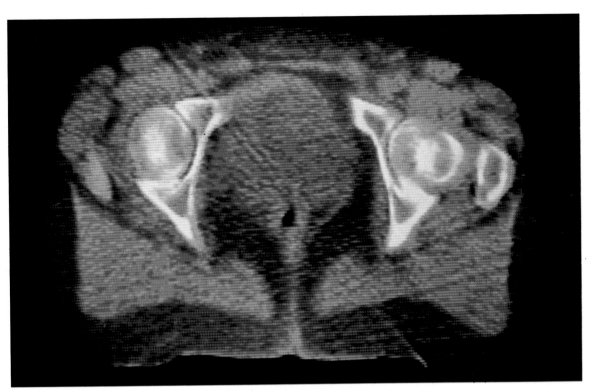

8.31 Color CT scan at the level of the uterine cervix. Note also the appearance of the bladder and rectum, partially surrounded by the musculature of the pelvic floor.

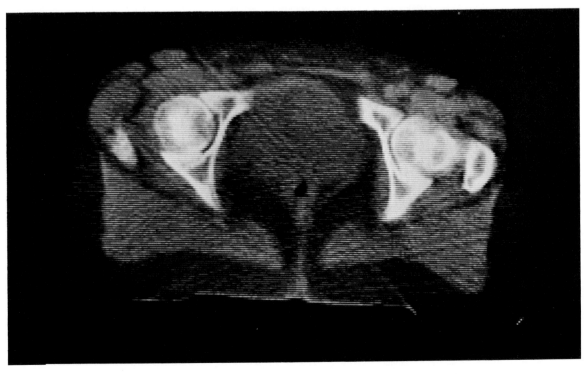

8.32 Black and white CT scan illustrating the musculature surrounding the hip joint

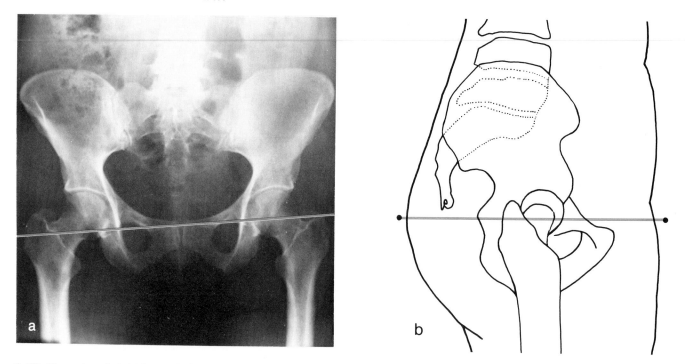

8.33 Scan level. (a) Normal A-P pelvic roentgenogram; red line shows cross-section level. (b) Schematic diagram of scan level.

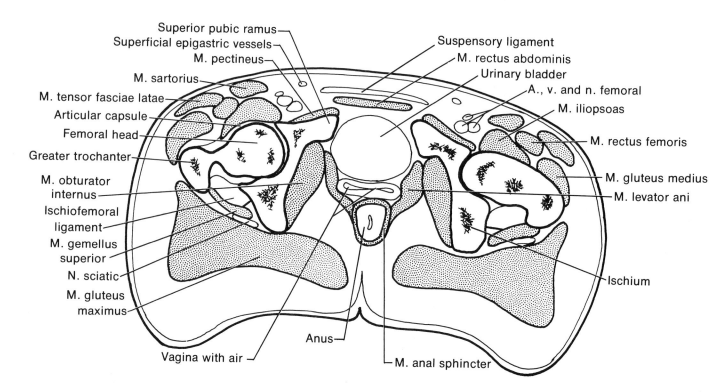

8.34 Anatomical diagram through the inferior portion of the hip joint.

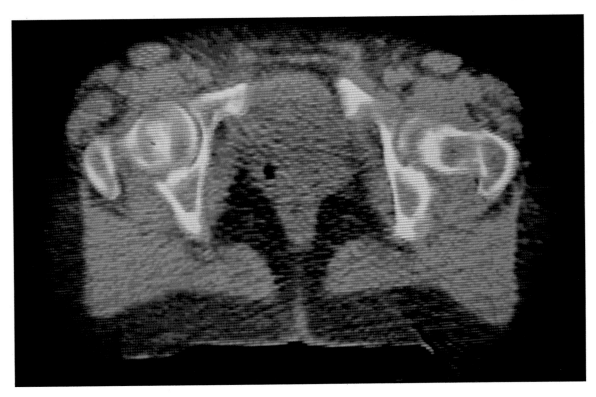

8.35 Color CT scan. Note the presence of air in the right side of the vagina.

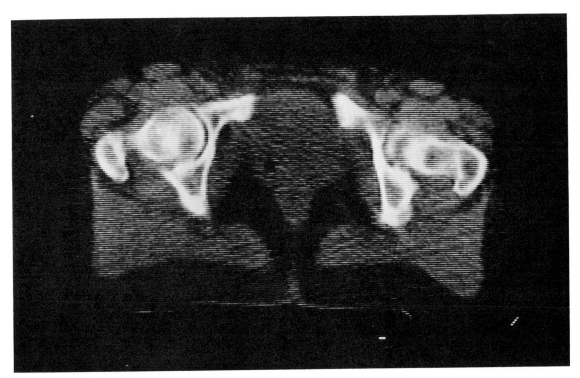

8.36 Black and white CT scan demonstrating the musculature of the hip joint as well as its articular capsule.

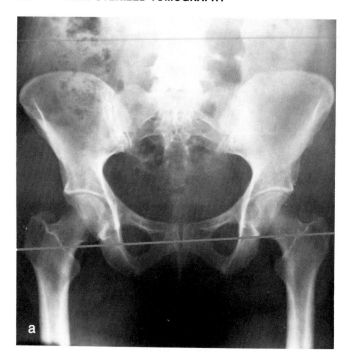
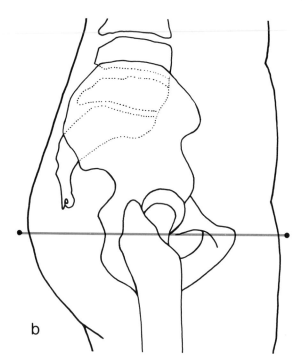

8.37 Scan level. (a) Normal A-P pelvic roentgenogram; red line shows cross-section level. (b) Schematic diagram of scan level.

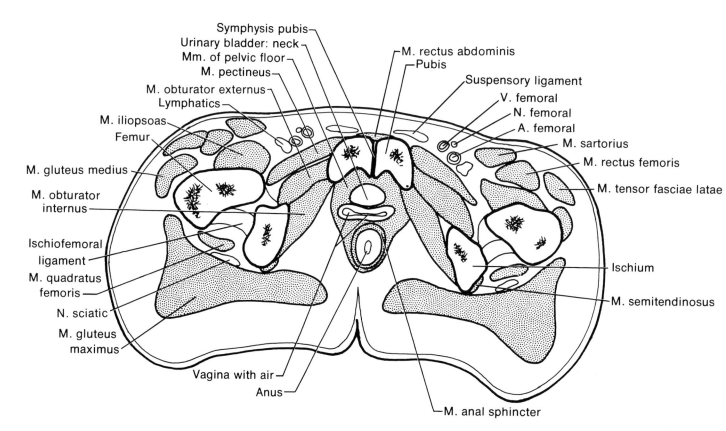

8.38 Anatomical diagram through the superior portion of the symphysis pubis.

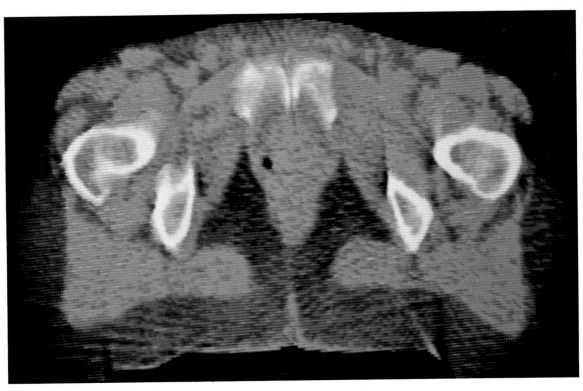

8.39 Color CT scan. Note the appearance of air on the right side of the vagina.

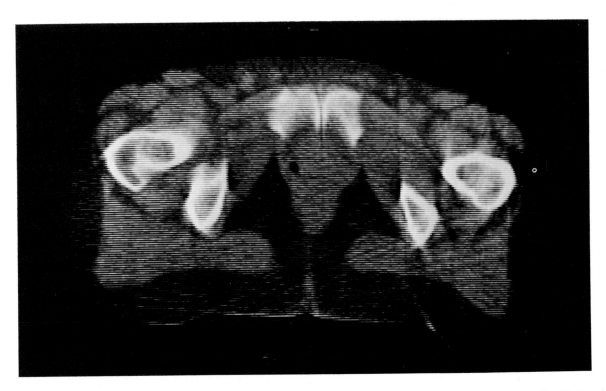

8.40 Black and white CT scan illustrating the musculature of the hip joint and anterior thigh. Note also the appearance of the femoral vessels and nerves.

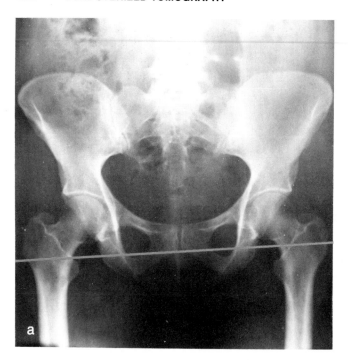
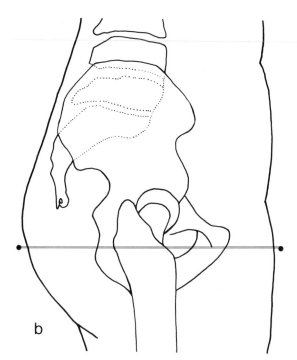

8.41 Scan level. (a) Normal A-P pelvic roentgenogram; red line shows cross-section level. (b) Schematic diagram of scan level.

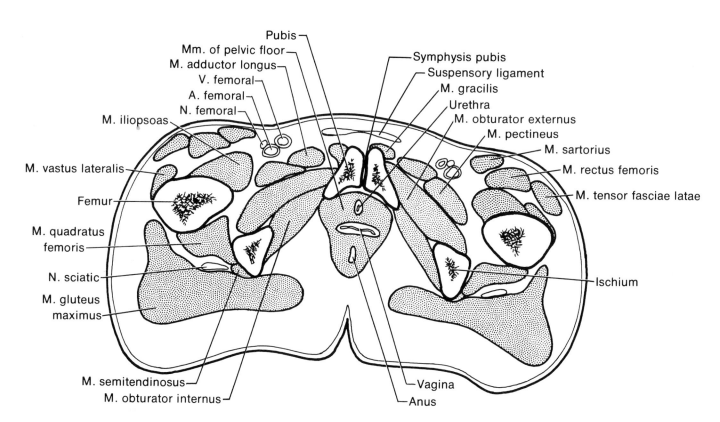

8.42 Anatomical diagram at the level of the obturator foramen.

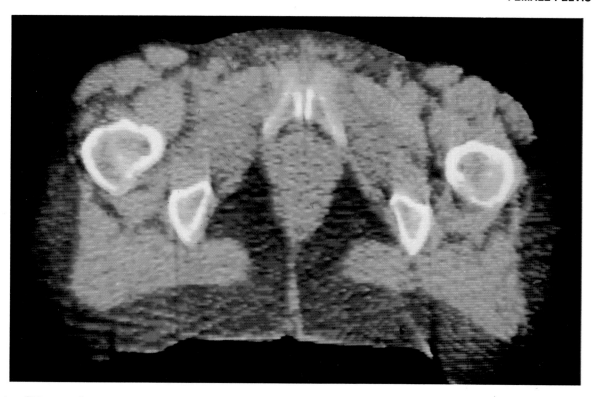

8.43 Color CT scan demonstrating the musculature of the hip joint. Note the appearance of the retropubic space.

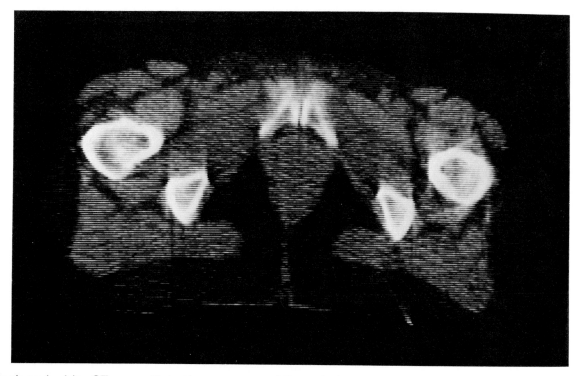

8.44 Black and white CT scan. Note the presence of the sciatic nerves.

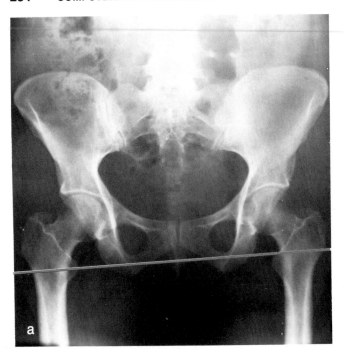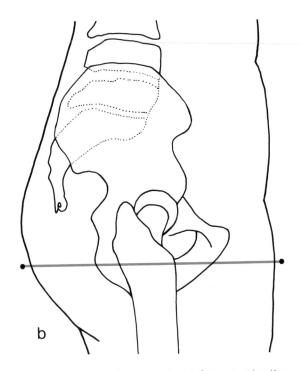

8.45 Scan level. (a) Normal A-P pelvic roentgenogram; red line shows cross-section level. (b) Schematic diagram of scan level.

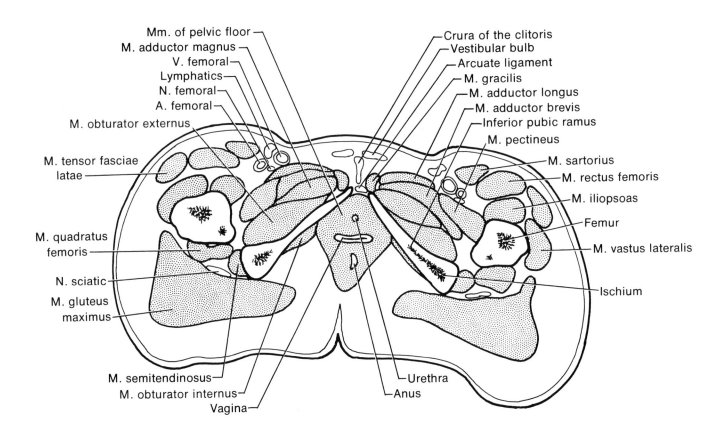

8.46 Anatomical diagram at the level of the inferior pubic ramus.

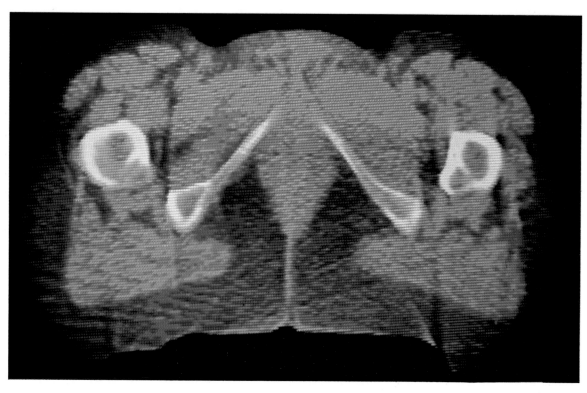

8.47 Color CT scan. Note the prominence of the adductor musculature of the thigh.

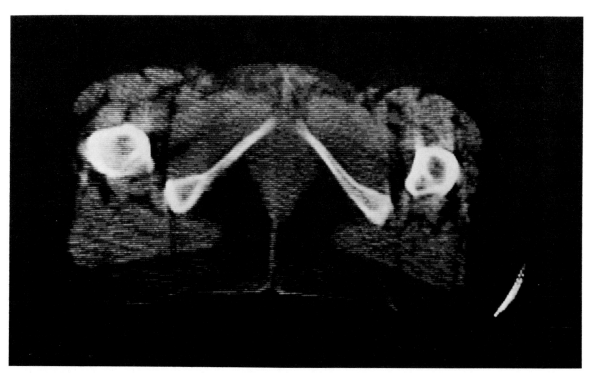

8.48 Black and white CT scan demonstrating some flattening of the dorsal structures due to the presence of the examining table under the subject.

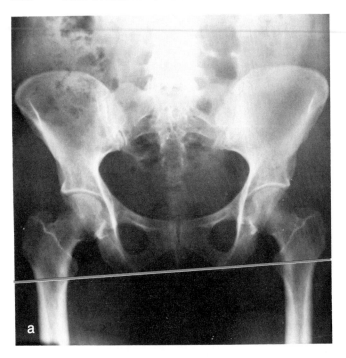
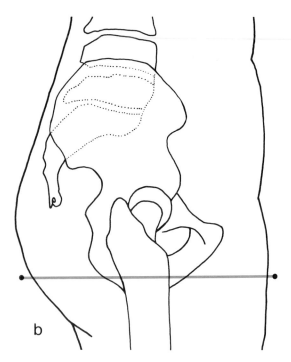

8.49 Scan level. (a) Normal A-P pelvic roentgenogram; red line shows cross-section level. (b) Schematic diagram of scan level.

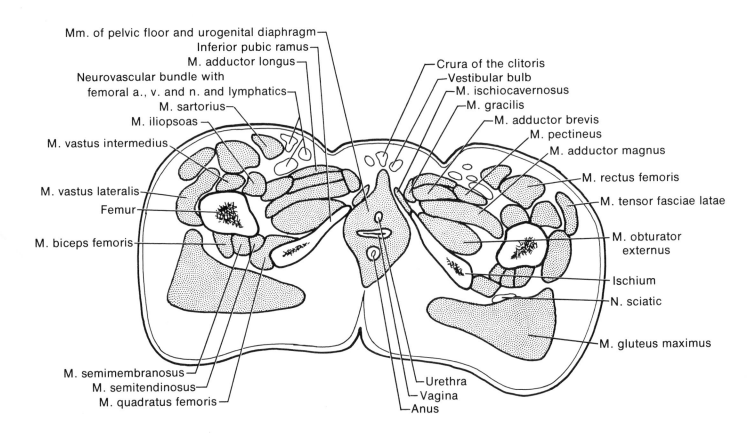

Mm. of pelvic floor and urogenital diaphragm
Inferior pubic ramus
M. adductor longus
Neurovascular bundle with
femoral a., v. and n. and lymphatics
M. sartorius
M. iliopsoas
M. vastus intermedius
M. vastus lateralis
Femur
M. biceps femoris
M. semimembranosus
M. semitendinosus
M. quadratus femoris

Crura of the clitoris
Vestibular bulb
M. ischiocavernosus
M. gracilis
M. adductor brevis
M. pectineus
M. adductor magnus
M. rectus femoris
M. tensor fasciae latae
M. obturator externus
Ischium
N. sciatic
M. gluteus maximus

Urethra
Vagina
Anus

8.50 Anatomical diagram at the level of the inferior pubic ramus.

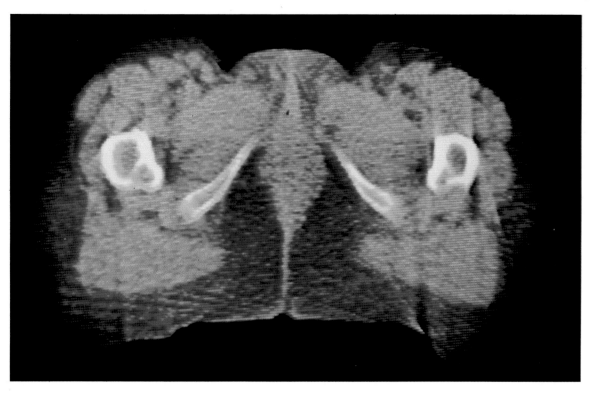

8.51 Color CT scan. Note the appearance of the muscles of the anterior thigh.

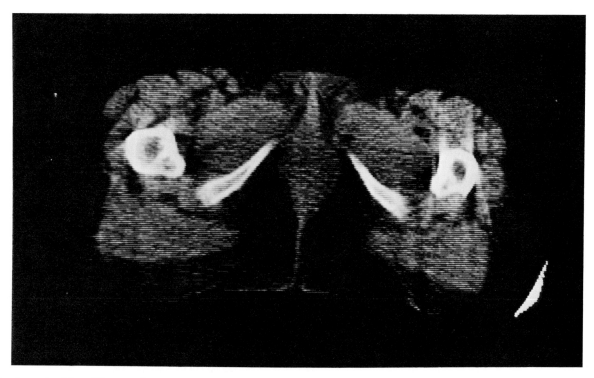

8.52 Black and white CT scan illustrating the femoral vessels and nerves as well as the structure of the perineum.

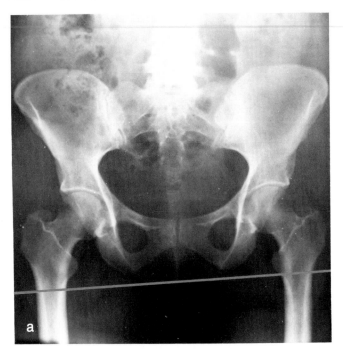
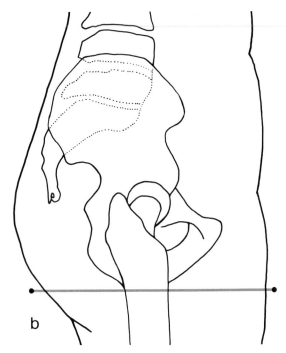

8.53 Scan level. (a) Normal A-P pelvic roentgenogram; red line shows cross-section level. (b) Schematic diagram of scan level.

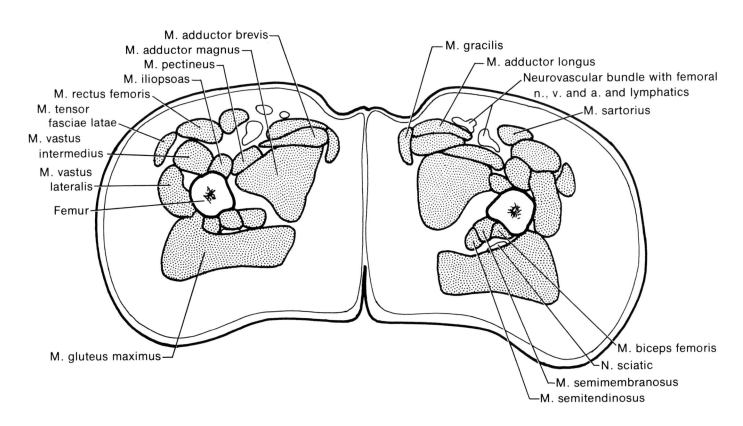

M. adductor brevis
M. adductor magnus
M. pectineus
M. iliopsoas
M. rectus femoris
M. tensor fasciae latae
M. vastus intermedius
M. vastus lateralis
Femur
M. gluteus maximus

M. gracilis
M. adductor longus
Neurovascular bundle with femoral n., v. and a. and lymphatics
M. sartorius
M. biceps femoris
N. sciatic
M. semimembranosus
M. semitendinosus

8.54 Anatomical diagram at the level of the upper thigh.

ERRATA

On page 261 a list is printed that provides a guide to locating cross-sections of interest within Chapter 9. The list incorrectly states the figure numbers of these cross-sections. Below is the correct list, printed to facilitate attachment to page 261 without compromise of the existing text. We apologize for this inconvenience.

THE PUBLISHER

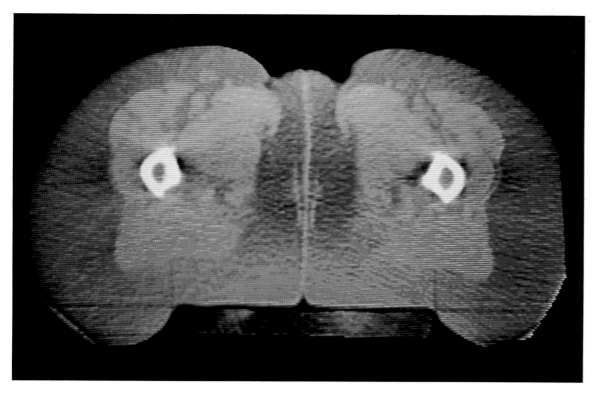

8.55 Color CT scan. Note the presence of the large adductor muscle group.

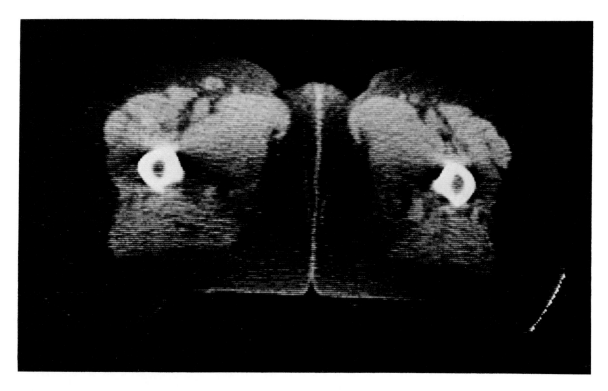

8.56 Black and white CT scan illustrating the femoral vessels and nerves as well as their associated lymphatics.

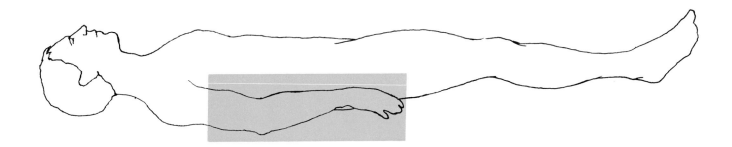

chapter nine

Upper Extremity

This section of the ATLAS contains views of the upper extremity with special emphasis on the elbow and wrist joints.

CT scanning of the limbs provides detailed cross-section and flexed transverse views of the bone structure, joint architecture, and soft tissue anatomy. Using these techniques provides additional information not normally obtainable by conventional radiographic techniques.

Extended transverse scans are provided of the right elbow, forearm, wrist, and hand; flexed transverse scans are provided for the right elbow. The orientation is depicted on both a conventional radiograph and a line drawing accompanying each scan.

All the scans were made using a 7.5-mm section thickness, a 0° gantry tilt, and a 1-cm scan interval. The flexed transverse view of the elbow was obtainable by flexing the joint to approximately 100° and placing it in the left lateral position with the joint surface roughly perpendicular to the scanning plane.

The elbow joint, which is difficult to examine accurately using conventional radiography, is clearly demonstrated with CT scans. The flexed transverse

sections give views of the whole joint, unobscured by overlying bone shadows. The method provides a means for the close study of fractures involving the joint, and it is also useful in the study of inflammatory and degenerative diseases.

The cross-sectional views at the distal portion of the forearm demonstrate the normal relationship of the soft tissues, and provide details of bone structure. The CT scan series of the normal wrist and hand illustrates the complex bony and soft tissue anatomy of these regions. The carpal tunnel is well shown in this transverse view.

The following list will provide a useful guide for locating cross-sections of interest in this chapter:

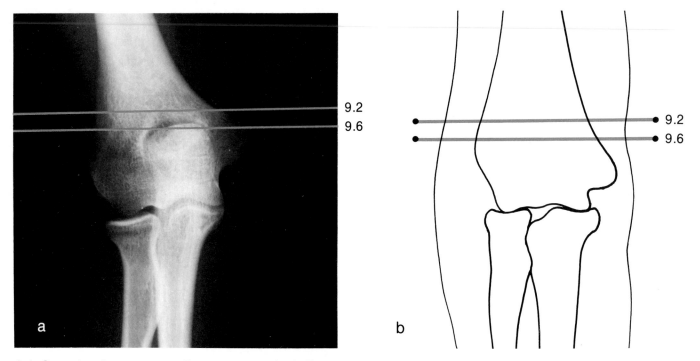

9.1 Scan levels corresponding to anatomical diagrams seen in Figures 9.2 and 9.6. (a) Roentgenogram of a normal extended elbow joint; red lines show cross-section levels. (b) Schematic diagram of scan levels.

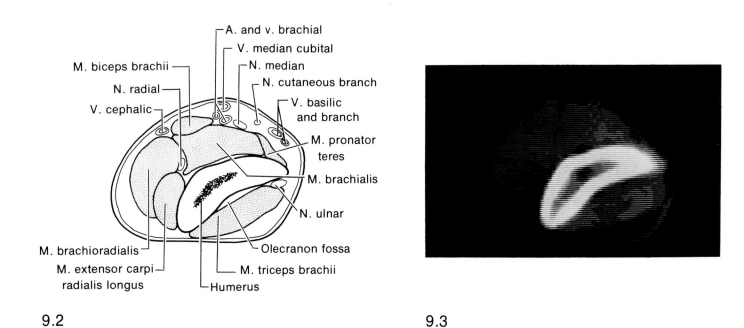

9.2

9.3

9.2 Anatomical diagram of an extended transverse section through the proximal elbow joint.
9.3 Black and white CT scan corresponding to the diagram in Figure 9.2.

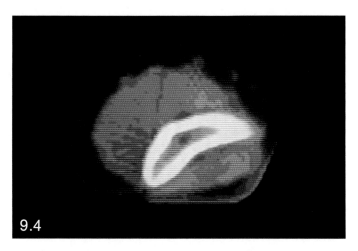

9.4

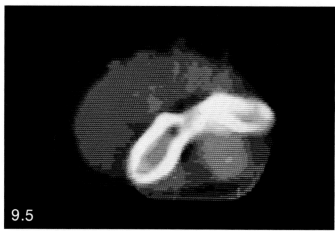

9.5

9.4 Color CT scan corresponding to the diagram in Figure 9.2. Note the appearance of the olecranon fossa just posterior to the humerus.

9.5 Color CT scan corresponding to the diagram in Figure 9.6 and illustrating the appearance of the proximal portion of the olecranon process.

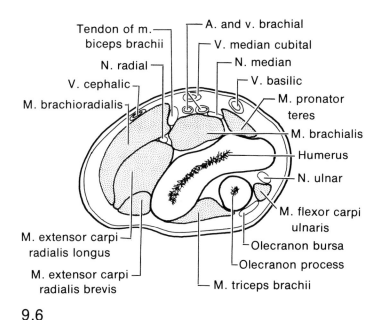

Tendon of m. biceps brachii
N. radial
V. cephalic
M. brachioradialis
A. and v. brachial
V. median cubital
N. median
V. basilic
M. pronator teres
M. brachialis
Humerus
N. ulnar
M. flexor carpi ulnaris
Olecranon bursa
Olecranon process
M. triceps brachii
M. extensor carpi radialis longus
M. extensor carpi radialis brevis

9.6

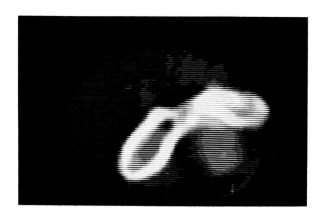

9.7

9.6 Anatomical diagram of an extended transverse section through the proximal elbow joint. Note the appearance of the musculature of the forearm at this level.

9.7 Black and white CT scan corresponding to the diagram in Figure 9.6.

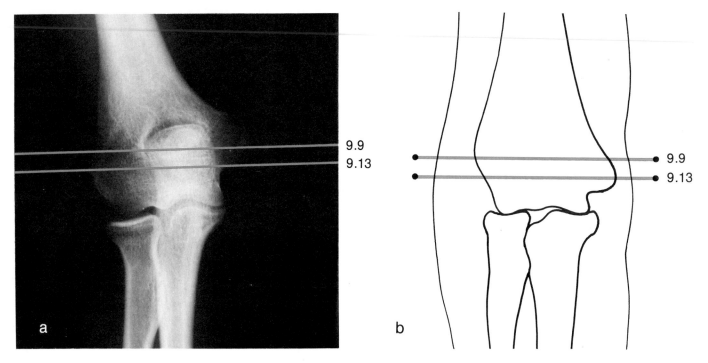

9.8 Scan levels corresponding to the anatomical diagrams in Figures 9.9 and 9.13. (a) Roentgenogram of a normal extended elbow joint; red lines show cross-section levels. (b) Schematic diagram of scan levels.

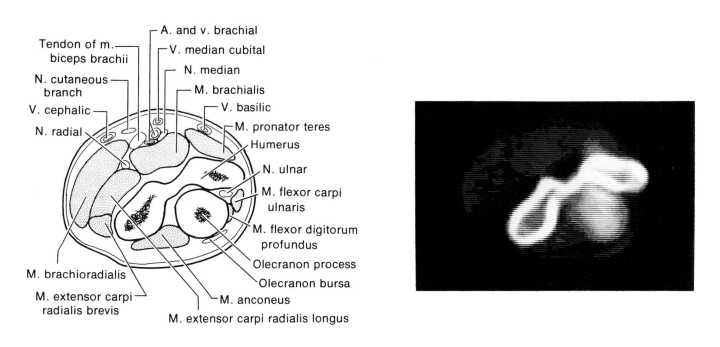

9.9

9.10

9.9 Anatomical diagram of an extended transverse section through the mid-portion of the elbow joint.
9.10 Black and white CT scan corresponding to the diagram in Figure 9.9. Note the appearance of the distal portion of the humerus in this section.

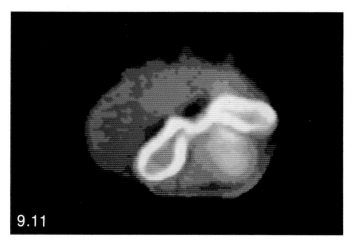

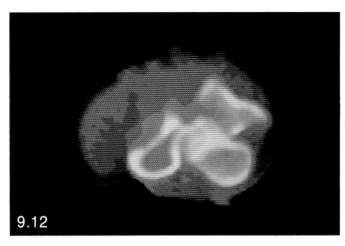

9.11 Color CT scan corresponding to the diagram in Figure 9.9. Note the relationship between the olecranon process and the humerus.
9.12 Color CT scan corresponding to the diagram in Figure 9.13. Note the prominent appearance of the musculature on the radial side of the forearm.

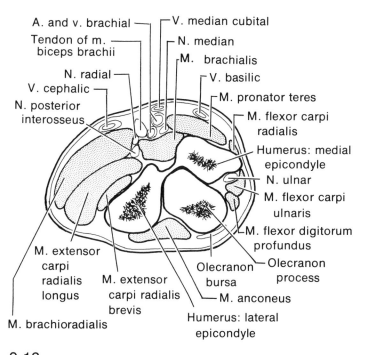

A. and v. brachial — ⌐V. median cubital
Tendon of m. — ⌐N. median
  biceps brachii
N. radial — ⌐M. brachialis
V. cephalic — ⌐V. basilic
N. posterior — ⌐M. pronator teres
  interosseus
— M. flexor carpi radialis
Humerus: medial epicondyle
N. ulnar
M. flexor carpi ulnaris
M. flexor digitorum profundus
M. extensor carpi radialis longus
M. extensor carpi radialis brevis
Olecranon bursa
Olecranon process
M. anconeus
M. brachioradialis
Humerus: lateral epicondyle

9.13

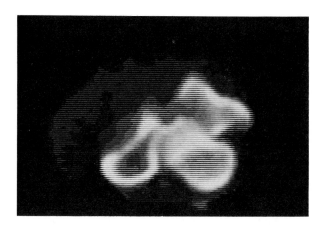

9.14

9.13 Anatomical diagram of an extended transverse section through the mid-portion of the elbow joint demonstrating the position of the olecranon bursa and the neurovascular supply to the forearm.
9.14 Black and white CT scan corresponding to the diagram in Figure 9.13 and illustrating the appearance of the superficially located veins.

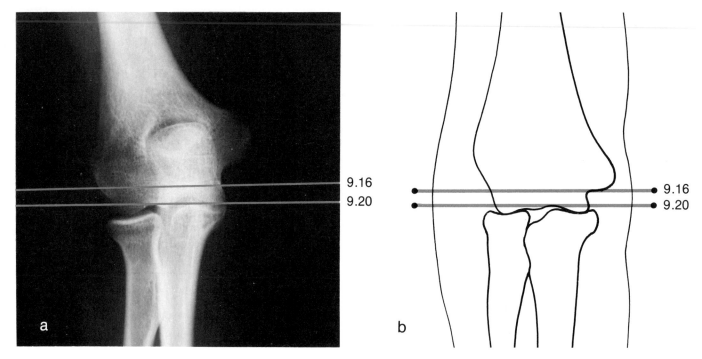

9.16
9.20

9.16
9.20

9.15 Scan levels corresponding to the anatomical diagrams seen in Figures 9.16 and 9.20. (a) Roentgenogram of a normal extended elbow joint; red lines show cross-section levels. (b) Schematic diagram of scan levels.

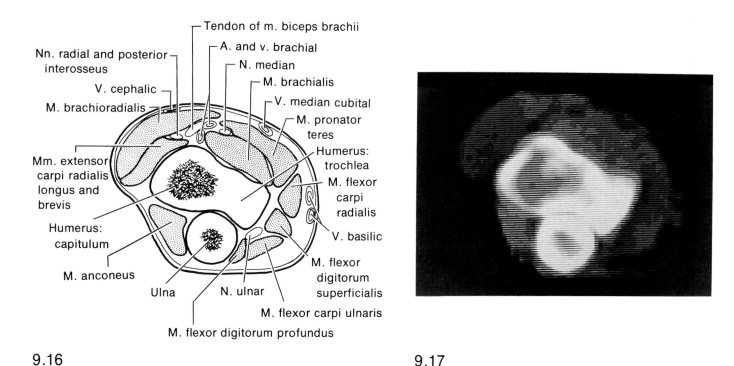

Tendon of m. biceps brachii
Nn. radial and posterior interosseus
A. and v. brachial
N. median
V. cephalic
M. brachialis
M. brachioradialis
V. median cubital
M. pronator teres
Mm. extensor carpi radialis longus and brevis
Humerus: trochlea
M. flexor carpi radialis
Humerus: capitulum
V. basilic
M. anconeus
M. flexor digitorum superficialis
Ulna
N. ulnar
M. flexor carpi ulnaris
M. flexor digitorum profundus

9.16   9.17

9.16 Anatomical diagram of an extended transverse section through the mid-portion of the elbow joint. Note the relationships of the musculature of the forearm.
9.17 Black and white CT scan corresponding to the diagram in Figure 9.16 and demonstrating the joint space between the distal humerus and the olecranon process.

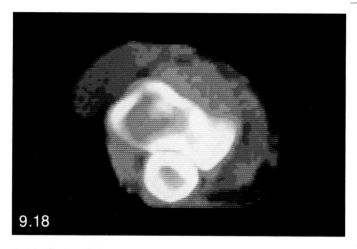

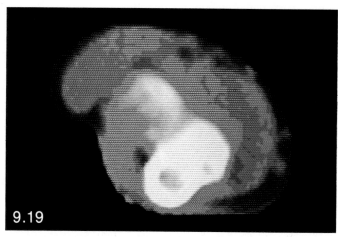

9.18 Color CT scan corresponding to the diagram in Figure 9.16 and illustrating the appearance of the trochlea and capitulum of the distal humerus.

9.19 Color CT scan corresponding to the diagram in Figure 9.20. Note the prominent musculature on the volar side of the joint.

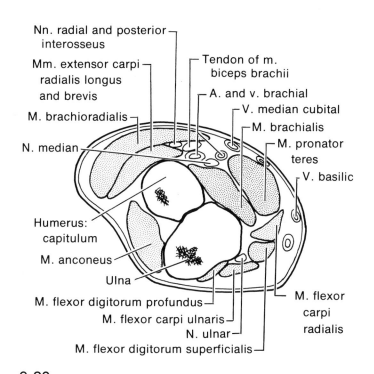

Nn. radial and posterior interosseus

Mm. extensor carpi radialis longus and brevis

M. brachioradialis

N. median

Tendon of m. biceps brachii

A. and v. brachial

V. median cubital

M. brachialis

M. pronator teres

V. basilic

Humerus: capitulum

M. anconeus

Ulna

M. flexor digitorum profundus

M. flexor carpi ulnaris

N. ulnar

M. flexor digitorum superficialis

M. flexor carpi radialis

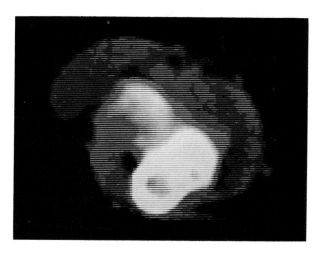

9.20

9.21

9.20 Anatomical diagram of an extended transverse section through the distal portion of the elbow joint.

9.21 Black and white CT scan corresponding to the diagram in Figure 9.20 and illustrating the peripherally situated veins of the forearm.

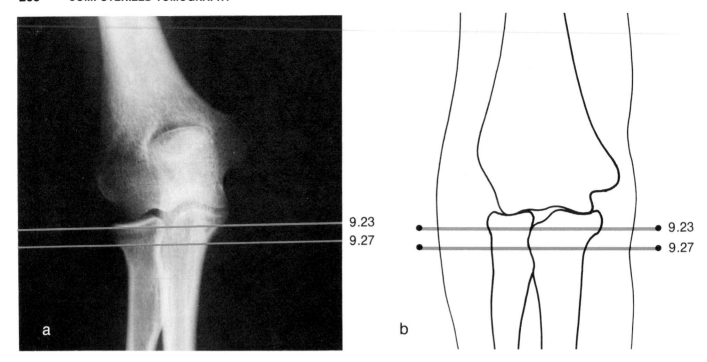

9.22 Scan levels corresponding to the anatomical diagrams seen in Figures 9.23 and 9.27. (a) Roentgenogram of a normal extended elbow joint; red lines show cross-section levels. (b) Schematic diagram of scan levels.

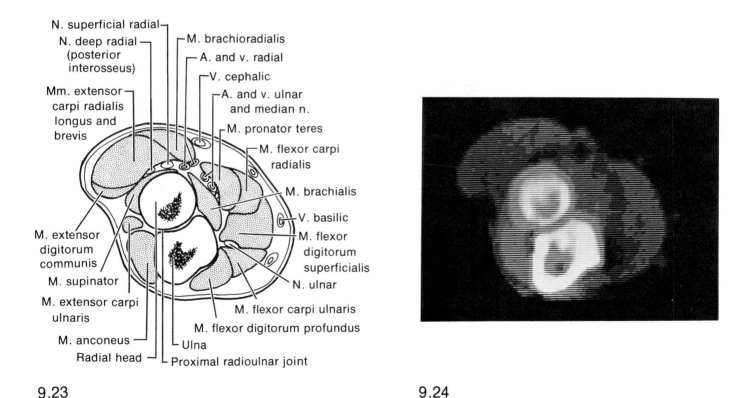

9.23

9.24

9.23 Anatomical diagram of an extended transverse section through the distal elbow joint. Note the complex musculature leading to the ulnar side of the forearm.

9.24 Black and white CT scan corresponding to the diagram in Figure 9.23. Note the appearance of the radioulnar joint at this level.

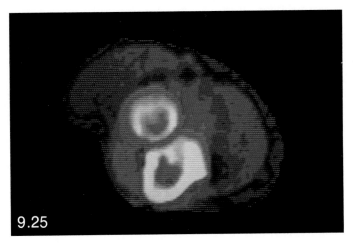

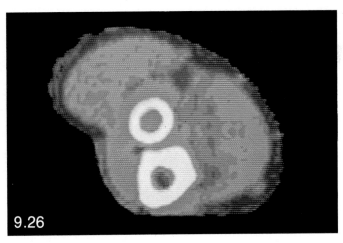

9.25

9.26

9.25 Color CT scan corresponding to the diagram in Figure 9.23. Note the separation of the musculature in the region of the neurovascular bundles to the forearm.

9.26 Color CT scan corresponding to the diagram in Figure 9.27. Note the appearance of the radioulnar joint at this level.

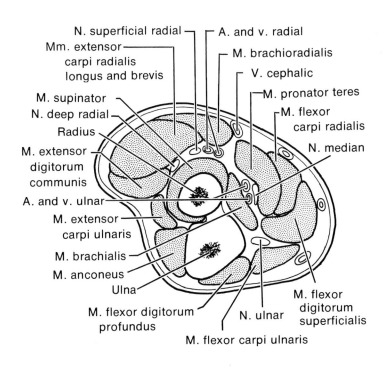

N. superficial radial ─┐ ┌─ A. and v. radial

Mm. extensor ─────
carpi radialis
longus and brevis

┌─ M. brachioradialis

┌─ V. cephalic

M. supinator ─
N. deep radial ─
Radius ─

┌─M. pronator teres

┌M. flexor
carpi radialis

M. extensor ─
digitorum
communis

N. median

A. and v. ulnar ─

M. extensor ─
carpi ulnaris

M. brachialis ─
M. anconeus ─
Ulna ─

M. flexor
digitorum
superficialis

M. flexor digitorum
profundus

N. ulnar

M. flexor carpi ulnaris

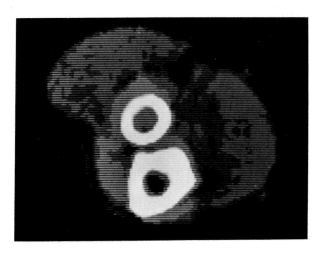

9.27

9.28

9.27 Anatomical diagram of an extended transverse section through the distal elbow joint and demonstrating the position of the three main nerve supplies to the forearm at this level.

9.28 Black and white CT scan corresponding to the diagram in Figure 9.27 and demonstrating the close adherence of the supinator muscle to the proximal portion of the radius.

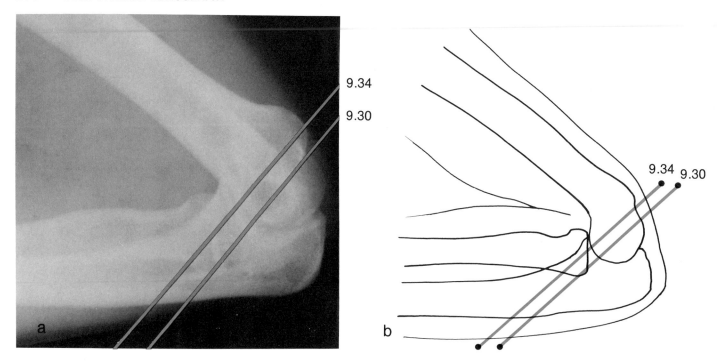

9.29 Scan levels corresponding to the anatomical diagrams seen in Figures 9.30 and 9.34. (a) Roentgenogram of a normal flexed elbow joint; red lines show cross-section levels. (b) Schematic diagram of scan levels.

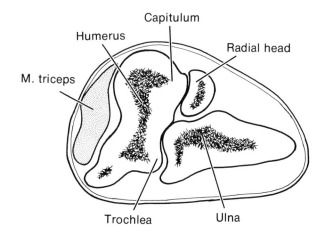

9.30

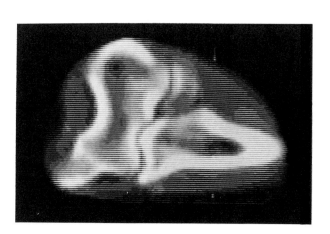

9.31

9.30 Anatomical diagram of a flexed transverse section through the elbow joint. Note the presence of the dorsally situated triceps muscle.

9.31 Black and white CT scan corresponding to the diagram in Figure 9.30 and illustrating the presence of all three bones of the elbow joint at this level.

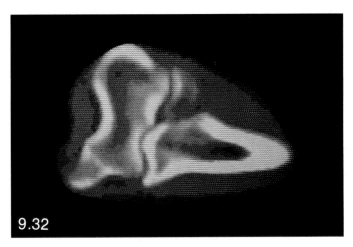

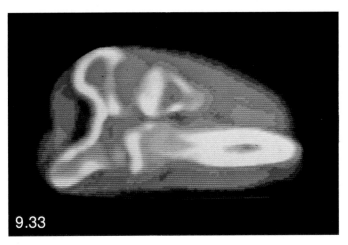

9.32 Color CT scan corresponding to the diagram in Figure 9.30. Note the appearance of the joint space between the humerus, and the radius and ulnar bones.

9.33 Color CT scan corresponding to the diagram in Figure 9.34. Note the appearance of the radioulnar joint at this level.

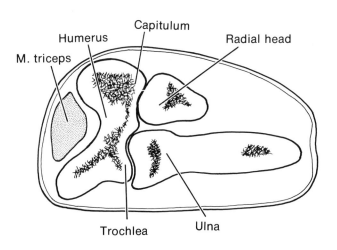

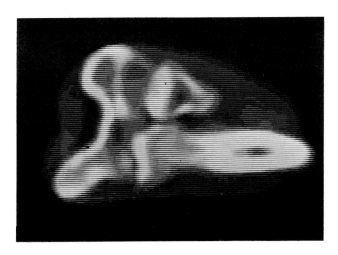

9.34 Anatomical diagram of a flexed transverse section through the elbow joint.

9.35 Black and white CT scan corresponding to the diagram in Figure 9.34. Note the appearance of the triceps muscle just dorsal to the distal humerus.

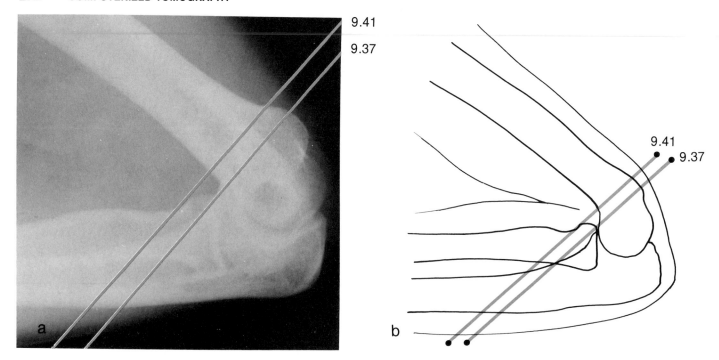

9.36 Scan levels corresponding to the anatomical diagrams seen in Figures 9.37 and 9.41. (a) Roentgenogram of a normal flexed elbow joint; red lines show cross-section levels. (b) Schematic diagram of scan levels.

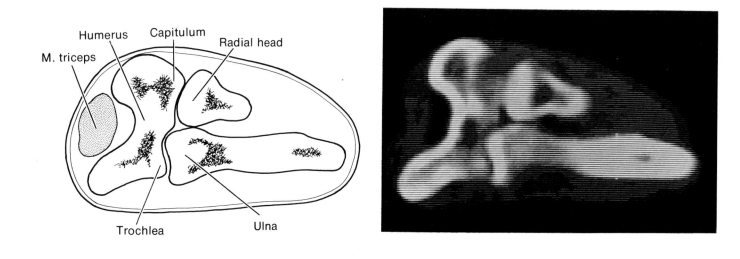

9.37

9.38

9.37 Anatomical diagram of a flexed transverse section through the elbow joint.
9.38 Black and white CT scan corresponding to the diagram in Figure 9.37. Note the well-defined proximal radioulnar joint in this scan.

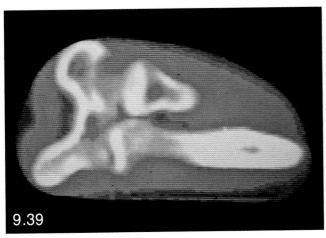

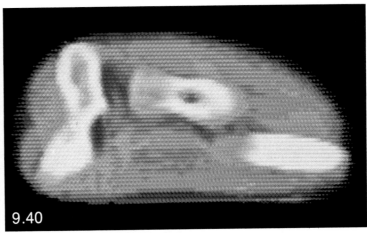

9.39 Color CT scan corresponding to the diagram in Figure 9.37. Note the appearance of the olecranon fossa, demonstrated in dark green in this scan.

9.40 Color CT scan corresponding to the diagram in Figure 9.41. Note the appearance of the ulna and radius cut obliquely at this level.

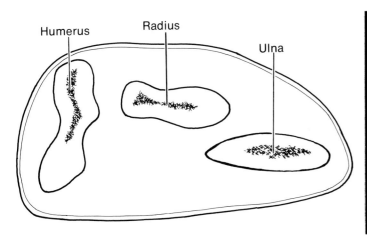

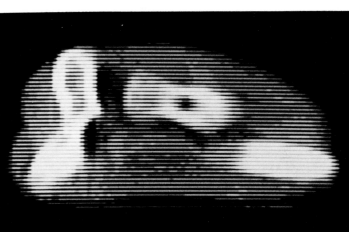

9.41

9.42

9.41 Anatomical diagram of a flexed transverse section through the elbow joint.

9.42 Black and white CT scan corresponding to the diagram in Figure 9.41.

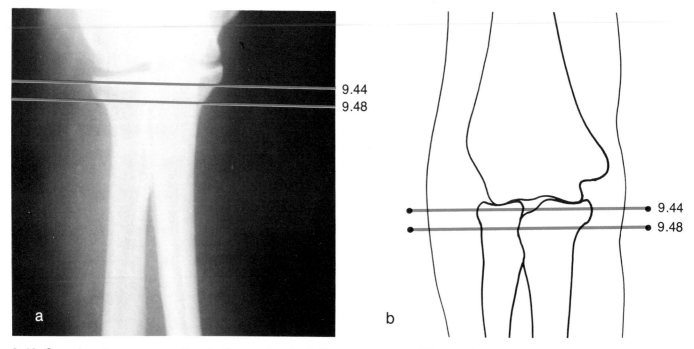

a

b

9.44
9.48

9.44
9.48

9.43 Scan levels corresponding to the anatomical diagrams seen in Figures 9.44 and 9.48. (a) Roentgenogram of a normal supine forearm; red lines show cross-section levels. (b) Schematic diagram of scan levels.

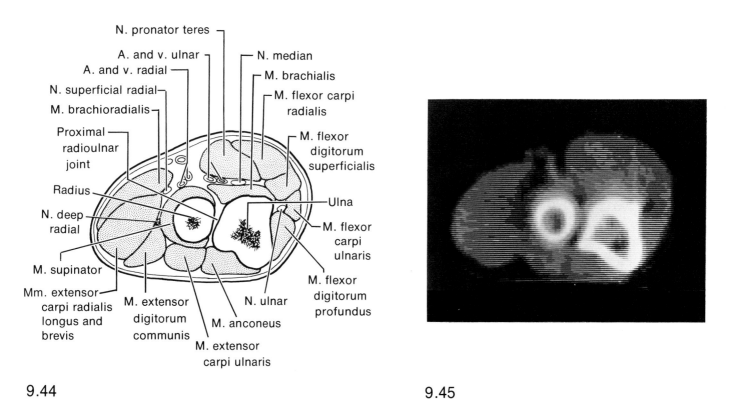

N. pronator teres
A. and v. ulnar
A. and v. radial
N. superficial radial
M. brachioradialis
Proximal radioulnar joint
Radius
N. deep radial
M. supinator
Mm. extensor carpi radialis longus and brevis
M. extensor digitorum communis
M. extensor carpi ulnaris
M. anconeus
N. ulnar
N. median
M. brachialis
M. flexor carpi radialis
M. flexor digitorum superficialis
Ulna
M. flexor carpi ulnaris
M. flexor digitorum profundus

9.44

9.45

9.44 Anatomical diagram of an extended transverse section through a supine forearm at the level of the proximal radioulnar joint.
9.45 Black and white CT scan corresponding to the diagram in Figure 9.44 and demonstrating the proximal radioulnar joint.

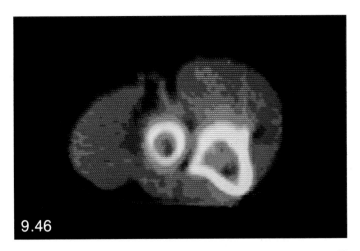

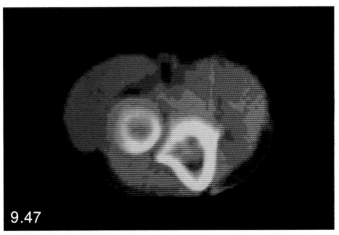

9.46 Color CT scan corresponding to the diagram in Figure 9.44. Note that there is some dorsal flattening of the musculature due to the presence of the examining table underneath the limb.

9.47 Color CT scan corresponding to the diagram in Figure 9.48. Note the appearance of the proximal radioulnar joint and the brachioradialis muscle.

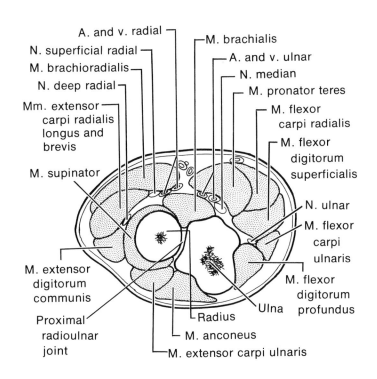

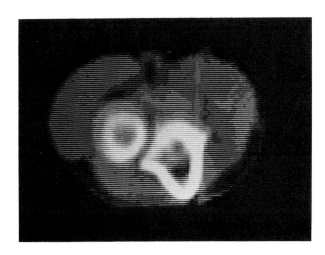

9.48   9.49

9.48 Anatomical diagram of a supine extended transverse section through the proximal radioulnar joint and illustrating the complex musculature of the forearm at this level.

9.49 Black and white CT scan corresponding to the diagram in Figure 9.48. Note the appearance of the dorsal musculature at this level, including the anconeus and extensor carpi ulnaris muscles just dorsal to the radioulnar joint.

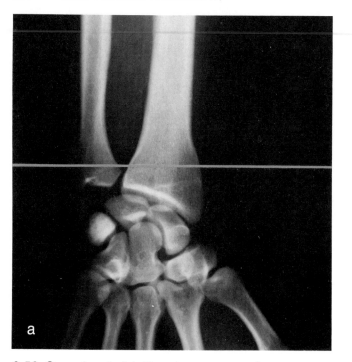
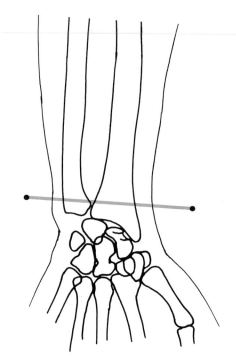

9.50 Scan level. (a) Roentgenogram of a normal pronated forearm; red line shows corss-section level. (b) Schematic diagram of scan level.

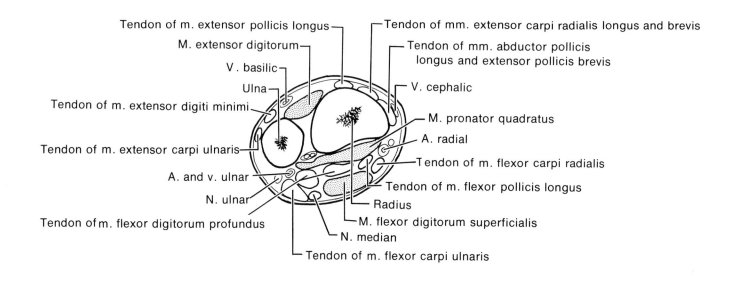

9.51 Anatomical diagram of an extended transverse section through the distal radioulnar joint in a pronated forearm. Note the complex musculature of the volar surface of the forearm at this level.

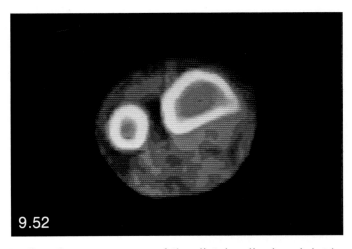

9.52 Color CT scan demonstrating the appearance of the distal radioulnar joint in a pronated forearm.

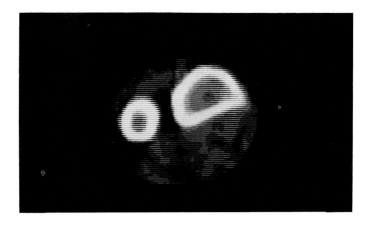

9.53 Black and white CT scan. Note the appearance of the extensor digitorum muscle on the dorsal surface of the forearm at this level.

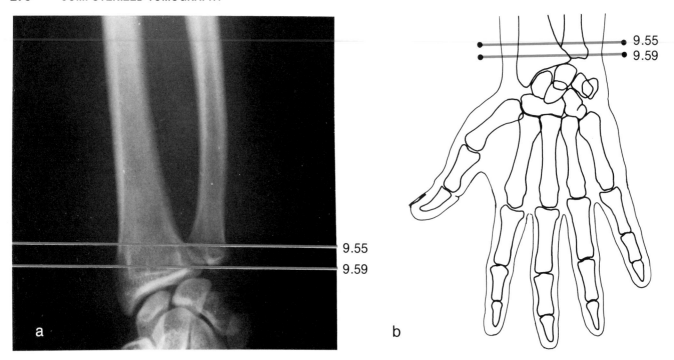

9.54 Scan levels corresponding to the anatomical diagrams seen in Figures 9.55 and 9.59. (a) Roentgenogram of a normal supine forearm; red lines show cross-section levels. (b) Schematic diagram of scan levels.

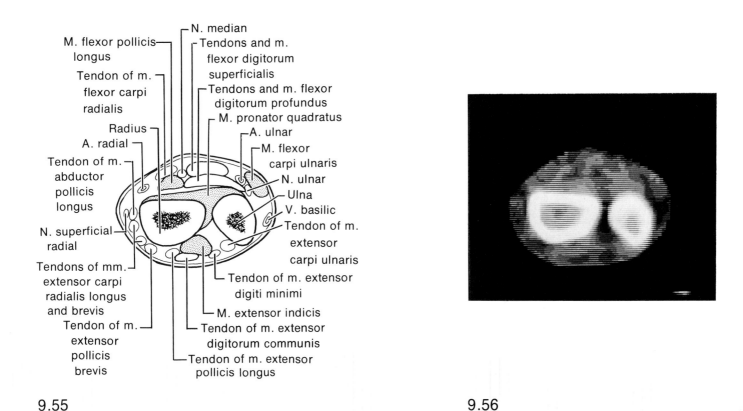

9.55

9.56

9.55 Anatomical diagram of an extended transverse section through the supine distal radioulnar joint. Note the many tendons on the radial side of this joint.

9.56 Black and white CT scan corresponding to the diagram in Figure 9.55.

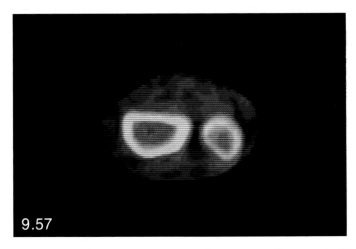

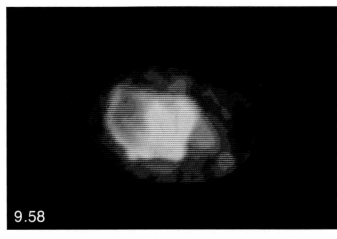

9.57 Color CT scan corresponding to the diagram in Figure 9.55. Note the appearance of the radioulnar joint at this level.

9.58 Color CT scan corresponding to the diagram in Figure 9.59. Note the presence of the styloid process of the ulna in this scan.

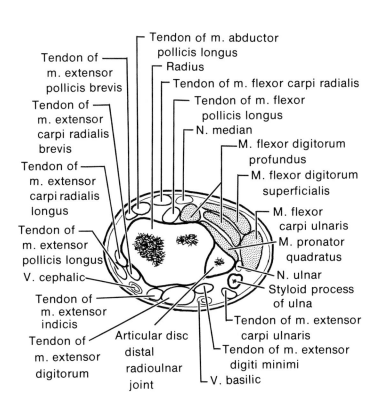

Tendon of m. abductor pollicis longus

Radius

Tendon of m. flexor carpi radialis

Tendon of m. flexor pollicis longus

N. median

M. flexor digitorum profundus

M. flexor digitorum superficialis

M. flexor carpi ulnaris

M. pronator quadratus

N. ulnar

Styloid process of ulna

Tendon of m. extensor carpi ulnaris

Tendon of m. extensor digiti minimi

V. basilic

Tendon of m. extensor pollicis brevis

Tendon of m. extensor carpi radialis brevis

Tendon of m. extensor carpi radialis longus

Tendon of m. extensor pollicis longus

V. cephalic

Tendon of m. extensor indicis

Tendon of m. extensor digitorum

Articular disc distal radioulnar joint

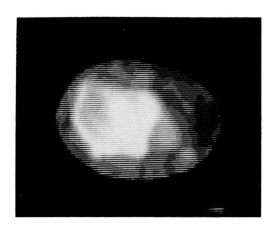

9.59   9.60

9.59 Anatomical diagram of an extended transverse section through the distal supine radio-ulnar joint. Note the presence of the many tendon sheaths surrounding the wrist at this level.

9.60 Black and white CT scan corresponding to the diagram in Figure 9.59.

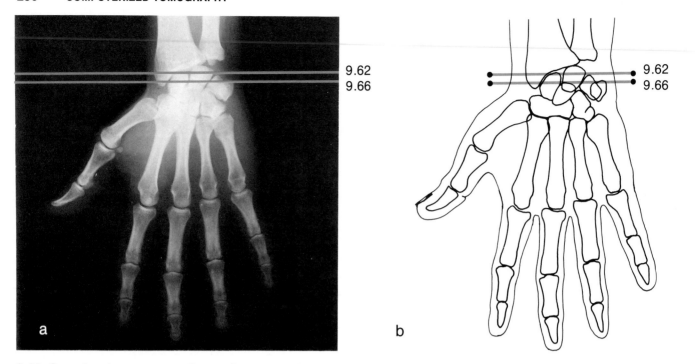

9.61 Scan levels corresponding to the anatomical diagrams seen in Figures 9.62 and 9.66. (a) Roentgenogram of a normal extended supine wrist joint; red lines show cross-section levels. (b) Schematic diagram of scan levels.

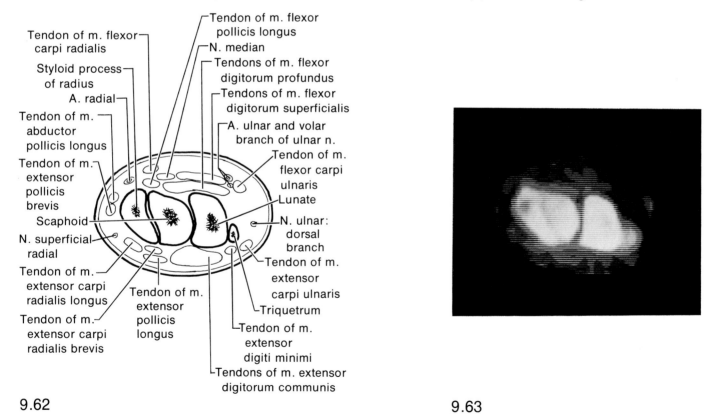

9.62

9.63

9.62 Anatomical diagram of an extended transverse section through the supine wrist joint demonstrating the relationships of the proximal carpal bones.

9.63 Black and white CT scan corresponding to the diagram in Figure 9.62. Note the prominent appearance of the joint space between the scaphoid and the lunate bones in this scan.

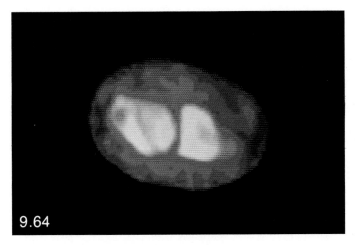

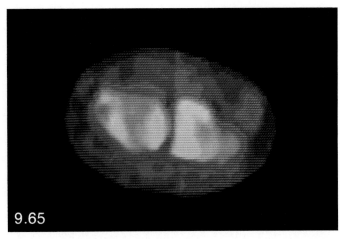

9.64 Color CT scan corresponding to the diagram in Figure 9.62. Note the appearance of the many tendons surrounding the joints at this level.

9.65 Color CT scan corresponding to the diagram in Figure 9.66. Note the appearance of the carpal bones at this level.

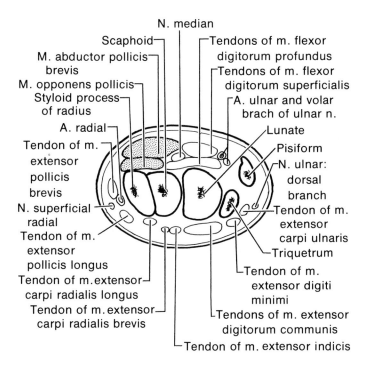

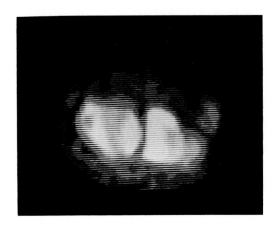

9.66   9.67

9.66 Anatomical diagram of an extended transverse section through the supine wrist joint. Note the position of the median nerve at this level.

9.67 Black and white CT scan corresponding to the diagram in Figure 9.66. Note the tendons on the radial side of the wrist joint at this level.

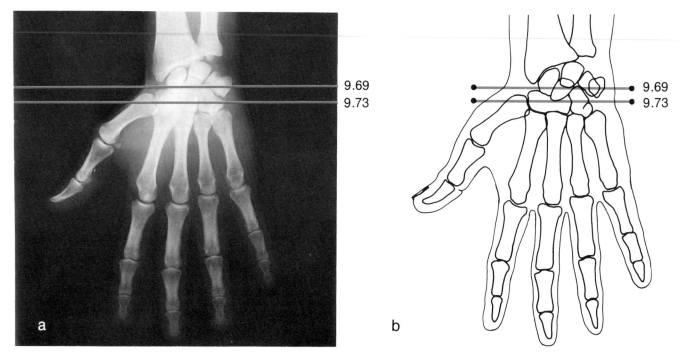

9.68 Scan levels corresponding to the anatomical diagrams seen in Figures 9.69 and 9.73. (a) Roentgenogram of a normal extended supine wrist joint; red lines show cross-section levels. (b) Schematic diagram of scan levels.

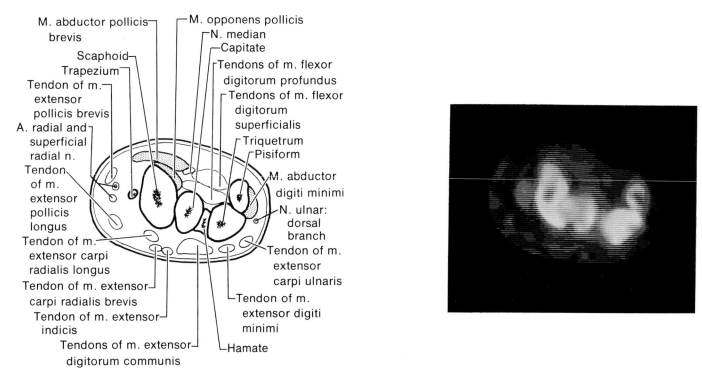

9.69

9.70

9.69 Anatomical diagram of an extended transverse section through the supine wrist joint. Note the presence of the median nerve in the carpal tunnel at this level.

9.70 Black and white CT scan corresponding to the diagram in Figure 9.69 and illustrating the relationships of the carpal bones at this level.

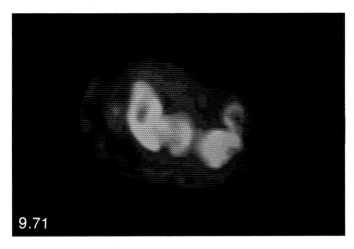

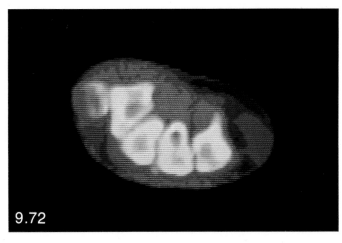

9.71

9.72

9.71 Color CT scan corresponding to the diagram in Figure 9.69. Note the small and peripherally situated pisiform bone in this scan.

9.72 Color CT scan corresponding to the diagram in Figure 9.73 and illustrating the appearance of the hamulus of the hamate bone in this scan.

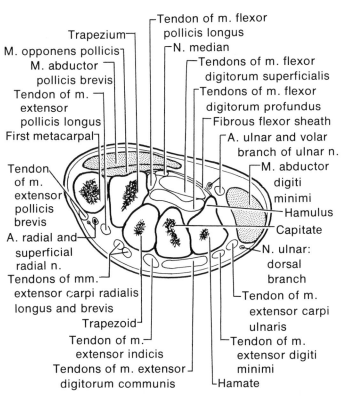

Trapezium
M. opponens pollicis
M. abductor pollicis brevis
Tendon of m. extensor pollicis longus
First metacarpal
Tendon of m. extensor pollicis brevis
A. radial and superficial radial n.
Tendons of mm. extensor carpi radialis longus and brevis
Trapezoid
Tendon of m. extensor indicis
Tendons of m. extensor digitorum communis

Tendon of m. flexor pollicis longus
N. median
Tendons of m. flexor digitorum superficialis
Tendons of m. flexor digitorum profundus
Fibrous flexor sheath
A. ulnar and volar branch of ulnar n.
M. abductor digiti minimi
Hamulus
Capitate
N. ulnar: dorsal branch
Tendon of m. extensor carpi ulnaris
Tendon of m. extensor digiti minimi
Hamate

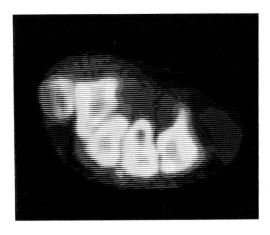

9.73

9.74

9.73 Anatomical diagram of an extended transverse section through the supine wrist joint. Note the well developed abductor digiti minimi muscle.

9.74 Black and white CT scan corresponding to the diagram in Figure 9.73. Note the appearance of the first metacarpal bone.

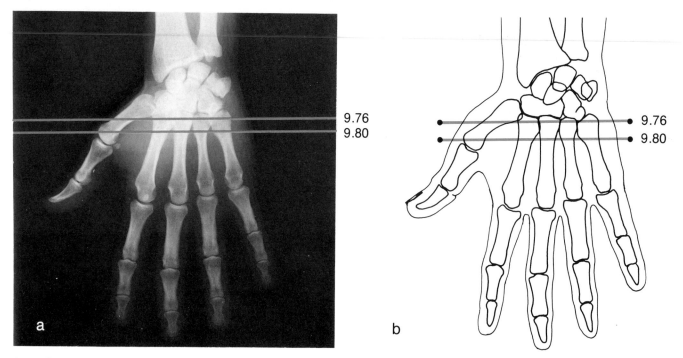

9.75 Scan levels corresponding to the anatomical diagrams seen in Figures 9.76 and 9.80. (a) Roentgenogram of a normal extended supine wrist joint; red lines show cross-section levels. (b) Schematic diagram of scan levels.

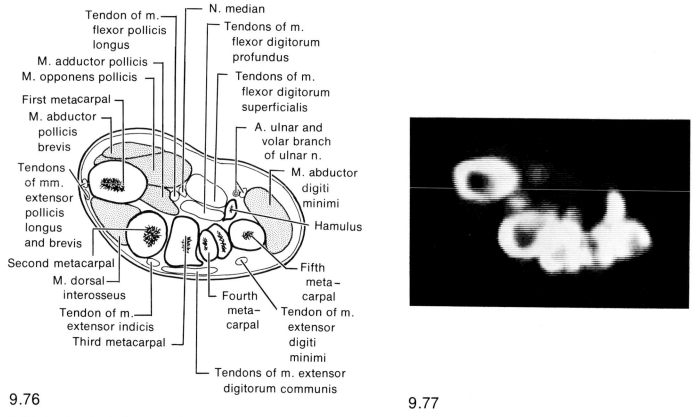

Tendon of m. flexor pollicis longus
N. median
Tendons of m. flexor digitorum profundus
M. adductor pollicis
M. opponens pollicis
Tendons of m. flexor digitorum superficialis
First metacarpal
M. abductor pollicis brevis
A. ulnar and volar branch of ulnar n.
Tendons of mm. extensor pollicis longus and brevis
M. abductor digiti minimi
Hamulus
Second metacarpal
M. dorsal interosseus
Fifth metacarpal
Tendon of m. extensor indicis
Fourth metacarpal
Tendon of m. extensor digiti minimi
Third metacarpal
Tendons of m. extensor digitorum communis

9.76

9.77

9.76 Anatomical diagram of an extended transverse section through a supine wrist joint. Note the first three metacarpals are visible at this level.

9.77 Black and white CT scan corresponding to the diagram in Figure 9.76. Note the prominent appearance of the hamulus process of the hamate bone.

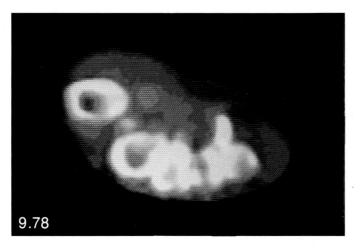

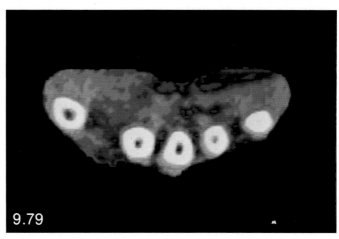

9.78 Color CT scan corresponding to the diagram in Figure 9.76 and demonstrating the appearance of the first three metacarpal bones at this level.

9.79 Color CT scan corresponding to the diagram in Figure 9.80 and demonstrating the five metacarpal bones at this level.

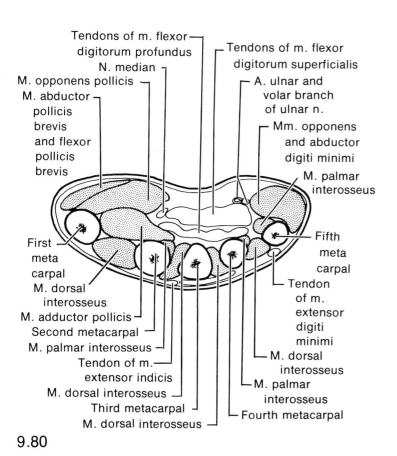

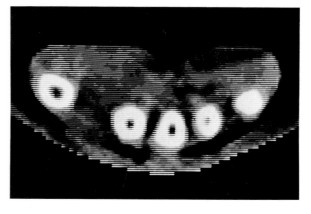

Tendons of m. flexor digitorum profundus

N. median

M. opponens pollicis

M. abductor pollicis brevis and flexor pollicis brevis

Tendons of m. flexor digitorum superficialis

A. ulnar and volar branch of ulnar n.

Mm. opponens and abductor digiti minimi

M. palmar interosseus

Fifth meta carpal

Tendon of m. extensor digiti minimi

M. dorsal interosseus

M. palmar interosseus

Fourth metacarpal

First meta carpal

M. dorsal interosseus

M. adductor pollicis

Second metacarpal

M. palmar interosseus

Tendon of m. extensor indicis

M. dorsal interosseus

Third metacarpal

M. dorsal interosseus

9.80   **9.81**

9.80 Anatomical diagram of an extended transverse section through the proximal protion of the hand. Note the position of the muscles of the thumb as well as the wide flexon tendon sheaths to the fingers.

9.81 Black and white CT scan corresponding to the diagram in Figure 9.80. Note that the palmer surface of the hand in this scan appears flattened; this was due to the presence of immobilization padding.

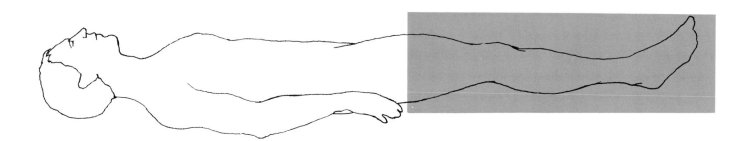

chapter ten

Lower Extremity

This section of the ATLAS illustrates the CT imaging of the lower extremity.

Transverse scans are provided of the left thigh and left mid-calf. Extended transverse and flexed transverse scans are provided for the left knee; plantar-flexed transverse scans are provided for the left ankle and foot. The orientation is depicted on both a conventional radiograph and a line drawing, which accompany each scan. All the scans were made using a 7.5-mm section thickness, a 0° gantry tilt and a 1-cm scan interval. The flexed transverse knee views were obtained by placing the joint, flexed to 100° in the left lateral position, with the joint surface roughly perpendicular to the scanning plane. The plantar-flexed transverse ankle views were obtained by seating the subject on the scanning table with the soles of the feet pressed firmly on the table top with 45° of plantar flexion.

CT flexed transverse scanning techniques give a new perspective to the study of the knee joint. The flexed transverse sections enable a thorough study of the complex relationship involving the patella and the femoral condyles to be made, and will be extremely useful in the assessment of the dislocating patella syndrome. The pathological changes associated with degenerative disease will also be easily recognized.

The extended transverse section taken at the level of the knee joint gives an excellent view of the medial and lateral menisci. This scan, combined with the flexed transverse view, may well provide a reliable noninvasive means of diagnosing meniscal tears.

The CT scans of the ankle provide clear views of both the ankle and subtalar joints, as well as the calcaneous bone. The scans will be useful in the study of calcaneal fractures involving the subtalar joint.

The scans of the foot through the tarsal and metatarsal bones illustrate clearly the transverse and longitudinal arches of the foot, and provide an excellent view of the complex musculoskeletal anatomy of the sole of the foot. These views could well find a place in the investigation of the common foot disorders, as well as in the study of the anatomical distortions secondary to paralytic foot disorders and congenital talipes equinovarus.

The following list will provide a useful guide for locating cross-sections of interest in this chapter:

Upper and lower thigh	Figs. 10.1–10.8
Extended supine knee	Figs. 10.9–10.50
Flexed knee	Figs. 10.51–10.71
Mid-calf	Figs. 10.72–10.75
Plantar-flexed ankle	Figs. 10.76–10.96

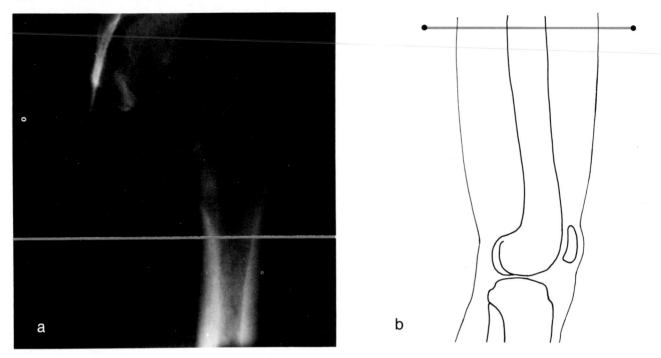

10.1 Scan level. (a) Roentgenogram of a normal pelvis, red line shows cross-section level; (b) Schematic diagram of scan level.

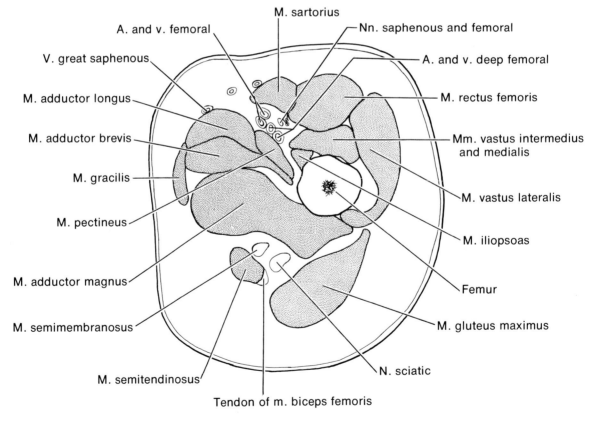

10.2 Anatomical diagram of a transverse section through the upper thigh. Note the large adductor muscle group.

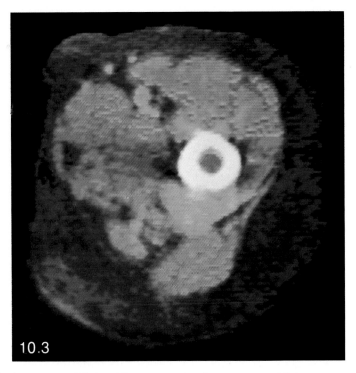

10.3 Color CT scan through the upper thigh with contrast enhancement. This scan was obtained with the patient in the prone position, thereby producing some flattening of the anterior structures of the leg at this level.

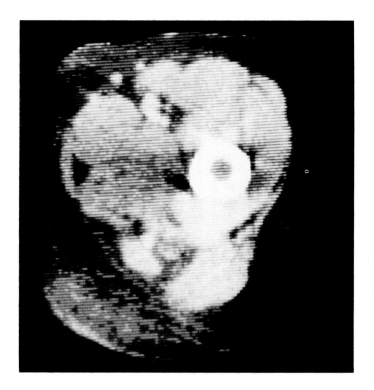

10.4 Black and white CT scan with contrast enhancement of the upper thigh. Note the uptake of contrast material by the muscles of the upper leg and the density of the vascular structures.

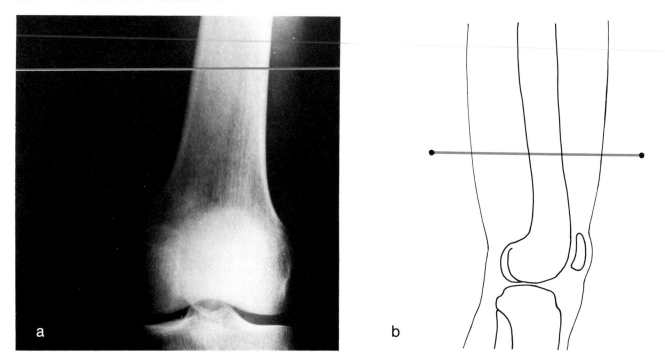

10.5 Scan levels. (a) Roentgenogram of a normal extended leg, red line shows cross-section level; (b) Schematic diagram of scan level.

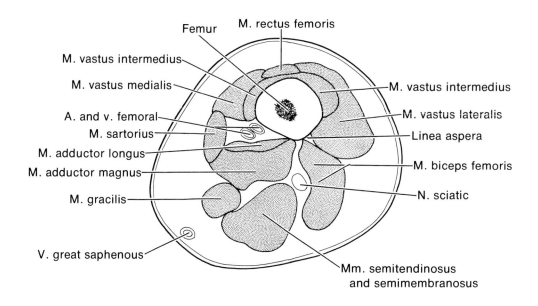

10.6 Anatomical diagram of a transverse section through the lower thigh. Note the change in muscular relationships relative to the diagram in Figure 10.2.

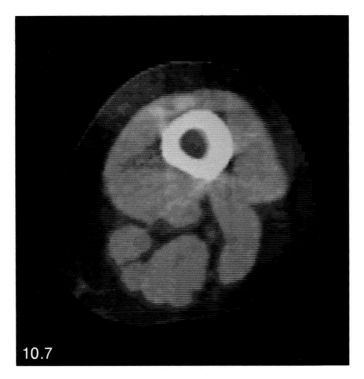

10.7 Color CT scan through the lower thigh. Note the prominent appearance of the sciatic nerve in this scan.

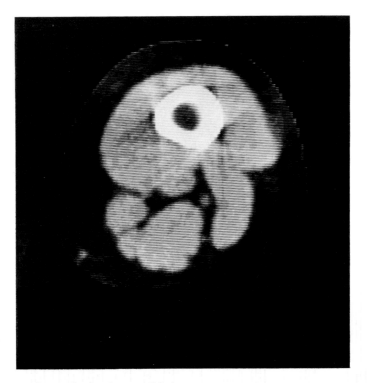

10.8 Black and white CT scan through the lower thigh.

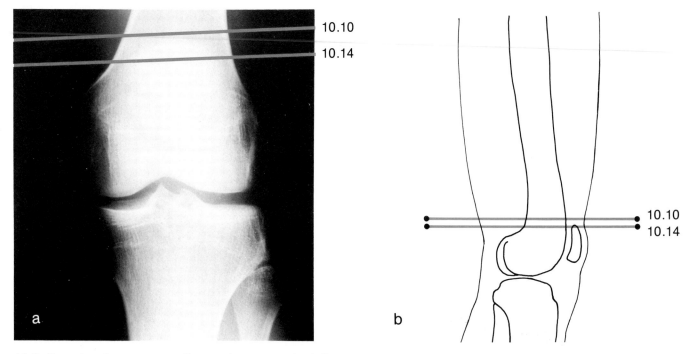

10.9 Scan levels corresponding to the anatomical diagrams seen in Figures 10.10 and 10.14. (a) Roentgenogram of a normal extended knee joint; red lines show cross-section levels; (b) Schematic diagram of scan levels.

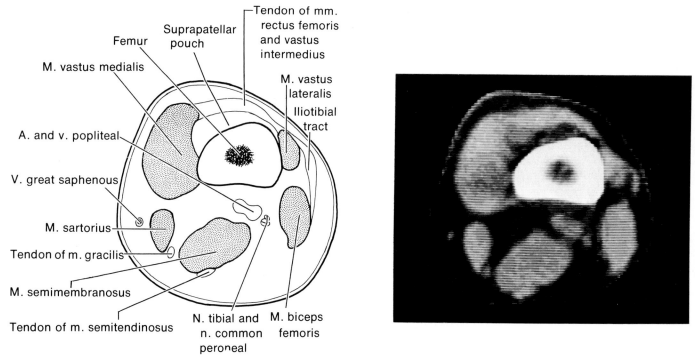

10.10

10.11

10.10 Anatomical diagram of an extended transverse section through the distal thigh. Note the position of the popliteal artery and vein.

10.11 Black and white CT scan corresponding to the diagram in Figure 10.10 and demonstrating the suprapatellar pouch just anterior to the femur.

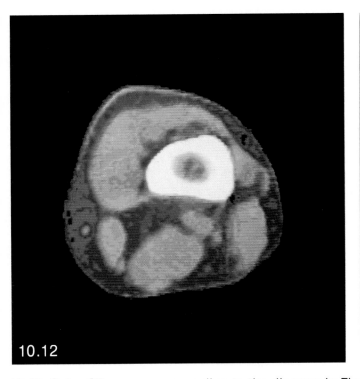

10.12

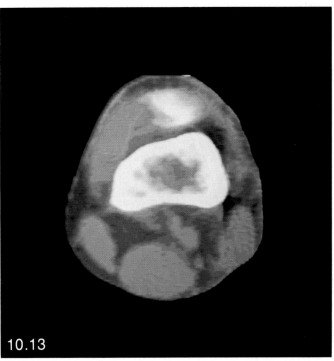

10.13

10.12 Color CT scan corresponding to the diagram in Figure 10.10 and clearly demonstrating the neurovascular supply to the lower leg, seen just posterior to the femur.

10.13 Color CT scan corresponding to the anatomical diagram in Figure 10.14 and illustrating the superior portion of the patella.

Tendon of m.
quadriceps femoris

Patella

M. vastus
medialis

M. vastus lateralis

A. popliteal

Iliotibial tract

M. sartorius

Femur

V. great
saphenous

V. popliteal

Tendon
of m. gracilis

M. biceps
femoris

Tendon of
m. semitendinosus

N. tibial   N. common
peroneal

M. semimembranosus

10.14

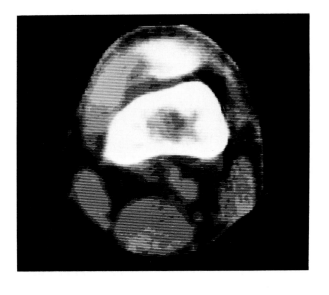

10.15

10.14 Anatomical diagram of an extended transverse section through the distal femur.

10.15 Black and white CT scan corresponding to the anatomical diagram in Figure 10.14. Note the presence of the popliteal vessels in this scan.

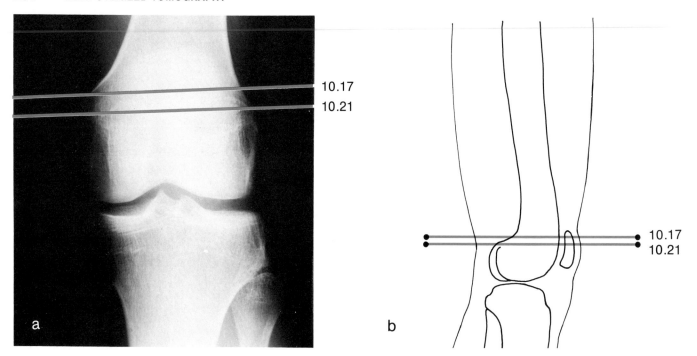

10.16 Scan levels corresponding to the anatomical diagrams seen in Figures 10.17 and 10.21. (a) Roentgenogram of a normal extended knee joint; red lines show cross-section levels; (b) Schematic diagram of scan levels.

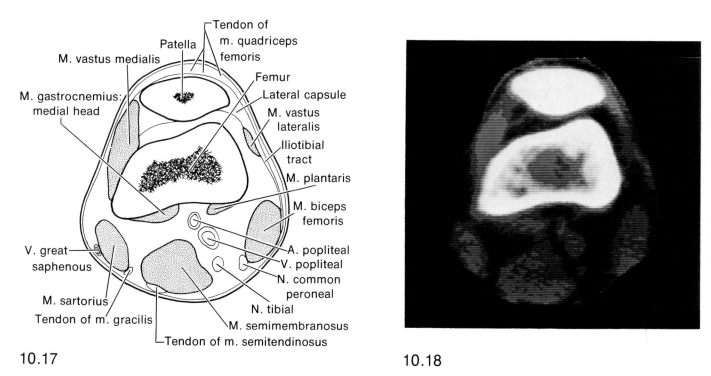

10.17

10.18

10.17 Anatomical diagram of an extended transverse section through the distal femur and demonstrating the origin of the gastrocnemius muscle.

10.18 Black and white CT scan corresponding to the diagram in Figure 10.17. Note the appearance of the gastrocnemius and plantaris muscles.

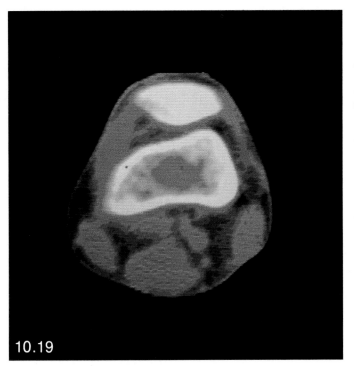

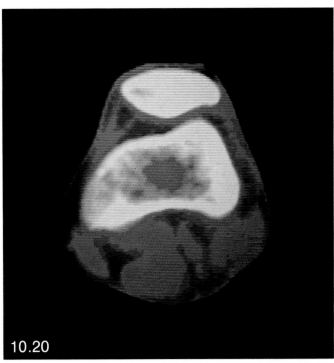

10.19 Color CT scan corresponding to the anatomical diagram in Figure 10.17. Note the appearance of the dense cortical bone of the femur, shown in white.

10.20 Color CT scan corresponding to the diagram in Figure 10.21 and illustrating the superior portion of the patellofemoral joint.

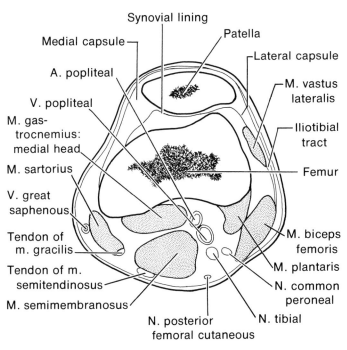

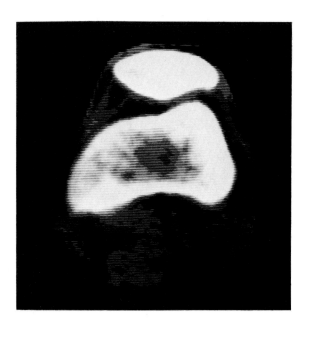

10.21

10.22

10.21 Anatomical diagram of an extended transverse section through the distal femur. Note the presence of three nerves in the posterior compartment of the leg at this level.

10.22 Black and white CT scan corresponding to the diagram in Figure 10.21.

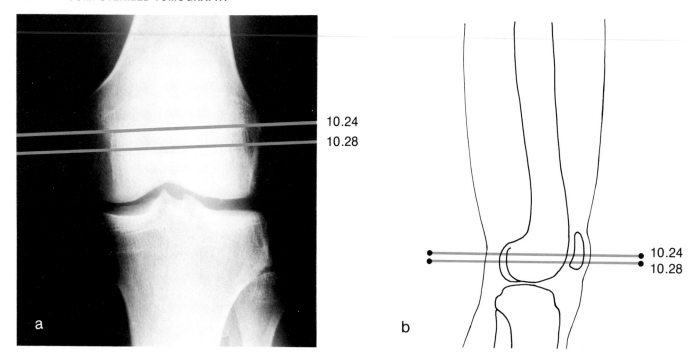

10.23 Scan levels corresponding to the anatomical diagrams seen in Figures 10.24 and 10.28. (a) Roentgenogram of a normal extended knee joint; red lines show cross-section levels; (b) Schematic diagram of scan levels.

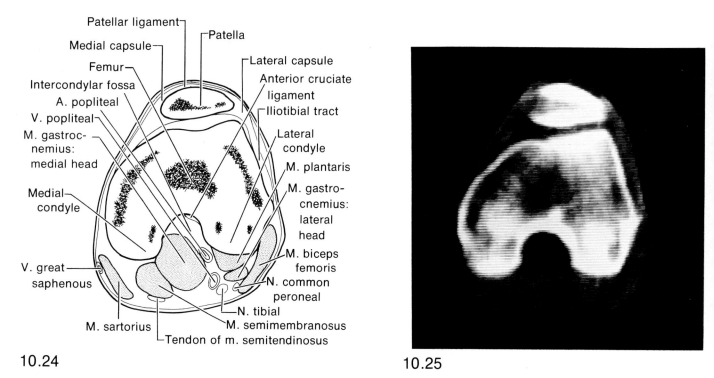

10.24

10.25

10.24 Anatomical diagram of an extended transverse section through the distal femur.
10.25 Black and white CT scan corresponding to the diagram in Figure 10.24 and demonstrating the appearance of the condyles of the femur.

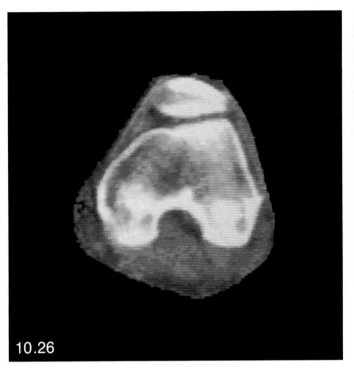
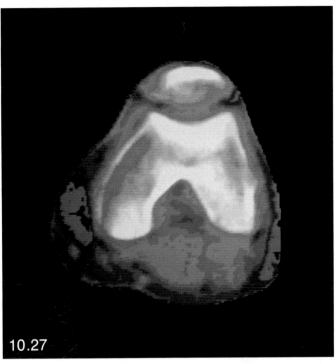

10.26

10.27

10.26 Color CT scan corresponding to the diagram in Figure 10.24 and illustrating the mid-portion of the patellofemoral joint.

10.27 Color CT scan corresponding to the diagram in Figure 10.28. Note the appearance of the patellofemoral joint space as well as the retinaculum, which serves as the medial and lateral boundaries of this joint.

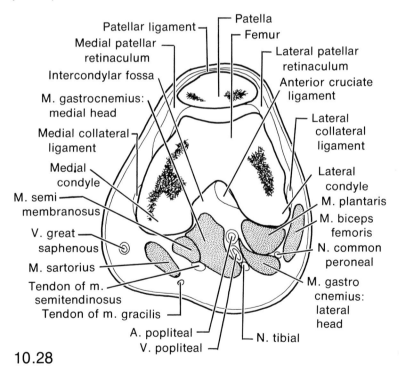
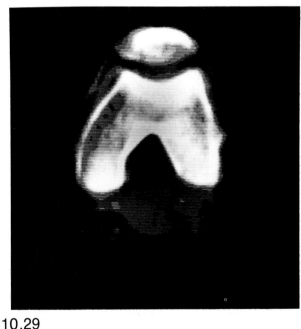

10.28

10.29

10.28 Anatomical diagram of an extended transverse section through the distal femur. Note the absence of anterior musculature at this level.

10.29 Black and white CT scan corresponding to the diagram in Figure 10.28. Note the presence of the great saphenous vein in this scan.

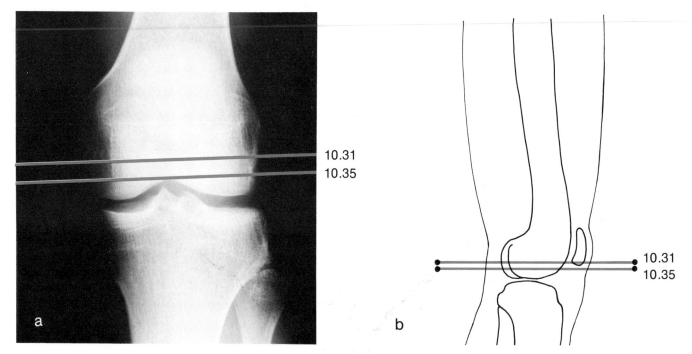

10.30 Scan levels corresponding to the anatomical diagrams seen in Figures 10.31 and 10.35. (a) Roentgeno-gram of a normal extended knee joint; red lines show cross-section levels; (b) Schematic diagram of scan levels.

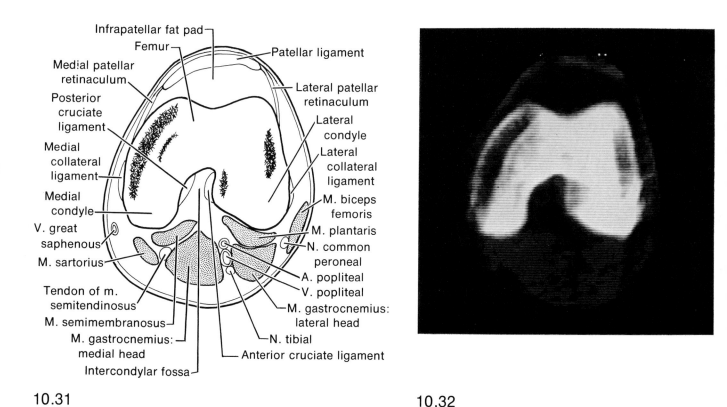

Infrapatellar fat pad
Femur
Patellar ligament
Medial patellar retinaculum
Lateral patellar retinaculum
Posterior cruciate ligament
Lateral condyle
Lateral collateral ligament
Medial collateral ligament
Medial condyle
M. biceps femoris
V. great saphenous
M. plantaris
N. common peroneal
M. sartorius
A. popliteal
Tendon of m. semitendinosus
V. popliteal
M. semimembranosus
M. gastrocnemius: lateral head
M. gastrocnemius: medial head
N. tibial
Intercondylar fossa
Anterior cruciate ligament

10.31

10.32

10.31 Anatomical diagram of an extended transverse section through the superior portion of the knee joint.
10.32 Black and white CT scan corresponding to the diagram in Figure 10.31. Note the dense cortical bone that serves as the inferior extent of the femoral condyles.

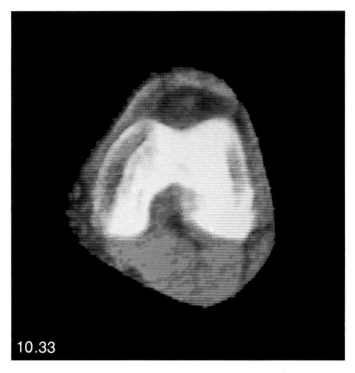

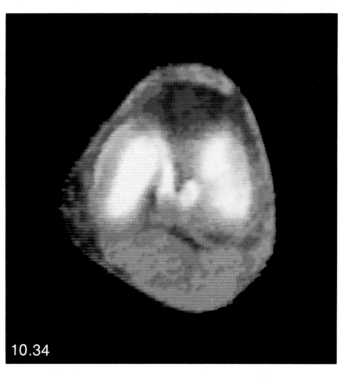

10.33

10.34

10.33 Color CT scan corresponding to the diagram in Figure 10.31 and illustrating the appearance of the cruciate ligaments in the intercondylar fossa.
10.34 Color CT scan corresponding to the diagram in Figure 10.35. Note the appearance of the tibial spines between the femoral condyles.

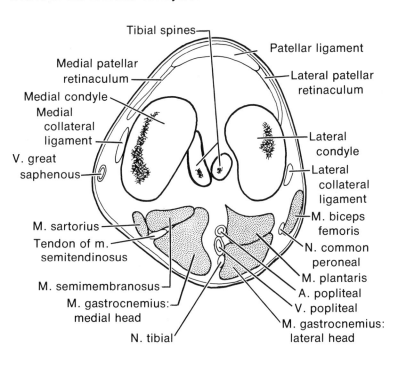

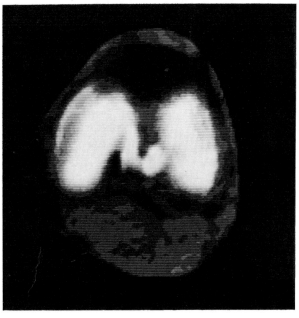

Tibial spines
Medial patellar retinaculum
Medial condyle
Medial collateral ligament
V. great saphenous
M. sartorius
Tendon of m. semitendinosus
M. semimembranosus
M. gastrocnemius: medial head
N. tibial
Patellar ligament
Lateral patellar retinaculum
Lateral condyle
Lateral collateral ligament
M. biceps femoris
N. common peroneal
M. plantaris
A. popliteal
V. popliteal
M. gastrocnemius: lateral head

10.35

10.36

10.35 Anatomical diagram of an extended transverse section through the superior portion of the knee joint.
10.36 Black and white CT scan corresponding to the diagram in Figure 10.35 and illustrating the inferior portion of the femoral condyles.

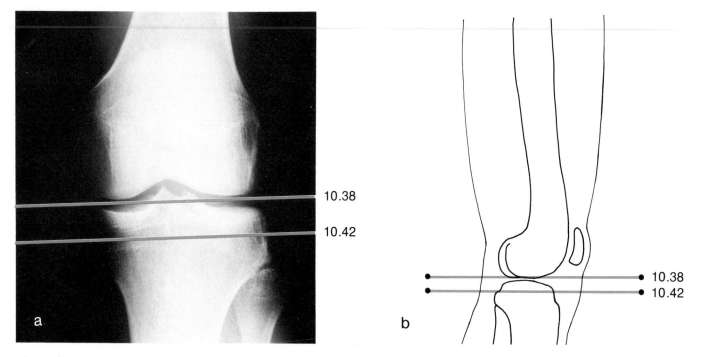

10.37 Scan levels corresponding to the anatomical diagrams seen in Figure 10.38 and 10.42. (a) Roentgenogram of a normal extended knee joint; red lines show cross-section levels; (b) Schematic diagram of scan levels.

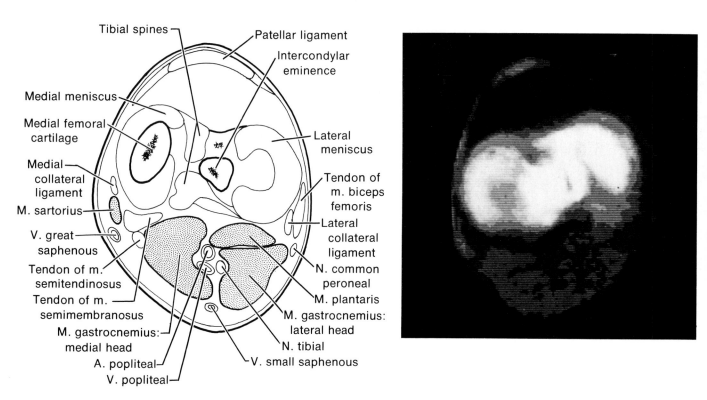

10.38   **10.39**

10.38 Anatomical diagram of an extended transverse section through the mid-portion of the knee joint and demonstrating the appearance of the medial and lateral menisci.

10.39 Black and white CT scan corresponding to the diagram in Figure 10.38.

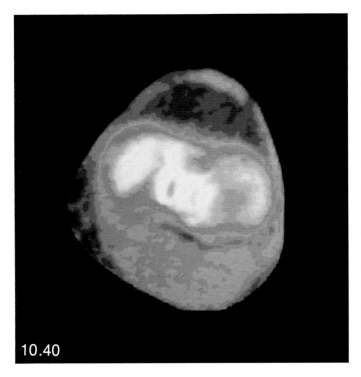

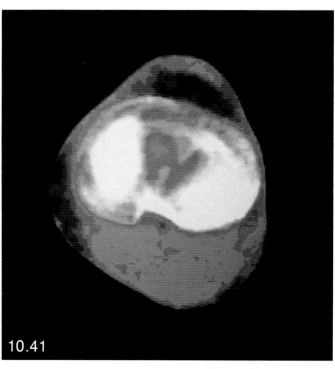

10.40 Color CT scan corresponding to the diagram in Figure 10.38. Note the appearance of the tibial spines medially and the menisci laterally in this scan.

10.41 Color CT scan corresponding to the diagram in Figure 10.42 and demonstrating the relatively dense appearance of the tibial plateau at this level.

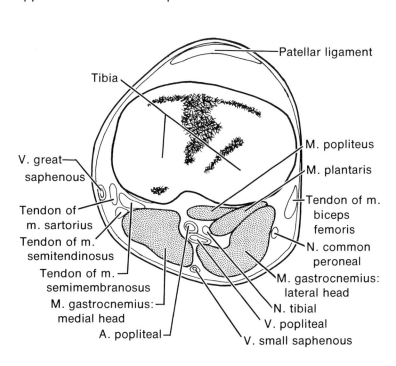

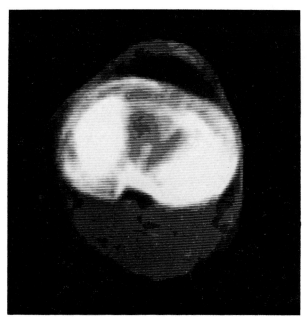

10.42

10.43

10.42 Anatomical diagram of an extended transverse section through the inferior portion of the knee joint.

10.43 Black and white CT scan corresponding to the diagram in Figure 10.42.

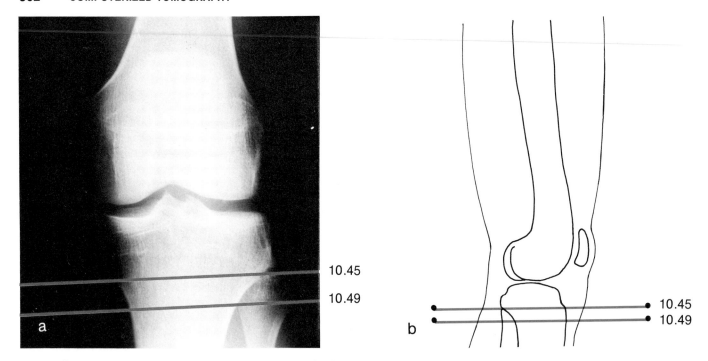

10.45
10.49

10.45
10.49

a

b

10.44 Scan levels corresponding to the anatomical diagrams seen in Figures 10.45 and 10.49. (a) Roentgenogram of a normal extended knee joint; red lines show cross-section levels; (b) Schematic diagram of scan levels.

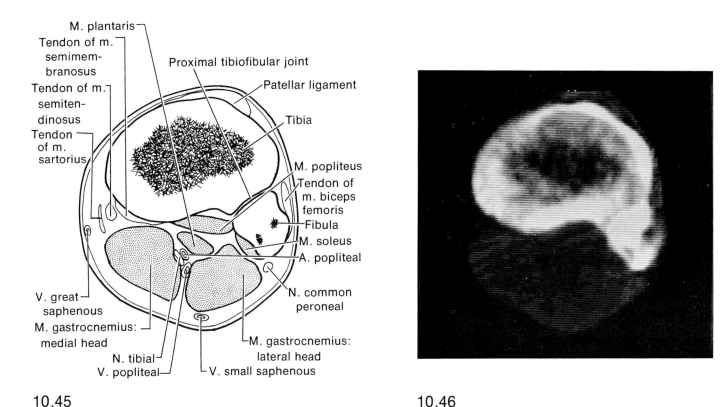

M. plantaris
Tendon of m. semimembranosus
Tendon of m. semitendinosus
Tendon of m. sartorius

Proximal tibiofibular joint
Patellar ligament
Tibia
M. popliteus
Tendon of m. biceps femoris
Fibula
M. soleus
A. popliteal
N. common peroneal

V. great saphenous
M. gastrocnemius: medial head
N. tibial
V. popliteal
V. small saphenous
M. gastrocnemius: lateral head

10.45

10.46

10.45 Anatomical diagram of an extended transverse section through the inferior portion of the knee joint. Note the appearance of the proximal portion of the tibiofibular joint.

10.46 Black and white CT scan corresponding to the diagram in Figure 10.45. Note the close proximity of the fibula to the tibia at this scan level.

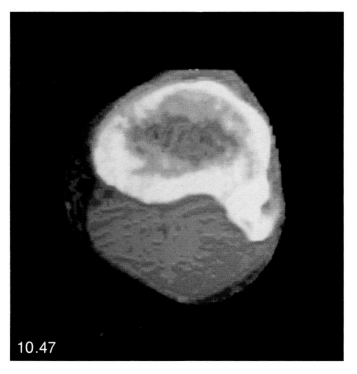

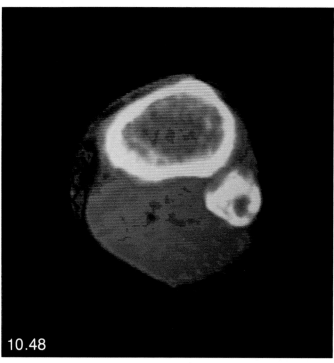

10.47 Color CT scan corresponding to the diagram in Figure 10.45 and illustrating the close adherence of the fibula to the tibia.

10.48 Color CT scan corresponding to the diagram in Figure 10.49. Note the appearance of the proximal tibiofibular joint at this level.

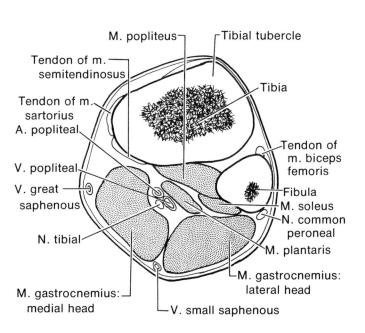

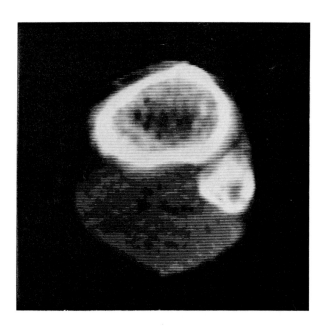

10.49   **10.50**

10.49 Anatomical diagram of an extended transverse section through the inferior portion of the knee joint. Note the appearance of the musculature of the proximal portion of the lower leg.

10.50 Black and white CT scan corresponding to the anatomical diagram in Figure 10.49 and demonstrating the appearance of the proximal tibiofibular joint.

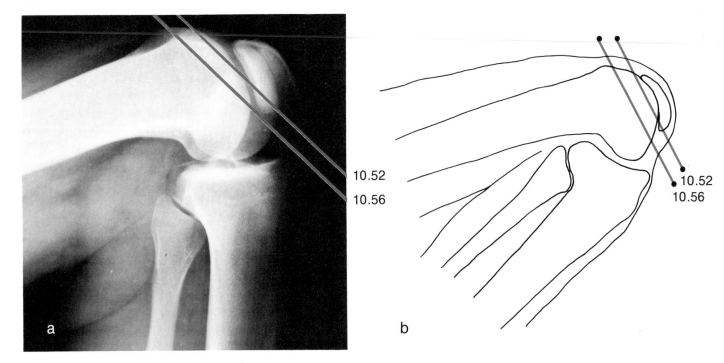

10.51 Scan levels. (a) Normal lateral roentgenogram of a knee joint flexed to approximately 90°; red lines show cross-section levels; (b) Schematic diagram of a knee joint flexed to approximately 100° and demonstrating the scan levels corresponding to the anatomical diagrams in Figures 10.52 and 10.56.

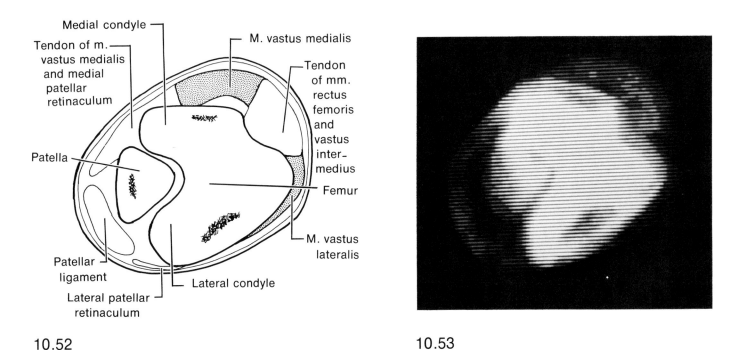

10.52   10.53

10.52 Anatomical diagram of a flexed (100°) transverse section through the knee joint.
10.53 Black and white CT scan corresponding to the anatomical diagram in Figure 10.52. Note the appearance of the patellofemoral joint in this scan.

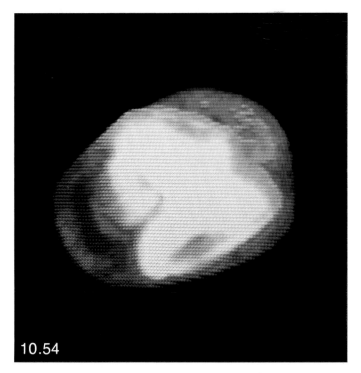

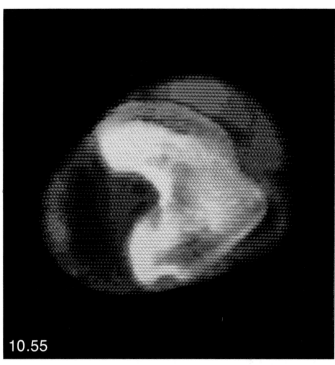

10.54 Color CT scan corresponding to the diagram in Figure 10.52 and illustrating the relatively dense tendon of the rectus femoris muscle.

10.55 Color CT scan corresponding to the anatomical diagram in Figure 10.56. Note the appearance of the intercondylar fossa in this scan.

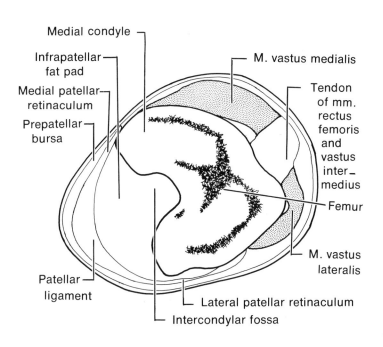

Medial condyle

Infrapatellar fat pad

Medial patellar retinaculum

Prepatellar bursa

M. vastus medialis

Tendon of mm. rectus femoris and vastus intermedius

Femur

M. vastus lateralis

Patellar ligament

Lateral patellar retinaculum

Intercondylar fossa

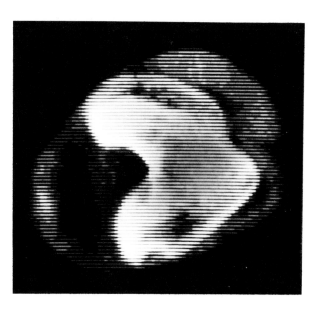

10.56

10.57

10.56 Anatomical diagram of a flexed (100°) transverse section through the knee joint.

10.57 Black and white CT scan corresponding to the diagram in Figure 10.56 and illustrating the anterior musculature of the distal thigh.

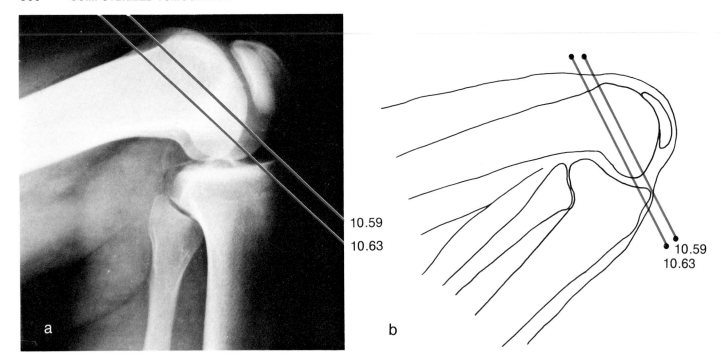

10.58 Scan levels. (a) Normal lateral roentgenogram of a knee flexed to approximately 90°; red lines show cross-section levels; (b) Schematic diagram of a knee flexed to approximately 100° and demonstrating the scan levels corresponding to the anatomical diagrams seen in Figures 10.59 and 10.63.

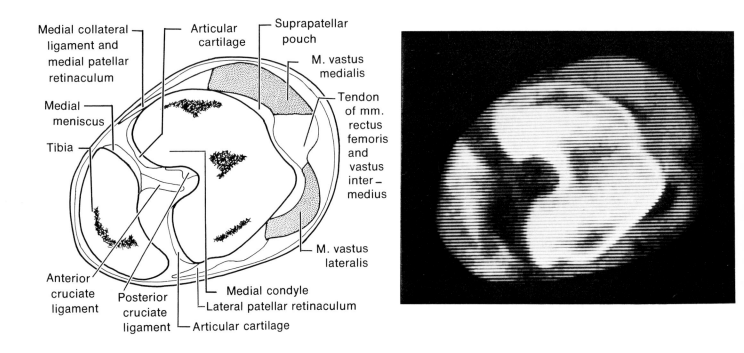

10.59   10.60

10.59 Anatomical diagram of a flexed (100°) transverse section through the knee joint. Note the appearance of the cruciate ligaments at this level.
10.60 Black and white CT scan corresponding to the diagram in Figure 10.59. Note the appearance of the proximal portion of the tibia and its relationship to the femoral condyle.

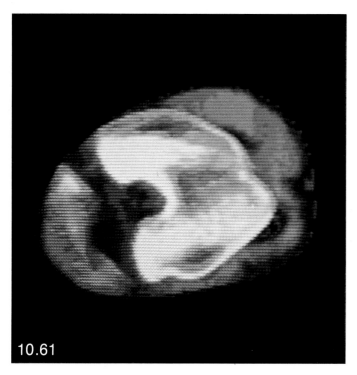

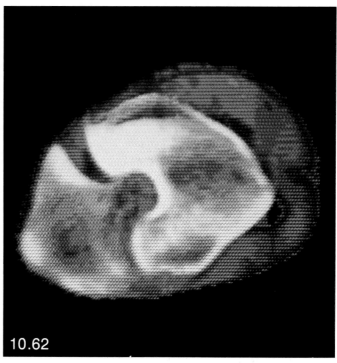

10.61 Color CT scan corresponding to the diagram in Figure 10.59 and demonstrating the appearance of the anterior musculature of the distal thigh.

10.62 Color CT scan corresponding to the diagram in Figure 10.63. Note the appearance of the joint space of the knee and the presence of the menisci within this joint space.

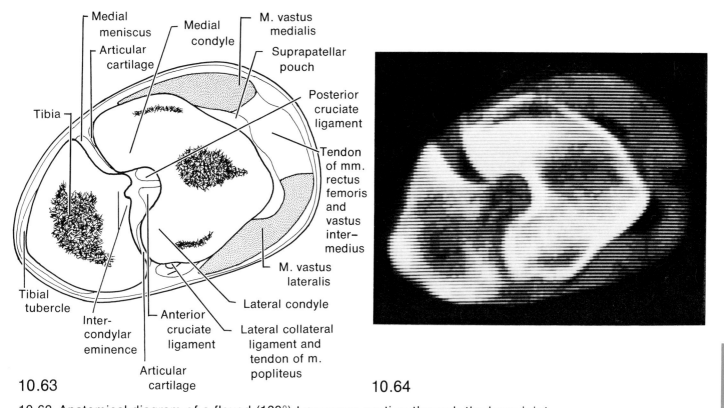

10.63 Anatomical diagram of a flexed (100°) transverse section through the knee joint.

10.64 Black and white CT scan corresponding to the diagram in Figure 10.63. Note the appearance of the tendon of the rectus femoris muscle in this scan.

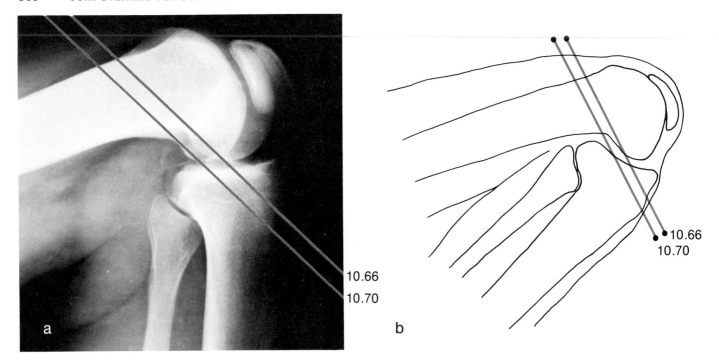

10.65 Scan levels. (a) Normal lateral roentgenogram of a knee joint flexed to approximately 90°; red lines show cross-section levels; (b) Schematic diagram of a knee flexed to approximately 100° and demonstrating the scan levels corresponding to the diagrams seen in Figures 10.66 and 10.70.

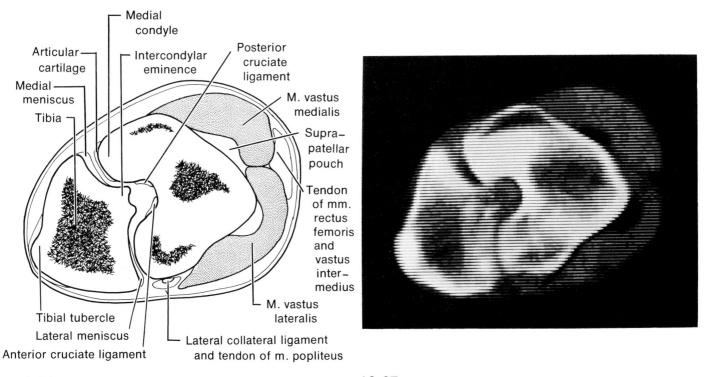

10.66

10.67

10.66 Anatomical diagram of a flexed (100°) transverse section through the knee joint.
10.67 Black and white CT scan corresponding to the diagram in Figure 10.66 and demonstrating the joint space between the tibial plateau and the femoral condyles.

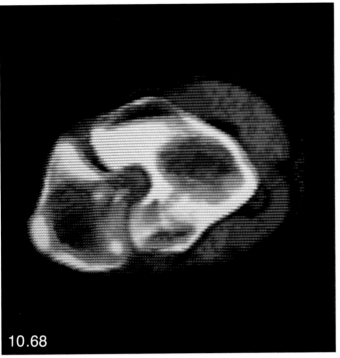

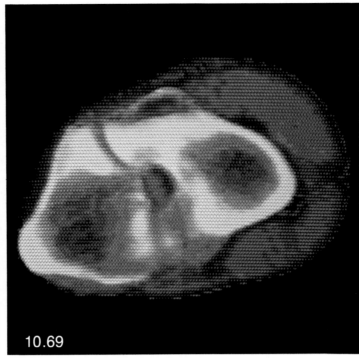

10.68 Color CT scan corresponding to the diagram in Figure 10.66. Note the appearance of both the cruciate ligaments as well as the lateral collateral ligament.

10.69 Color CT scan corresponding to the diagram in Figure 10.70. Note the appearance of the suprapatellar pouch, the intercondylar fossa and the tibial tubercle.

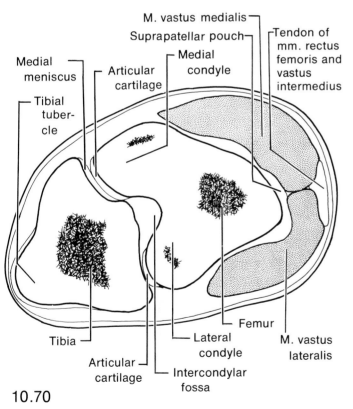

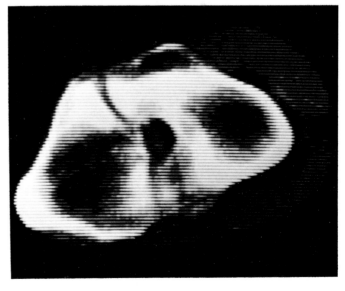

10.70

10.71

10.70 Anatomical diagram of a flexed (100°) transverse section through the knee joint.

10.71 Black and white CT scan corresponding to the diagram in Figure 10.70.

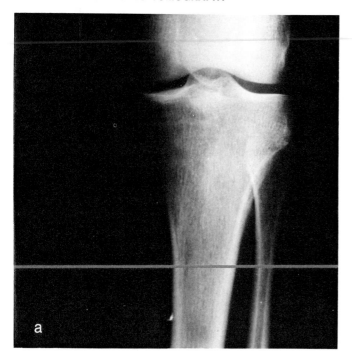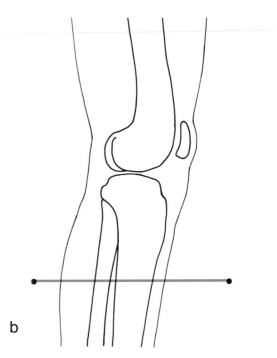

10.72 Scan level. (a) Roentgenogram of a normal extended leg; red line shows cross-section level; (b) Schematic diagram of scan level.

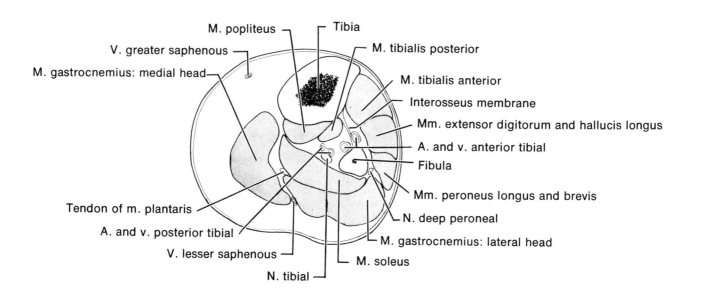

10.73 Anatomical diagram of a transverse section through the mid-portion of the lower leg.

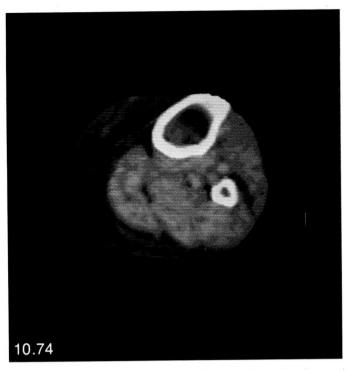

10.74

10.74 Color CT scan clearly demonstrating the neurovascular supply to the lower leg and foot.

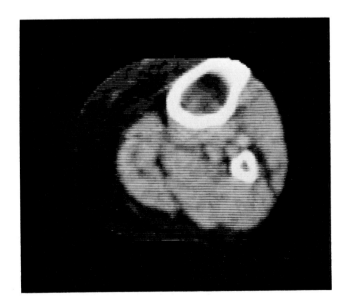

10.75 Black and white CT scan illustrating the musculature of the lower leg and the close proximity of the neurovascular supplies of the lower leg and foot with the fibula.

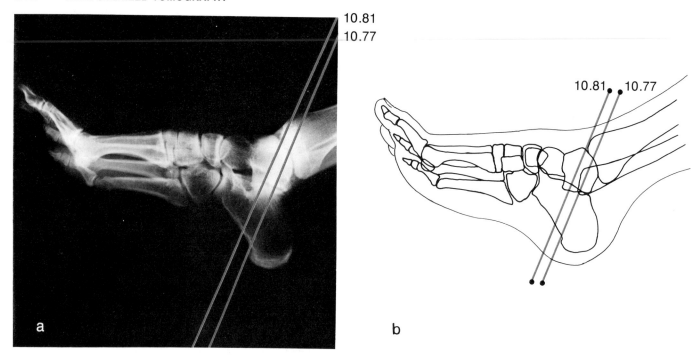

10.76 Scan levels. (a) Roentgenogram of a normal ankle joint with approximately 45° of plantar flexion; red lines show cross-section levels; (b) Schematic diagram of a flexed ankle joint, demonstrating scan levels corresponding to the diagrams in Figures 10.77 and 10.81.

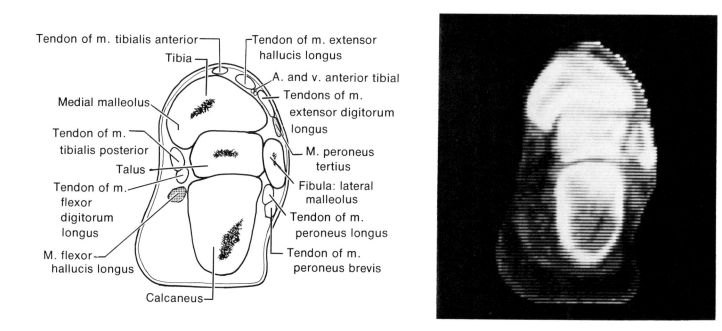

10.77   **10.78**

10.77 Anatomical diagram of a plantar-flexed (45°) transverse section through the ankle joint. Note the position of the multiple tendons surrounding this joint.

10.78 Black and white CT scan corresponding to the diagram in Figure 10.77 and illustrating the joint spaces between the tibia, the talus, the fibula and the calcaneus bones.

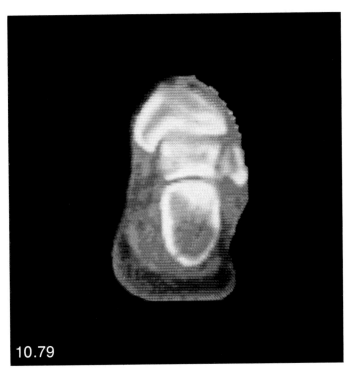

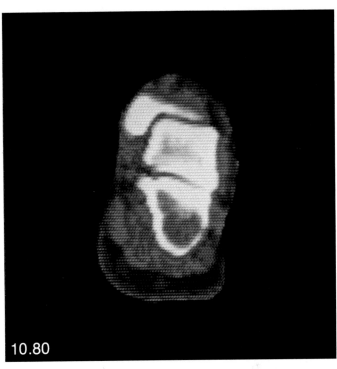

10.79 Color CT scan corresponding to the diagram in Figure 10.77. Note the presence of the peroneus tendon just posterior to the fibula in this view.

10.80 Color CT scan corresponding to the diagram in Figure 10.81 and demonstrating the musculature of the foot, particularly in the posterior compartment, at this level.

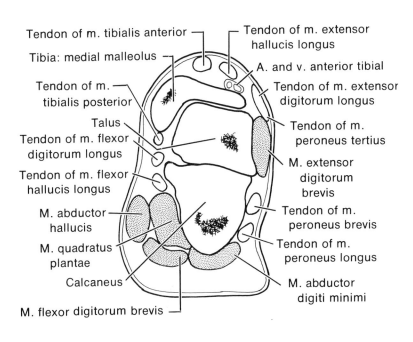

Tendon of m. tibialis anterior

Tibia: medial malleolus

Tendon of m. tibialis posterior

Talus

Tendon of m. flexor digitorum longus

Tendon of m. flexor hallucis longus

M. abductor hallucis

M. quadratus plantae

Calcaneus

M. flexor digitorum brevis

Tendon of m. extensor hallucis longus

A. and v. anterior tibial

Tendon of m. extensor digitorum longus

Tendon of m. peroneus tertius

M. extensor digitorum brevis

Tendon of m. peroneus brevis

Tendon of m. peroneus longus

M. abductor digiti minimi

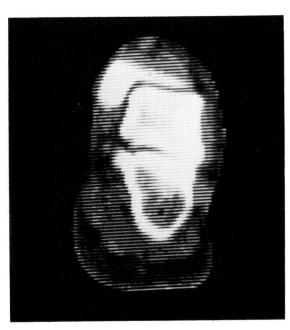

10.81

10.82

10.81 Anatomical diagram of a plantar-flexed (45°) transverse section through the ankle joint.
10.82 Black and white CT scan corresponding to the diagram in Figure 10.81.

10.88   10.84

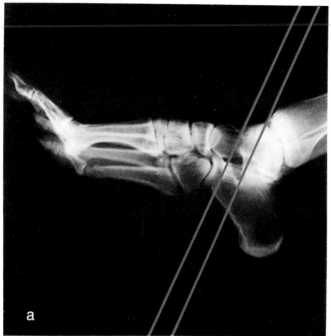

10.88   10.84

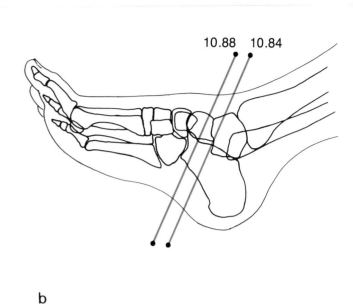

a

b

10.83 Scan levels. (a) Normal lateral roentgenogram of an ankle joint with approximately 45° of plantar flexion; red lines show cross-section levels; (b) Schematic diagram of the scan levels corresponding to the diagrams in Figure 10.84 and 10.88.

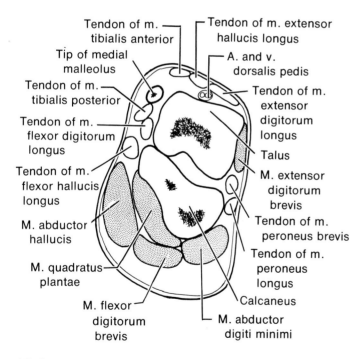

Tendon of m. tibialis anterior
Tip of medial malleolus
Tendon of m. tibialis posterior
Tendon of m. flexor digitorum longus
Tendon of m. flexor hallucis longus
M. abductor hallucis
M. quadratus plantae
M. flexor digitorum brevis

Tendon of m. extensor hallucis longus
A. and v. dorsalis pedis
Tendon of m. extensor digitorum longus
Talus
M. extensor digitorum brevis
Tendon of m. peroneus brevis
Tendon of m. peroneus longus
Calcaneus
M. abductor digiti minimi

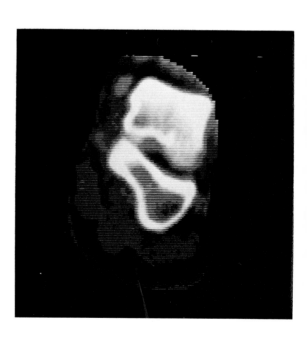

10.84

10.85

10.84 Anatomical diagram of a plantar-flexed (45°) transverse section through the ankle joint.
10.85 Black and white CT scan corresponding to the diagram in Figure 10.84 and illustrating the abundant posterior musculature leading to the foot.

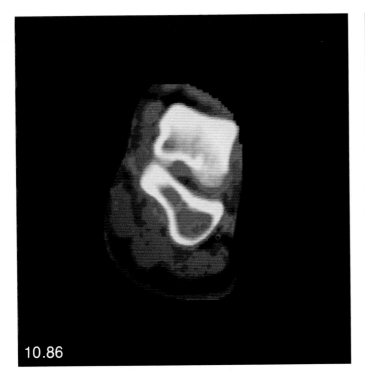

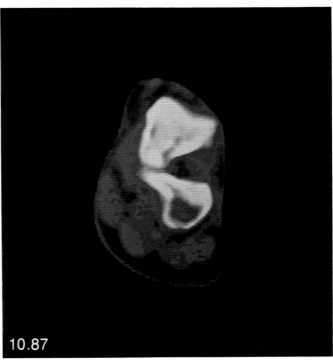

10.86 Color CT scan corresponding to the diagram in Figure 10.84. Note the appearance of the posterior muscles and the more anterior and lateral tendons leading to the foot at this scan level.

10.87 Color CT scan corresponding to the diagram in Figure 10.88. Note the abundant musculature on the medial side of the ankle, depicted in green in this scan.

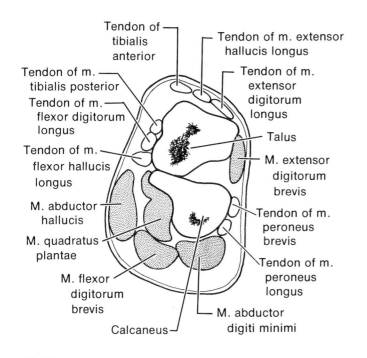

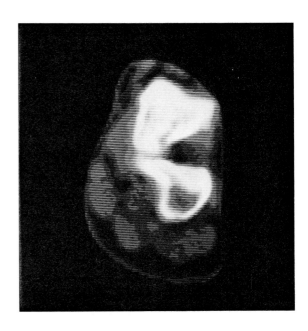

10.88

10.89

10.88 Anatomical diagram of a plantar-flexed (45°) transverse section through the ankle joint.

10.89 Black and white CT scan corresponding to the diagram in Figure 10.88.

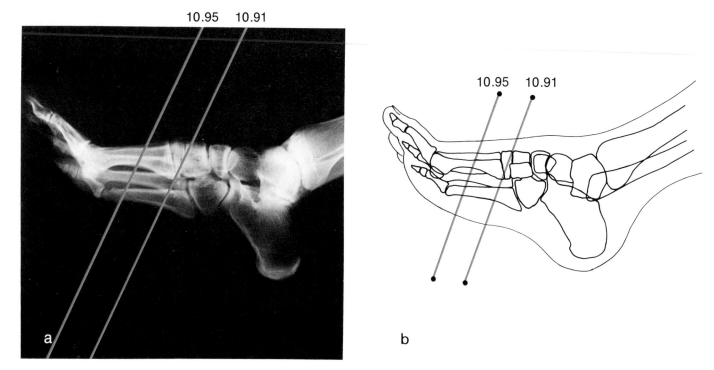

10.90 Scan levels. (a) Normal lateral roentgenogram of an ankle joint with approximately 45° of plantar flexion; red lines show cross-section levels; (b) Schematic diagram of scan levels corresponding to the diagrams in Figures 10.91 and 10.95.

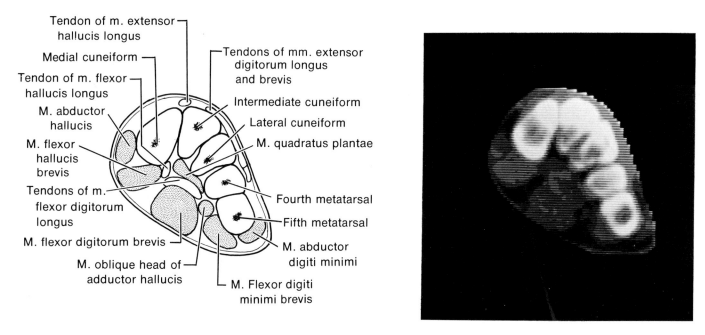

10.91

10.92

10.91 Anatomical diagram of a flexed (45°) transverse section through the proximal portion of the foot.
10.92 Black and white CT scan corresponding to the diagram in Figure 10.91. Note the appearance of the cuneiform bones as well as the fourth and fifth metatarsal bones at this level.

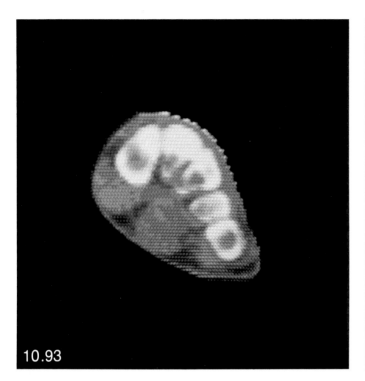

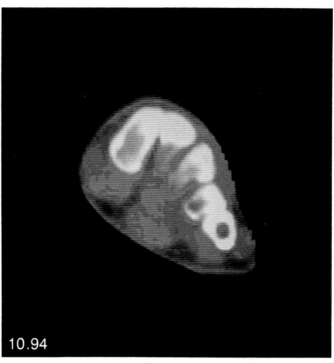

10.93 Color CT scan corresponding to the diagram in Figure 10.91. Note the joint spaces between the cuneiform and metatarsal bones as well as the abundant musculature of the foot, inferior to these bony densities.

10.94 Color CT scan corresponding to the diagram in Figure 10.95 and demonstrating the appearance of the metatarsal bones of the foot.

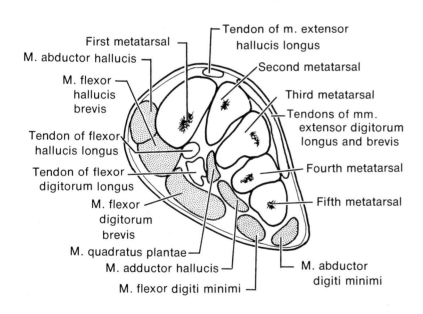

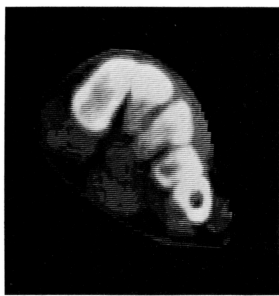

10.95

10.96

10.95 Anatomical diagram of a plantar-flexed (45°) transverse section through the mid-portion of the foot.

10.96 Black and white CT scan corresponding to the diagram in Figure 10.95 and demonstrating the metatarsal bones as well as the appearance of the musculature of the plantar surface of the foot.

references

Eycleshymer, A. C., Schoemaker, D. M. *A Cross-Section Anatomy.* Appleton-Century-Crofts, New York, New York, 1939.

One of the few complete cross-sectional anatomy texts of the whole body, prepared from drawings of cadaver specimens.

Grant, J. C. B. *An Atlas of Anatomy.* Sixth Edition, The Williams & Wilkins Company, Baltimore, Maryland, 1972.

A classical anatomical text, organized by body region and containing a few cross-sectional views.

Hanaway, J., Scott, W. R., Strother, C. M. *Atlas of the Human Brain and the Orbit for Computed Tomography.* Warren H. Green, II, Inc., St. Louis, Missouri, 1977.

Contains labeled photographs of cadaver heads cut at 0°, 25° and 35° to the orbital-meatal line. Corresponding CT scans are also provided with labels of the more prominent features.

International Anatomical Nomenclature Committee. *Nomina Anatomica.* Third Edition, Excerpta Medica, Amsterdam, Princeton, London, 1972.

Prepared in order to standardize international anatomical nomenclature, this text was used as a basis for the anglicized terms which appear in this ATLAS. In addition, we have occasionally substituted clinical nomenclature in place of the anatomical terms when it seemed appropriate.

Matsui, T., Kawamoto, K., Iwata, M., Kurent, J. E., Imai, T., Osugi, T., Hirano, A. "Anatomical and Pathological Study of the Brain by CT Scanner—1: Anatomical Study of Normal Brain," *Computerized Tomography.* Volume 1, pp. 3–43, 1977.

Contains photographs and diagrams of cut brain sections as well as corresponding CT scans. Cross-section orientation based on the shape of the ventricular and cisternal spaces is provided.

Pernkopf, E. (Editors: Ferner, H., Mansen, H.). *Atlas of Topographic and Applied Human Anatomy.* Volumes I & II. W. B. Saunders Company, Philadelphia, Pennsylvania, 1964.

English version of this classic European anatomical text which represents the human body via artists' drawings. Included in this work are some excellent cross-sectional illustrations.

Roberts, M., Hanaway, J. *Atlas of the Human Brain in Section.* Lea and Febiger, London, 1970.

A labeled photographic atlas of cut cadaver brain sections. The sections in this atlas are oriented at the classic neuroanatomical horizontal, coronal and sagittal angles.

Takahaski, S. *An Atlas of Axial Transverse Tomography and its Clinical Application.* Springer-Verlag, New York, New York, 1969.

A whole-body atlas of labeled diagrams and the corresponding conventional tomograms, prepared using cadavers and including some specialized contrast studies.

index

(Numbers enclosed in parentheses indicate figure numbers.)

(Numbers enclosed in parentheses indicate figure numbers.)

(Numbers enclosed in parentheses indicate figure numbers.)

(Numbers enclosed in parentheses indicate figure numbers.)

(Numbers in parentheses indicate figure numbers.)

(Numbers in parentheses indicate figure numbers.)

(Numbers in parentheses indicate figure numbers.)

(Numbers in parentheses indicate figure numbers.)

(Numbers in parentheses indicate figure numbers.)

ANATOMICAL STRUCTURE INDEX

VERTEBRAL LEVEL

The indicated vertebral levels are within normal anatomical ranges and are based on the subjects scanned in preparing this text.

STRUCTURE	PAGE	GREATER TROCHANTER	COCCYX	SACRUM	L5	L4	L3	L2	L1	T12	T11	T10	T9	T8	T7	T6	T5	T4	T3	T2	T1	C7	C6	C5	C4	C3	C2	C1	OCCIPITAL PROTUBERANCE	VERTEX
CEREBRUM	4–29																													■
CEREBELLUM	16–29																												■	
SPHENOID SINUS	40–51 58–59																												■	■
FRONTAL SINUS	24–29 34–35																												■	
MAXILLARY SINUS	48–53 58–65																											■	■	
EPIGLOTTIS	74–81																								■	■				
LARYNX	78–83																							■	■					
THYROID	84–93																				■	■	■							
TRACHEAL BIFURCATION	108–109																■													
AORTIC ARCH	102–107																	■												
HEART	118–133											■	■	■																
LEFT LUNG	94–143										■	■	■	■	■	■	■	■	■											
RIGHT LUNG	92–143										■	■	■	■	■	■	■			■										
DIAPHRAGM	124–155							■	■	■	■	■																		
STOMACH	132–149								■	■																				